A Clinical Guide for the Treatment of Schizophrenia

A Clinical Guide for the Treatment of Schizophrenia

Edited by

ALAN S. BELLACK

Medical College of Pennsylvania at EPPI
Philadelphia, Pennsylvania

PLENUM PRESS • NEW YORK AND LONDON

Library of Congress Cataloging in Publication Data

A Clinical guide for the treatment of schizophrenia.

   Includes bibliographies and index.
   1. Schizophrenia—Treatment. I. Bellack, Alan S. [DNLM: 1. Schiozphrenia—therapy.
WM 203 C64115]
RC514.C56   1989   616.89′8206   88-32137
ISBN 0-306-43064-9

© 1989 Plenum Press, New York
A Division of Plenum Publishing Corporation
233 Spring Street, New York, N.Y. 10013

To Barbara, Jonathan, and Adam —

They provide a reason to work, and

pleasure when the work is done.

Contributors

ALAN S. BELLACK, Department of Psychiatry, Medical College of Pennsylvania at EPPI, Philadelphia, Pennsylvania

JOHN F. CLARKIN, Department of Psychology, New York Hospital-Cornell Medical Center, 21 Bloomingdale Road, White Plains, New York

C. WESLEY DINGMAN, Chestnut Lodge Hospital, 500 West Montgomery Avenue, Rockville, Maryland

MAXINE HARRIS, Community Connections, 1512 Pennsylvania Avenue, S.E., Washington, DC

JOHN M. KANE, Department of Psychiatry, Hillside Hospital, Division of Long Island Jewish Medical Center, 75-59 263rd Street, Glen Oaks, New York, and School of Medicine, Health Sciences Center, State University of New York at Stony Brook, Stony Brook, New York

MARGARET W. LINN, Social Science Research Department, Veterans Administration Medical Center, and Department of Psychiatry, University of Miami School of Medicine, Miami, Florida

CHRISTINE W. McGILL, University of California San Francisco, Department of Psychiatry, San Francisco General Hospital, 1001 Potrero Avenue, San Francisco, California

THOMAS H. McGLASHAN, Chestnut Lodge Hospital, 500 West Montgomery Avenue, Rockville, Maryland

RANDALL L. MORRISON, Department of Psychiatry, Medical College of Pennsylvania at EPPI, Philadelphia, Pennsylvania

LOREN R. MOSHER, Associate Director, Addiction, Victim and Mental Health Services for Montgomery County, 401 Hungerford Drive #500, Rockville, Maryland

KIM T. MUESER, Department of Psychiatry, Medical College of Pennsylvania at EPPI, Philadelphia, Pennsylvania

PHILIP T. NINAN, Department of Psychiatry, Emory University Clinic, Atlanta, Georgia

JANET S. ST. LAWRENCE, Department of Psychology, Jackson State University, Jackson, Mississippi, and University of Mississippi Medical Center, 2500 North State Street, Jackson, Mississippi

ROBERT W. SURBER, Department of Psychiatry, San Francisco General Hospital, 1001 Potrero Avenue, San Francisco, California

GILBERT K. WEISMAN, 1107 Park Hills, Berkeley, California

JOHN T. WIXTED, Department of Psychology, University of California, San Diego, La Jolla, California

Preface

Research on the nature and treatment of schizophrenia has undergone a revival and metamorphosis in the last decade. For a long while, the field had been moribund, weighed down by an unreliable diagnostic system, pessimism about the possibility of new discoveries, and a dearth of research funds. A number of factors have seemingly coalesced to change this situation, with the result that the field is now alive with excitement and optimism.

Four factors seem to have played important roles in the resurgence of interest. First, prior to the publication of DSM-III in 1980 there was no reliable diagnostic system for the disorder. Previous definitions were overly general and imprecise. Consequently, the label "schizophrenia" applied to a very heterogeneous group of severely disturbed patients. It was rarely clear whether two investigators had studied comparable samples, making it impossible to determine if new findings were generalizable or if failures to replicate were due to the unreliability of the results or the fact that the investigators had studied different disorders. DSM-III has not totally resolved this problem, but it has allowed scientists to reliably identify a much more homogeneous group. As a result, it is now possible to integrate the results of different studies, making it much more likely that we can make important advances.

The second important factor was the development of new technologies that promised to help uncover the nature and etiology of the disorder. The field was plagued by pessimism through the early 1970s as research seemed to be at a stalemate. This has changed in the last 10 years with the development and increasing availability of new brain-imaging procedures. Technological advances, such as new-generation CAT scans, PET, and MRI, as well as technology for measuring regional cerebral blood flow, have dramatically increased our ability to understand brain functioning. These procedures are making it possible to directly test previous hypotheses, such as the dopamine theory, as well as facilitating the development of new models.

The ability to "see" inside the brain and to measure its functioning more directly promises to unlock the neurological keys to the disorder.

The third factor was the development of new approaches to psychosocial treatment. The psychoanalytic and family models that had dominated the field in the 1960s had proven to be useless in the treatment of schizophrenia. Coupled with the realization that neuroleptics had only limited effectiveness, there was considerable pessimism about the prospect of treating the disorder. This situation began to change in the late 1970s as evidence began to accumulate on the effectivenss of new strategies, including social-skills training and some innovative forms of family therapy. It became apparent that psychosocial treatment was not sufficient by itself, but that it could play a vital role in the treatment process.

The fourth factor was more economic and political than scientific. Until recently, schizophrenia, and mental illness in general, has been something of a pariah in our society. One result of this negative societal reaction has been substantial underfunding for research and treatment. This situation began to change in the late 1970s, due in large part to the development of the National Alliance for the Mentally Ill (NAMI). Families of mentally retarded citizens have been an effective lobbying force for decades and have done much to generate public and private funds and secure legal rights for their handicapped relatives. The development of NAMI has now set the stage for a similar increase in public attention, acceptance, and financial support for the mentally ill. In just a few years, they have become a powerful force on both the national and the local level. Among the most immediate and important effects of their support is a substantial increase in research funds available for work on schizophrenia. In fact, schizophrenia has become one of the primary priority areas for the National Institute of Mental Health, the major source of research dollars in the United States.

The issues discussed above might not all seem to bear directly on the subject of this book: new developments in the treatment of schizophrenia. But there would not be enough new developments if it were not for that combination of circumstances. For the most part, the treatment strategies described in this volume are based on new information about the nature of the disorder, its etiology, its course, and the special aspects of the disorder that determine treatment needs. Neither the treatment procedures themselves nor the more basic research that stimulated them would have eventuated without a resurgence of enthusiasm and resources. Regrettably, this book does not provide the "final" answers about treatment of schizophrenia. It does not provide any miracle cures or promise definitive help for every patient. However, it does provide a state-of-the-art picture. It outlines programs that can be of help to a great many patients, and it also identifies limitations and misuses of some popular current strategies. The procedures discussed in this book offer the best that is available until the next major breakthrough.

This book is a product of a great many people. I would like to thank my contributors, who were kind enough to share their expertise. As always, Eliot Werner from Plenum Press made it easy to produce a first-class product. Last, but certainly not least, is Florence Levito. Nothing comes out of my office that does not depend upon her at some level.

Contents

A Comprehensive Model for Treatment of Schizophrenia

ALAN S. BELLACK

SCHIZOPHRENIA AND THE COMMUNITY MENTAL HEALTH REVOLUTION

The treatment of schizophrenia in the United States during the twentieth century has been a national embarrassment. The (approximately) 2 million schizophrenics in the United States have received short shrift from the government, mental health professionals, and the public at large. In contrast to citizens with severe physical illnesses or mental retardation, schizophrenics have generally been segregated and either mistreated or ignored. This situation first attracted significant public and governmental attention in the late 1950s and early 1960s as a function of the community mental health (CMH) movement. Referred to as the "third mental health revolution" (Hobbs, 1964), the CMH movement had as one of its primary goals the development of new and more effective treatment programs and the improvement of the quality of life for schizophrenics and for the chronic mentally ill in general. The culmination of CMH efforts was the 1963 Community Mental Health Centers Act, which funded the development of local facilities to provide a range of needed services in the community. To be sure, the CMH movement has led to dramatic changes in the pattern of mental health care and the structure of the mental health system. But, like most revolutions, it has not worked out precisely as planned. To the contrary, it has been

ALAN S. BELLACK • Department of Psychiatry, Medical College of Pennsylvania at EPPI, 3200 Henry Avenue, Philadelphia, Pennsylvania 19129.

argued that in many respects the chronic mentally ill are as victimized and ignored by society today as they were before the erstwhile revolution (Gralnick, 1985).

The designated villain in the treatment of schizophrenics before the advent of community care was the state psychiatric hospital system. In the first half of this century state hospitals were transformed from a series of small, therapeutic asylums to a network of large, unmanageable warehouses in which society imprisoned many of its indigent and distasteful members. By the mid-1950s state hospitals provided nearly 50% of all psychiatric care in the country (Sharfstein, 1984). Close to one-half of these institutions housed over 3,000 patients; several had as many as 20,000. Forty-five percent of the residents had been hospitalized for more than 10 years (Yolles, 1977). Given the low priority afforded these hospitals by the public sector, they were almost all overcrowded, underfunded, and understaffed. As a result, they placed greater emphasis on "management" than on "treatment." The result was often mistreatment, and the so-called institutionalization syndrome of withdrawal, apathy, and infantile behavior (Paul & Lentz, 1977).

The role of the state hospital in the overall mental health service delivery system has changed substantially in the last 30 years. Stimulated by the development of phenothiazines and the 1961 report of the President's Joint Commission on Mental Illness and Health, there has been a dramatic shift from primary reliance on long-term hospitalization in state facilities to short stays and community-based treatment. This process has led to the *ad hoc* policy of "deinstitutionalization," in which large numbers of long-term patients have been discharged to community care, and new admissions have been severely restricted. The number of state hospital beds decreased from a high of 559,000 in 1955 to 138,000 in the late 1970s, and the average length of stay dropped from 6 months to 3 weeks. By 1977 state hospitals provided only 9% of all mental health care in the country (Sharfstein, 1984).

Unfortunately, these dramatic changes reflect differences in how and where treatment is provided, rather than changes in the prevalence or effects of chronic mental illness. In fact, the shift in service delivery is better reflected by the term *transinstitutionalization* than by *deinstitutionalization*. The decline in state hospital beds has been paralleled by an equally dramatic increase in psychiatric beds in local facilities, including general hospitals, Veterans Administration Hospitals, community mental health centers, and private psychiatric hospitals (Goldman, Adams, & Taube, 1983). It has been estimated that as many as 750,000 of the 2 million patients in nursing homes are chronic mentally ill; many were transferred directly from state hospitals, while others were denied admission owing to current admission policies (Goldman, 1984). Overall, there has been a 38% increase in inpatient episodes since 1955, resulting primarily from a tremendous increase in readmissions. Some 70% of all admissions involve patients with a previous history of hospitalization (Sharfstein, 1984). Whereas patients entering a psychiatric hospital in the 1950s could expect a multiyear stay, they now enter through a "revolving door" and can expect to have multiple admissions of several days to several weeks. Hospital charts detailing two or three admissions per year for 5 to 10 years are regrettably common. It has been suggested that schizophrenics alone account for some 500,000 hospital admissions per year (Goldman, 1984). Were current commitment laws more lenient, these figures would be even higher. There has also been a dramatic rise in emergency room visits that do not lead to hospitalization but that nonetheless reflect frequent acute exacerbations.

A major goal of deinstitutionalization and the CMH system was to provide treatment in patients' home communities, rather than in large, geographically isolated institutions. It was hypothesized that living in the community would allow patients to be reintegrated into family and peer groups, thereby facilitating adjustment, as well as restoring civil liberties and allowing patients to enjoy the many privileges and benefits our society has to offer. While these expectations were fulfilled for a minority of patients, the majority of chronic patients have traded the distressing conditions in state hospitals for marginal lives in the community (Klerman, 1977; Lehman, 1983).

Only a small proportion of ex-patients have been effectively reintegrated into the community. Most are ostracized or actively avoid social contacts. The vast majority are chronically unemployed, with little hope or desire to find work. As a result, they are dependent on the social service system for money, food, and shelter, and have poor nutrition and health. Comparatively few ex-patients are capable of living independently; the majority require supervised living arrangements (Goldstrom & Manderscheid, 1981). Of those living on their own, a great many live in run-down apartments or rooming houses in decaying areas of cities. Many others have no residence whatsoever; as many as one-half of the 2 million homeless people in our country are mentally ill (Cordes, 1984). It is also thought that a significant number of mentally ill individuals find shelter in prisons, having been arrested rather than brought to psychiatric facilities by police.

The NIMH-sponsored Community Support Program (Goldstrom & Manderscheid, 1981) has yielded the most comprehensive data to date on the community adjustment of chronic mental patients. The data document that most chronic patients have a poor quality of life even aside from housing. They are easy prey for street criminals, and thus they are frequent crime victims. The majority are unable to perform the tasks of daily living: Fewer than 60% are able independently to perform household chores, prepare meals, or maintain an adequate diet; fewer than 50% can manage their own money or take medication as prescribed. They suffer from poor physical health and have shortened life expectancies. Chronic patients also fail to take advantage of social and recreational opportunities, lacking the money, skills, and motivation to participate in society. Less than half engage in recreational activities other than watching television or listening to the radio. Many are socially isolated, spending endless hours sleeping, walking the streets, or sitting in community mental health center day rooms.

While the practice of long-term hospitalization employed through the early 1960s created the institutionalization syndrome, the policy of deinstitutionalization has created a new syndrome, that of the aftercare client. It is characterized by revolving door rehospitalization, poor physical health, social isolation, inadequate housing, dependence on others, chronic unemployment, and poverty. In many respects, this new syndrome is just as pernicious and has an equally poor prognosis.

FACTORS CONTRIBUTING TO FAILURE

How could such a well-intentioned policy have led to such disappointing results? With 20/20 hindsight, three factors now seem apparent. First, expectations about the effectiveness of the then newly discovered phenothiazines were overly optimistic. It was assumed that medication not only would control psychotic symptoms in the vast majority of patients but would allow them to take advantage of community programs and develop constructive lives. It is now apparent that as many as 50% of schizophrenics may not benefit from antipsychotics (Gardos & Cole, 1976). A significant minority do not have a notable clinical response to the medication, while others will not take it as prescribed. Of those who do respond, 25% to 30% can be expected to relapse within 1 year and 50% within 2 years (Hogarty et al., 1979).

The overall effect of medication is also more circumscribed than had been thought. Antipsychotics have a demonstrable effect on positive symptoms, such as thought disorder, hallucinations, and delusions. However, they often do not appreciably reduce negative symptoms, such as apathy, anergia, and withdrawal (Carpenter, Heinrichs, & Alphs, 1985). Similarly, they do not develop skills of daily living or enhance quality of life (Diamond, 1985). Moreover, 15% to 50% of patients experience significant side effects, including akinesia, akathisia, and tardive dyskinesia (Johnson, 1985). These side effects can be as disruptive and distressing as core psychotic symptoms (Drake & Ehrlich, 1985; Van Putten & May, 1978). It is now apparent that antipsychotic medication is a necessary part of treatment for the majority of patients, but that it is far from a panacea.

The second factor was unrealistic expectations about the effectiveness of the community mental health system. It was assumed that CMH centers would be able to provide the diversity of treatment and support functions needed to help patients maintain themselves in the community. Unfortunately, the broad range of needed services was not anticipated, and the centers were never given adequate funding to accomplish this goal. For all their failures, the state hospitals were integrated institutions that provided shelter, food, clothing, and medical care as well as psychiatric treatment. The major needs confronting chronic psychiatric patients in the community include housing, economic support, and medical care, none of which CMH centers are able to provide (Talbott, 1981; Tessler & Manderscheid, 1982).

Yet another problem is that the limited resources available to CMH centers have been disproportionately utilized by the "worried well," rather than by schizophrenics and other chronic patients. One reason state hospitals now provide only 9% of overall psychiatric care is that the CMH program has attracted large numbers of less disturbed individuals who did not previously seek treatment because of the cost or lack of availability (Goldman et al., 1983). State hospitals still account for 64% of all inpatient care.

In a related vein, many CMH staff members have not been adequately trained to deal with schizophrenics, and the services provided by CMH centers often are not suited to the needs of chronic psychiatric patients. There continues to be an overemphasis on group and individual psychotherapy, despite evidence that these interventions are not particularly effective for these patients (Mosher & Keith, 1980). The primary therapeutic modality at most CMH centers is day treatment, yet there are few data to document the efficacy of such treatment or to suggest appropriate content or intensity (Linn, 1988). Moreover, because of severe underfunding, case loads at most CMH centers are so high that staff members cannot provide the individual support and continuity that schizophrenics require. In many cases, no one knows whether a patient is attending treatment programs or receiving medication, and no one is available to do anything about it even if the patient's absence is recognized. Too often, day treatment is a euphemism for day camp, where the primary therapeutic goal seems to be securing *per diem* reimbursement from the county or state.

The third factor leading to the current situation was an unrealistic model of illness. Stimulated by the writings of Freud, the mental health community has subscribed to an infectious disease model of illness, in which treatment is viewed as a short-term process for dealing with a circumscribed, temporary disturbance. This model is not suited to a disease such as schizophrenia, which is characteristically a multiply handicapping, lifelong disorder. Only a minority of patients will have a full recovery with a return to premorbid levels of functioning (Strauss & Carpenter, 1981). The majority will have residual handicaps even when the primary symptoms are under control. As many as one-third of schizophrenics will have only a minimal recovery and will remain substantially dysfunctional for their entire lives. Most will be dependent on the social service system and mental health establishment for some services throughout their lives. Periodic relapse is a natural part of the illness, rather than a sign of treatment failure.

In some respects, the mental health system has been frustrated by the fact that schizophrenics do not get better and "go away." Yet the "up and out" philosophy of treatment resulting from an infectious disease model not only is ineffective for schizophrenics but may actually increase stress and precipitate relapse (Schooler & Spohn, 1982). Schizophrenia is better represented by a chronic illness model, akin to that employed for individuals suffering from renal disease, juvenile diabetes, and Down syndrome. Treatment for these disorders is multidimensional, mutidisciplinary, and long-term. The goal is management of symptoms, teaching living and coping skills, and enhancing patients' quality of life, rather than "curing" the illness. We must adopt a similar approach for the treatment of schizophrenia if we are to progress beyond the current, unsatisfactory state of affairs.

A COMPREHENSIVE MODEL OF CARE

The chronic illness model implies a dramatically different conception of the needs of the schizophrenic patient. We can no longer think of "treatment" in the traditional manner of the patient coming to the clinic for a brief visit to receive a single intervention for a limited period of time. Treatment *per se* is only one element of a multicomponent system of services, each of which serves an essential role in the overall care or management of the patient (Anthony & Nemec, 1984; Test, 1984). Such a system is presented in Table 1. It is representative of the range and types of services required, but it is not all-inconclusive. We believe that the specific elements subsumed under each category of service are essential, but other elements may also prove to be needed. Many of the elements of the program are discussed in detail in the subsequent chapters of this book. In the following sections we will highlight some of the most important elements.

TREATMENT

A Model for Understanding Schizophrenia

The elements of our treatment program have been selected on the basis of Zubin and Spring's (1977) stress-vulnerability model of schizophrenia.

Table 1. A Comprehensive Program
of Care

Treatment
  Medication
  Family therapy
  Social skills training
  Medical care
  Crisis intervention
Rehabilitation
  Housekeeping
  Nutrition and hygiene
  Job training
  Transportation
Social services
  Income support
  Housing
  Social support
  Recreation
Continuity of care
  Active coordination of above services

According to this model, the emergence of schizophrenic symptoms results from the combined influence of psychobiological vulnerability and environmental stress. Vulnerability is a sensitivity or predisposition to decompensate under stress and experience the range of schizophrenic symptoms. The degree of vulnerability varies among individuals, determined largely by genetic and developmental factors. The factors mediating vulnerability may be structural anomalies in the brain, such as enlarged cerebral ventricles (Weinberger, Wagner, & Wyatt, 1983), or biochemical dysfunctions, such as excessive dopaminergic activity and/or hypersensitivity of dopamine receptors (Haracz, 1982). The degree of vulnerability may be reflected by such factors as genetic loading (Gottesman, 1968), reduced information-processing capacity (Nuechterlein & Dawson, 1984), heightened autonomic reactivity (Dawson & Nuechterlein, 1984), and schizotypal personality.

Stressors are environmental events or contingencies that have a negative impact upon an individual, such as life events (Rabkin, 1980), negative ambient family emotion (Koenigsberg & Handley, 1986), or an unstructured, improvished environment (Wing & Brown, 1970; Wong et al., 1987). They can also include "internal" events, such as physical illness and the implication of psychostimulants or hallucinogens. The greater an individual's vulnerability, the less stress is required for schizophrenic symptoms to appear.

The impact of environmental stressors on biological vulnerability is mediated by a person's coping skills. Coping skills are those abilities and resources that enable an individual to reduce stress and achieve instrumental or socioemotional goals that maximize adaptation. They include social skills, such as the ability to perceive relevant social stimuli and emit effective verbal and paralinguistic responses; problem-solving skills, such as the ability to identify problems and generate and evaluate effective solutions; skills needed for daily living, such as using public transportation and money management; and basic self-care skills, such as personal hygiene and grooming. Coping skills can help to minimize the negative effect of a stressor on the individual by circumventing potential stressors entirely, as well as by decreasing the severity and duration of their impact.

Medication. We have previously indicated that medication is far from a panacea in the treatment of schizophrenia. A significant number of patients do not respond to medication, and many who do respond can be expected to relapse. Nevertheless, it is generally agreed that antipsychotic medications play an essential role in the treatment of acutely ill patients. Relapse rates on placebo are at least two to three times higher than on active medication (Davis & Gierl, 1984), and the majority of patients are simply unable to function without it. Since there is, as yet, no method to reliably distinguish those patients who will not be medication responders or who will improve without active medication, antipsychotics are the initial treatment of choice for all patients experiencing an acute exacerbation of symptoms (Johnson, 1985; Kessler & Waletzky, 1981).

There is less agreement about the role of medication in maintenance treatment than there is about its role in treatment of the acute episode. Standard practice is to maintain patients on moderate doses of antipsychotics for as long as possible, since relapse rates increase dramatically once medication is terminated (Johnson, 1985). Conversely, the incidence of negative side effects increases as dosage and duration of use increase (Kane, 1985). In light of the risk of harmful side effects and the clinical observation that some patients do not seem to require maintenance medication, there has been considerable interest in the last few years in alternative medication strategies. The goal of many of these efforts is to administer as little medication as possible in order to maintain an adequate level of functioning in the community. Several recent studies have demonstrated that a sizable minority of patients can be maintained without constant medication, or on much lower doses than had heretofore been employed (i.e., one-tenth to one-fifth regular dose) (Herz, Szymanski, & Simon, 1982; Kane, 1983; Marder et al., 1984).

In contrast to standard dose regimens, these dose-reduction strategies are not static. They require careful monitoring of the patient in order to identify prodromal signs of impending relapse. Medication is then initiated or increased until the patient restabilizes. In the absence of such early intervention, relapse rates on low doses or no medication are unacceptably high. Consequently, these new strategies may not be suitable for the typical CMH center or outpatient clinic, where case loads are so high that patients cannot be carefully monitored and the clinical staff do not get to know patients well enough to identify prodromal changes. Use of these strategies will require changes in the way we structure clinical settings, as well as the specific way in which medication is prescribed.

Family Therapy. One of the most exciting new findings about the course of schizophrenia concerns the role of expressed emotion (EE) in relapse (Hooley, 1985). EE is a construct that reflects the style of communication between family members and the schizophrenic relative. Family members are characterized as high or low EE on the basis of the manner in which they talk about the patient in a semistructured interview (Vaughn & Leff, 1976a). High EE relatives exhibit high levels of critical comments and hostility or are overly intrusive and infantalizing in their interactions with the patient (Miklowitz, Goldstein, Falloon, & Doane, 1984). This pattern of interactions is believed to be highly stressful for patients, resulting in a substantially increased risk of relapse. Patients living with high EE relatives are as much as four to six times more likely to relapse than patients living with a low EE relative or having no contact with a high EE relative. The impact of high EE relatives apparently can even vitiate the effects of medication (Vaughn & Leff, 1976b).

The research on EE has generated renewed interest in family therapy, and several new family interventions have been developed in the last few years (Goldstein, 1984). For the most part, they each attempt to alter the emotional climate within the family so as to reduce stress on the patient. These new programs all place considerable emphasis on psychoeducation. It is assumed that much of the conflict and stress in households with a schizophrenic member results from a lack of basic information about the illness and its consequences. Psychoeducational programs attempt to teach family members (and patients) about the nature of the illness and its probable causes, its major symptoms and course, the importance of medication and the nature of side effects, the role of the family in relapse and relapse prevention, and similar factors. Such education is intended to help enlist family members in the treatment process, as well as to reduce some of their negative feelings about the patient. Several studies have yielded very positive results for psychoeducational programs (Goldstein, Rodnick, Evans, May, & Steinberg, 1978; Hogarty et al., 1986; Leff, Kuipers, Berkowitz, Eberleim-Vries, & Sturgeon, 1982).

A second new family approach is behavioral family therapy, which attempts to alter family interactions more directly by teaching the family communication and problem-solving skills. In addition to didactic psycho-education, this approach places great emphasis on modeling, role-playing, and repeated practice of new behaviors. Notably, the treatment is conducted in the family's home rather than in the clinic, which seems to enhance participation of multiple family members. An initial clinical trial achieved highly positive results (Falloon et al., 1982), and the program is currently being evaluated more extensively in a multisite NIMH collaborative study.

The initial data evaluating these new family approaches are especially impressive in that similar results have been achieved by several different research groups in both the United States and England. These strategies would also appear to dovetail very well with the new medication strategies discussed above, as family members are enlisted to help increase medication compliance and identify prodromal symptoms. Given the apparent negative consequences of high EE behavior in the household and the significant gains that can be achieved by these new family treatment techniques, family therapy would appear to be an essential part of a comprehensive program.

Social Skills Training. Poor social functioning is one of the hallmarks of schizophrenia (Bellack & Hersen, 1978; Hersen & Bellack, 1976). While some schizophrenics are socially competent between acute episodes, most have significant social impairments. They tend to avoid social interactions, and when they do interact, their behavior is often disconcerting to the interpersonal partner. Most have a history of poor premorbid social compe-tence, and as adults they have significant social skill deficits. As a result, they are unable to develop positive interpersonal relationships or to perform essential social tasks. The inability to function adequately in social situations is a major factor in the poor quality of life experienced by many chronic patients. Their inability to effectively express feelings and achieve goals in social encounters is a frequent source of frustration, anxiety, and anger, and it appears to be a major factor in relapse.

Social skills training is a structured training program designed to teach more effective interpersonal behavior. It is based on the premise that schizo-phrenics can be taught the specific social skills needed to perform more effectively in social situations. Like behavioral family therapy, it employs modeling, role-playing, and *in vivo* practice, and is analogous to teaching a motor skill, such as tennis or piano playing. Numerous studies have docu-mented that the procedures are effective in teaching patients new skills, and that the behaviors are reasonably well maintained over time (Morrison & Bellack, 1984; Morrison & Wixted, 1988). A number of studies have found that the training is associated with symptomatic improvement and reduced rates of relapse (Bellack, Turner, Hersen, & Luber, 1984; Hogarty et al.,

1986; Wallace & Liberman, 1985). Questions still remain about the generalizability of the effects (e.g., the extent to which patients use their new skills in the natural environment). However, the existing data are positive enough to support inclusion of skills training in a comprehensive program.

Crisis Intervention. Given the nature of schizophrenia and the limitations of available treatments, most patients will need to be hospitalized, albeit briefly, periodically throughout their lives. While some of these admissions will be necessitated by the patient's condition, others will be a function of external circumstances (Franklin, Kittredge, & Thrasher, 1975; Miller & Willer, 1976). Prior hospitalizations, the availability of a bed, the willingness of the on call physician to complete the intake paperwork, insurance coverage, local attitudes about hospitalization, the patient's economic situation, and the tolerance of family members and police toward the patient's behavior are but some of the factors that determine whether a patient is brought to the emergency room and whether or not he or she is admitted.

It is widely agreed that hospitalization should be avoided when it is not absolutely necessary, since it has many negative consequences, including stigmatization and disruption of the patient's life (Kiesler, 1982). Many hospitalizations could be avoided if adequate crisis facilities were available in the community. As previously indicated, schizophrenics are highly vulnerable to stress, and they lack the skills and resources needed to cope with stressful circumstances. Even minor events, such as loss of a bus pass or arguments with strangers, have the capacity to precipitate a symptom exacerbation. However, many minor exacerbations can be easily managed before hospitalization is required if prompt support is available (Stein & Test, 1980). Often, the patient simply needs a place to sleep for one or two nights in order to be away from the family or other source of stress. At other times, the patient needs help in solving a problem, such as replacing the bus pass, finding a new apartment, or resolving a family argument. The critical issue seems to be availability of a flexible, 24-hour-a-day resource in the community. This should be a facility where patients can come of their own volition, or where family and police can bring them in lieu of the busy hospital emergency room (Gudeman, Dickey, Hellman, & Buffett, 1985). Such a system would ease the shortage of public hospital beds, as well as enhancing patients' adjustment in the community.

Medical Care. The term *medical care* here refers to treatment of somatic illness. As previously indicated, chronic parients frequently lack skills needed for daily living in the community, including the ability to maintain adequate hygiene and nutrition. They also lack the financial resources, information, and behavioral skills (e.g., ability to use public transportation) to secure regular medical and dental care. Further, they frequently have inadequate clothing and live in substandard housing, increasing their vulnerability to disease. These factors all contribute to poor health care, a disproportionately high prevalence of somatic illness, and shortened life-span (Babigian & Lehman, 1987; Tessler & Manderscheid, 1982). Between 30% and 60% of newly admitted psychiatric inpatients suffer from significant physical illnesses (Strickland & Kendall, 1983), and there is little reason to presume that the prevalence is lower in outpatients.

Physical illness is a significant source of stress and disrupts daily routines even in people without psychiatric illness. It seems likely to be even more disruptive to schizophrenics, who have difficulty coping with stress and meeting life's demands under the best of circumstances. Tessler and Manderscheid (1982) have hypothesized that poor physical health is one of the three most significant factors affecting the adjustment of chronic patients in the community. Consequently, a comprehensive program must ensure that patients receive adequate medical and dental care.

REHABILITATION

Self-Maintenance Skills. In addition to suffering from a broad range of social deficits that impede their ability to establish and maintain social supports, schizophrenics often lack the most rudimentary self-care skills, impeding their ability to survive independently in the community. In many areas of functioning, these patients are more disabled than are retarded persons living in comparable environments (Sylph, Ross, & Kedward, 1977). They often are poorly groomed, fail to wash regularly, lack table manners, and are unable to use public transportation to reach available community resources. Chronic schizophrenics typically have little knowledge about basic housekeeping skills, such as cleaning, cooking, shopping, and budgeting money. As previously indicated, they are unable to maintain adequate nutrition or secure good medical care. They often have poor personal hygiene and grooming, which predisposes them to social rejection even after they have developed interpersonal skills.

In a 3- to 4-year outcome study conducted by Presly, Grubb, and Semple (1982), successful transition into the community was related to self-maintenance skills such as care of clothes, money management, and cooking ability, whereas previous psychiatric history and measures of psychopathology were not related to outcome. In the absence of these basic life skills, even the best-intentioned community-oriented rehabilitation efforts are doomed to failure. Therefore, a comprehensive community treatment program for chronically disabled psychiatric patients must assure that these patients receive training in essential self-care skills (e.g., Brown & Munford,

1983) in addition to the interpersonal skills necessary for the establishment and maintenance of social supports.

Job Training. Inability to obtain adequate employment is a major problem for psychiatric patients living in the community, and it contributes substantially to their poor quality of life (Lehman, 1983). Unemployment rates in the United States for recently discharged psychiatric patients range as high as 70% (Goldstrom & Mandersheid, 1981). Chronic unemployment and the resulting poverty can be expected to affect schizophrenics in many of the same ways it affects nonpatients: lowered self-esteem, anger and frustration, excess spare time, increased use of alcohol and drugs. Unfortunately, the effects are magnified in schizophrenics owing to their otherwise poor coping skills and heightened reaction to stress.

Vocational training, including job finding and interviewing skills, are important ingredients of any comprehensive rehabilitation program. One promising method for teaching these skills is the establishment of a job-finding club (Azrin & Besalel, 1980; Jacobs, Kardashian, Kreinbring, Ponder, & Simpson, 1984), which provides a forum for learning the skills and engaging in the difficult process of searching for a job; it also provides social support from other patients undergoing the same process. Unfortunately, many patients are unable to retain their jobs after the arduous process of finding employment. Of approximately 30% of patients who returned to work within 6 months of leaving a psychiatric hospital, only half were employed by the time of a 1-year follow-up (Anthony, Cohen, & Vitalo, 1978). Many patients do not have the skills necessary to maintain their jobs, such as ability to adhere to a schedule, ability to interact effectively with co-workers and supervisors, or ability to solve problems and/or ask for help. Thus, rehabilitation efforts must not cease when the patient secures employment. Rather, ongoing support, training, and problem solving are necessary.

SOCIAL SERVICES

Inability to find employment, insufficient income to meet daily needs, and substandard housing are liabilities that would tax the coping resources of even healthy individuals. The effects on chronic schizophrenics can be devastating. No mental health service is sufficient to manage this environmental burden in addition to mental health needs *per se.* Rather, the broader social service network must become involved in providing support and resources.

Income and Housing. The staggering numbers of the homeless who are mentally ill and the abject poverty in which many chronically ill patients live in the United States is ample evidence of the failure of the current social service system to provide even the most basic life supports to severely disturbed persons: income and shelter. At least two misconceptions regarding the anticipated impact of the "third mental health revolution" are significant factors in the substandard conditions in which many chronic patients live today. The first was the assumption that deinstitutionalization and the transition of the locus of mental health care delivery to the community would enable essentially the same services to be provided at a cheaper cost. This expectation appears to have been based on the expectation that living in the community would promote psychiatric rehabilitation by exposing patients to social supports, role models, and learning and economic opportunities that they would not have had in an institution. However, this has not been the case. The cost of providing quality mental health services to schizophrenics in the community is actually greater than in hospitals (Kirk & Therrien, 1975). Thus, community services have been grossly underfunded. Moreover, direct economic supports to patients have been minimal, owing in part to the faulty expectation that most patients would eventually find employment, and in part to societal neglect.

The second misconception of how deinstitutionalization would promote rehabilitation stems from the previously discussed predominance of the infectious disease model of illness, rather than the more suitable chronic disease model. Community living arrangements for chronic patients have been oriented toward transitional live-in homes focused on rapid patient turnover, with the goal of independent living for all patients. This transition is often premature and overwhelms the patient's economic and psychological coping resources. The result has been that halfway houses and board-and-care homes, like hospitals, have frequently become gate houses through which patients cycle in and out on a periodic basis. Comprehensive care in the community must be based on the recognition that supportive living environments provide a stable social environment for psychiatric patients that is conducive to maintaining adequate functioning in the community, rather than as a transition to more independent living (Hewitt & Ryan, 1975). The need for long-term supportive living conditions for chronic patients should also not be confused with some community warehouse alternatives to hospitalization, such as large understaffed nursing homes, which result in even poorer clinical outcomes than psychiatric hospitalization (Linn et al., 1985).

Of course, many patients can move on to independent living after a transitional period. However, assignment to community homes is often based more on economic and pragmatic considerations than on a careful assessment of the patient's needs and goals. Furthermore, there is a dearth of adequate low-cost housing for patients who can live independently. Thus, continued economic support is necessary even for these higher-functioning patients.

Social Support. The significant role of social support in buffering the effects of stress has been well documented in both psychiatric and non-psychiatric populations (Cohen & Wills, 1985). Availability of an effective social network, as well as a strong relationship with one or two key people, appears to be essential for satisfactory life adjustment and the ability to deal with physical, environmental, and psychological stressors. Yet despite their greater need for social support, schizophrenics have severe disruptions in their social networks. They lack the skills needed to develop interpersonal relationships, and they often fear close ties. The stigma associated with their illness and the social disruption associated with hospitalization tends to erode even the few ties they manage to develop (Beels, 1981).

Thus, a central aspect of community-oriented treatment must be the development and strengthening of social support networks. This can best be accomplished by a multilevel approach, including teaching relevant inter-personal skills, working with the patient's family to enhance communication and problem-solving skills, provision of a social living environment with peers and involved paraprofessionals, and recreational and social activities where interpersonal contacts may be developed over time. Under the best of circumstances it is a slow and difficult process for these patients to get close to others and develop a sense of trust. Unfortunately, the current mental health system does not afford them the necessary time. The high case loads and high staff turnover in most facilities make it impossible for the patient to develop any stable relationships with primary caregivers. As discussed in a subsequent section, continuity of mental health staff is essential. It is also important to reduce the number of short-term hospital admissions and subsequent changes in community living arrangements, which prevent the patient from developing trusting relationships with staff and residents of a single board-and-care facility or group home.

Recreational Activities. It is now apparent that the negative symptoms of schizophrenia (e.g., anhedonia, anergia) can be as pernicious as the more apparent positive symptoms (Andreasen, 1982, 1985). They are apparently responsible for much of the asociality and lack of functional activity common to the disorder. Apparently, this lack of activity and understimulation leads to boredom, alcohol and drug abuse, increases in positive symptoms, and other negative consequences. Treatment planning for such patients requires identification of the amount of structure needed to minimize the symptoms of the illness and maximize functional behavior, while at the same time not imposing too high a level of demands. Recreational activities would appear to be an excellent option, which could help to minimize symptomatic behaviors and provide another arena for social interaction, as well as enhancing the quality of life. At present, however, the majority of psychiatric patients engage in no recreational activities other than watching TV or listening to the radio (Goldstrom & Manderscheid, 1981). Community mental health services must attempt to develop broad-based recreational programs geared toward attracting the widest possible range of participants. These activities should be geared to the age and developmental level of the participants, rather than be limited to the arts and crafts found at most community health center day programs. They should also involve excursions into the community, to teach patients how to use community resources as well as allowing them to take fuller advantage of the benefits that community living can offer.

CONTINUITY OF CARE

The hallmark of a successful comprehensive community treatment program is a continuity of services provided to patients. All too often over the course of their illness patients interact with a variety of mental health professionals from different treatment teams, who know relatively little about each other's treatment plans concerning the patient. A survey of schizophrenic patients 5 to 9 years after they were discharged from the hospital indicated that 27% had no contact at all with any medical or social services, despite considerable problems in symptoms, social functioning, and finances (Johnstone, Owens, Gold, Crow, & Macmillan, 1984).

Evidence suggests that the variety of services received in the community by recently discharged patients is an important determinant of their community tenure, whereas the extent of individual therapy and case management is not (Solomon, Davis, & Gordon, 1984). The continuity of social and medical services is essential to any comprehensive treatment program, since even if all the necessary services are available, only continuity of care can assure that these services will be appropriately utilized. It is clear that chronic psychiatric patients do not have the cognitive skills necessary to plan and coordinate their own continued care and rehabilitation. The challenge for the community mental health system is to assume the role of treatment coordinator, guiding patients to available resources as they are needed and maintaining contact during periods of stabilization.

Bachrach (1981) has outlined a multidimensional model of continuity of care that includes seven dimensions. First, the system must be longitudinal: Services provided to patients must vary in accordance to their changing needs over an extended period of time. Second, treatment programming must be *individualized*, oriented to a specific patient and his or her family rather than assigning everyone to a lock-step program. Care must be *comprehensive*, involving a multidisciplinary treatment approach. The program must be *flexible* and have the ability to respond rapidly to changes in life circumstances, symptomatology, and treatment needs. It must also be *accessible* in time and locations: Patients often have problems traveling to services, and their crises are not restricted to ordinary weekday business hours. Often, home visits or late-night meetings are the only way to resolve crises or ensure that a patient receives medication. Finally, the *relationship* between the patient and the care providers should be constant, and *communication* channels between them must remain open in order to build rapport and effectively provide appropriate social services.

CONCLUSION

Deinstitutionalization of the chronically mentally ill and the associated attempt to shift the major responsibility for their care to CMH centers has not resulted in significantly better treatment. It has been cogently argued that many of these patients are now worse off than before. Neither antipsychotic medications nor simple immersion in the community will enable chronic patients to overcome their pervasive social and functional deficits. A treatment strategy oriented to the chronically disabling nature of schizophrenia is needed to replace the current "quick-fix" approach.

A model for the comprehensive care of chronic psychiatric patients was outlined that covers treatment, rehabilitation, social services, and continuity. Some model programs have been developed that incorporate many of these features, such as the Community Living Program (Stein & Test, 1980) and Fountain House (Glascote, Cumming, Rutman, Sussex, & Glassman, 1971). However, these programs remain rare exceptions. Indeed, the very comprehensiveness of these model programs has been an obstacle to implementing similar programs in communities faced with severe financial constraints, lack of available resources, and differing organizational structures. In order to improve current treatment standards, substantial changes are required in the CMH service delivery system. A first step to accomplish this goal would be the development of a unified agency on the community level that would coordinate services and assure continuity of care. Chronic patients could be assigned to a regional mental health center for their life that would oversee their treatment and rehabilitation, and assure that their basic life needs were being met. Only by pooling the resources available in the community and orchestrating a unified approach can the CMH system effectively manage the long-term care and rehabilitation of these patients.

ACKNOWLEDGMENTS

Preparation of this paper was supported in part by grants MH 38636 and MH 39998 from the National Institute of Mental Health.

REFERENCES

Andreasen, N. C. (1982). Negative symptoms in schizophrenia: Definition and reliability. *Archives of General Psychiatry, 39*, 784–788.

Andreasen, N. C. (1985). Positive and negative schizophrenia: A critical evaluation. *Schizophrenia Bulletin, 11*, 380–389.

Anthony, W. A., Cohen, M. R., & Vitalo, R. (1978). The measurement of rehabilitation outcome. *Schizophrenia Bulletin, 4*, 365–389.

Anthony, W. A., & Nemec, P. B. (1984). Psychiatric rehabilitation. In A. S. Bellack (Ed.), *Schizophrenia: Treatment, management, and rehabilitation.* Orlando: Grune & Stratton.

Azrin, N. H., & Besalel, V. A. (1980). *Job club counselor's manual.* Baltimore: University Park Press.

Babigian, H. M., & Lehman, A. F. (1987). Functional psychoses in later life: Epidemiological patterns from the Monroe County Psychiatric Register. In N. E. Miller & G. D. Cohen (Eds.), *Schizophrenia and aging.* New York: Guilford Press.

Bachrach, L. L. (1981). Continuity of care for chronic mental patients: A conceptual analysis. *American Journal of Psychiatry, 138*, 1449–1456.

Beels, C. C. (1981). Social support and schizophrenia. *Schizophrenia Bulletin, 7*, 58–72.

Bellack, A. S., & Hersen, M. (1978). Chronic psychiatric patients: Social skills training. In M. Hersen & A. S. Bellack (Eds.), *Behavior therapy in the psychiatric setting.* Baltimore: Williams & Wilkins.

Bellack, A. S., Turner, S. M., Hersen, M., & Luber, R. F. (1984). An examination of the efficacy of social skills training for chronic schizophrenic patients. *Hospital and Community Psychiatry, 35*, 1023–1028.

Brown, M. A., & Munford, A. M. (1983). Life skills training for chronic schizophrenics. *Journal of Nervous and Mental Disease, 171*, 466–470.

Carpenter, W. T., Jr., Heinrichs, D. W., & Alphs, L. D. (1985). Treatment of negative symptoms. *Schizophrenia Bulletin, 11*, 440–452.

Cohen, S., & Wills, T. A. (1985). Stress, social support, and the buffering hypothesis. *Psychological Bulletin, 98*, 310–357.

Cordes, C. (1984). The plight of the homeless mentally ill. *APA Monitor, 15*, 1–13.

Davis, J. M., & Gierl, B. (1984). Pharmacological treatment in the care of schizophrenic patients. In A. S. Bellack (Ed.), *Treatment and care for schizophrenia.* New York: Grune & Stratton.

Dawson, M. E., & Neuchterlein, K. H. (1984). Psychophysiological dysfunctions in the developmental course of schizophrenic disorders. *Schizophrenia Bulletin, 10*, 204–232.

Diamond, R. (1985). Drugs and the quality of life: The patient's point of view. *Journal of Clinical Psychiatry, 46*, 29–35.

Drake, R. E., & Ehrlich, J. (1985). Suicide attempts associated with akathisia. *American Journal of Psychiatry, 142*, 499–501.

Falloon, I. R. H., Boyd, J. L., McGill, C. W., et al. (1982). Family management in the prevention of exacerbations of schizophrenia. *New England Journal of Medicine, 306*, 1437–1440.

Franklin, J. L., Kittredge, L. D., & Thrasher, J. H. (1975). A survey of factors related to mental hospital readmissions. *Hospital and Community Psychiatry, 26*, 749–751.

Gardos, G., & Cole, J. O. (1976). Maintenance antipsychotic therapy: Is the cure worse than the disease? *American Journal of Psychiatry, 133*, 32–36.

Glasscote, R. M., Cumming, E., Rutman, I. P., Sussex, J. N., & Glassman, S. M. (1971). *Rehabilitating the mentally ill in the community.* Washington, DC: Joint Information Service of the APA and the National Association for the Mentally Ill.

Goldman, H. H. (1984). Epidemiology. In J. A. Talbott (Ed.), *The chronic mental patient: Five years later.* Orlando: Grune & Stratton.

Goldman, H. H., Adams, N. H., & Taube, C. A. (1983). Deinstitutionalization: The data demythologized. *Hospital and Community Psychiatry, 34*, 129–134.

Goldstein, M. J. (1984). Family intervention programs. In A. S. Bellack (Ed.), *Schizophrenia: Treatment, management, and rehabilitation.* Orlando: Grune & Stratton.

Goldstein, M. J., Rodnick, E. H., Evans, J. R., May, P. R. A., & Steinberg, M. R. (1978). Drug and family therapy in the aftercare of acute schizophrenics. *Archives of General Psychiatry, 35*, 1169–1177.

Goldstrom, I. D., & Manderscheid, R. W. (1981). The chronically mental ill: A descriptive analysis from the uniform client data instrument. *Community Support Service Journal, 2*, 4–9.

Gottesman, I. I. (1968). Severity/concordance and diagnostic refinement in the Maudsley-Bethlem schizophrenic twin study. In D. Rosenthal & S. S. Kety (Eds.), *The transmission of schizophrenia.* New York: Pergamon Press.

Gralnick, A. (1985). Build a better state hospital. Deinstitutionalization has failed. *Hospital and Community Psychiatry, 36*, 738–741.

Gudeman, J. E., Dickey, B., Hellman, S., & Buffett, W. (1985). From patient to inn status: A new residential model. *Psychiatric Clinics of North America, 8*, 461–469.

Haracz, J. L. (1982). The dopamine hypothesis: An overview of studies with schizophrenic patients. *Schizophrenia Bulletin, 8*, 438–469.

Hersen, M., & Bellack, A. S. (1976). Social skills training for chronic psychiatric patients: Rationale, research findings, and future directions. *Comprehensive Psychiatry, 17*, 559–580.

Herz, M. I., Szymanski, H. V., & Simon, J. C. (1982). Intermittent medication for stable schizophrenic outpatients: An alternative to maintenance medication. *American Journal of Psychiatry, 139*, 918–922.

Hewitt, S., & Ryan, P. (1975). Alternatives to living in psychiatric hospitals—A pilot study. *British Journal of Medicine, 14*, 65–70.

Hobbs, N. (1964). Mental health's third revolution. *American Journal of Orthopsychiatry, 34*, 822–833.

Hogarty, G. E., Anderson, C. M., Reis, D. J., Kornblith, S. J., Greenwald, D. P., Javno, C. D., & Madonia, M. J. (1986). Family psycho-education, social skills training and maintenance chemotherapy I. One year effects of a controlled study on relapse and expressed emotion. *Archives of General Psychiatry, 43*, 633–642.

Hogarty, G. E., Schooler, N. R., Ulrich, R., et al. (1979). Fluphenazine and social therapy in the aftercare of schizophrenic patients. *Archives of General Psychiatry, 36*, 1283–1294.

Hooley, J. (1985). Expressed emotion: A review of the critical literature. *Clinical Psychology Review. 5*, 119–140.

Jacobs, H. E., Kardashian, S., Krienbring, P. K., Ponder, R., & Simpson, A. R. (1984). A skills oriented model for facilitating employment among psychiatrically disabled persons. *Rehabilitation Counseling Bulletin, 28*, 87–96.

Johnson, D. A. W. (1985). Antipsychotic medication: Clinical guidelines for maintenance therapy. *Journal of Clinical Psychiatry, 46*, 6–15.

Johnstone, E. C., Owens, D. G., Gold, A., Crow, T. J., & Macmillan, J. F. (1984). Schizophrenic patients discharged from hospital—A follow-up study. *British Journal of Psychiatry, 145,* 586–590.

Kane, J. M. (1983). Low dose medication strategies in the maintenance treatment of schizophrenia. *Schizophrenia Bulletin, 9,* 29–33.

Kane, J. M. (1985). Antipsychotic drug side effects: Their relationship to dose. *Journal of Clinical Psychiatry, 46,* 16–21.

Kessler, K. A., & Waletzky, J. P. (1981). Clinical use of the antipsychotics. *American Journal of Psychiatry, 138,* 202–209.

Kiesler, C. A. (1982). Mental hospitals and alternative care: Noninstitutionalization as potential public policy for mental patients. *American Psychologist, 37,* 349–360.

Kirk, S. A., & Therrien, M. E. (1975). Community mental health myths and the fate of former hospitalized patients. *Psychiatry, 38,* 209–217.

Klerman, G. L. (1977). Better but not well: Social and ethical issues in the deinstitutionalization of the mentally ill. *Schizophrenia Bulletin, 3,* 617–631.

Koenigsberg, H. W., & Handley, R. (1986). Expressed emotion: From predictive index to clinical construct. *American Journal of Psychiatry, 143,* 1361–1373.

Leff, J., Kuipers, L., Berkowitz, R., Eberlein-Vries, R., & Sturgeon, D. (1982). A controlled trail of social intervention in the families of schizophrenic patients. *British Journal of Psychiatry, 141,* 121–134.

Lehman, A. (1983). The well-being of chronic mental patients. *Archives of General Psychiatry, 40,* 369–373.

Linn, M. W. (1988). Partial hospitalization. In A. S. Bellack (Ed.), *A clinical guide for the treatment of schizophrenia.* New York: Plenum Press.

Linn, M. W., Gurel, L., Williford, W. O., Overall, J., Gurland, B., Laughlin, P., & Barchiesi, A. (1985). Nursing home care as an alternative to psychiatric hospitalization. *Archives of General Psychiatry, 42,* 544–551.

Marder, S. R., Van Putten, T., Mintz, J., McKenzie, J., Lebell, M., Faltico, G., & May, P. R. A. (1984). Costs and benefits of two doses of fluphenazine. *Archives of General Psychiatry, 41,* 1025–1029.

Miklowitz, D. J., Goldstein, M. J., Falloon, I. R. H., & Doane, J. A. (1984). Interactional correlates of expressed emotion in the families of schizophrenics. *British Journal of Psychiatry, 144,* 482–487.

Miller, G. H., & Willer, B. (1976). Predictors of return to a psychiatric hospital. *Journal of Consulting and Clinical Psychology, 44,* 898–900.

Morrison, R. L., & Bellack, A. S. (1984). Social skills training. In A. S. Bellack (Ed.), *Schizophrenia: Treatment, management, and rehabilitation* (pp. 247–279). Orlando: Grune & Stratton.

Morrison, R. L., & Wixted, J. T. (1988). Social skills training. In A. S. Bellack (Ed.), *A clinical guide for the treatment of schizophrenia.* New York: Plenum Press.

Mosher, L. R., & Keith, S. J. (1980). Psychosocial treatment: Individual, group, family, and community support approaches. *Schizophrenia Bulletin, 6,* 10–14.

Nuechterlein, K. H., & Dawson, M. E. (1984). A heuristic vulnerability/stress model of schizophrenic episodes. *Schizophrenia Bulletin, 10,* 300–312.

Paul, G. L., & Lentz, R. J. (1977). *Psychosocial treatment of chronic mental patients: Milieu versus social-learning programs.* Cambridge, MA: Harvard University Press.

Presly, A. S., Grubb, A. B., & Semple, D. (1982). Predictors of successful rehabilitation in long-stay patients. *Acta Psychiatrica Scandinavica, 66,* 83–88.

Rabkin, R. G. (1980). Stressful life events and schizophrenia: A review of the research literture. *Psychological Bulletin, 87,* 408–425.

Schooler, C., & Spohn, H. E. (1982). Social dysfunction and treatment failure in schizophrenia. *Schizophrenia Bulletin, 8,* 85–98.

Sharfstein, S. S. (1984). Sociopolitical issues affecting patients with chronic schizophrenia. In A. S. Bellack (Ed.), *Schizophrenia: Treatment, management, and rehabilitation.* Orlando: Grune & Stratton.

Solomon, P., Davis, J., & Gordon, B. (1984). Discharged state hospital patient's characteristics and use of aftercare: Effect on community tenure. *American Journal of Psychiatry, 141,* 1566–1570.

Stein, L. I., & Test, M. A. (1980). Alternative to mental hospital treatment. I. Conceptual model, treatment program, and clinical evaluation. *Archives of General Psychiatry, 37,* 392–397.

Strauss, J. S., & Carpenter, W. T., Jr. (1981). *Schizophrenia.* New York: Plenum Press.

Strickland, B. R., & Kendall, K. E. (1983). Psychological symptoms: The importance of assessing health status. *Clinical Psychology Review, 3,* 179–200.

Sylph, J. A., Ross, H. E., & Kedward, H. B. (1977). Social disability in chronic psychiatric patients. *American Journal of Psychiatry, 134,* 1391–1394.

Talbott, J. A. (1981). *The chronic mentally ill.* New York: Human Sciences Press.

Tessler, R. C., & Manderscheid, R. W. (1982). Factors affecting adjustment to community living. *Hospital and Community Psychiatry, 33,* 203–207.

Test, M. A. (1984). Community support programs. In A. S. Bellack (Ed.), *Schizophrenia: Treatment, management, and rehabilitation.* Orlando: Grune & Stratton.

Van Putten, T., & May, P. R. A. (1978). Akinetic depression in schizophrenia. *Archives of General Psychiatry, 35,* 1101–1107.

Vaughn, C., & Leff, J. (1976a). The measurement of expressed emotion in the families of psychiatric patients. *British Journal of Social and Clinical Psychology, 15,* 157–165.

Vaughn, C. E., & Leff, J. P. (1976b). The influence of family and social factors on the course of psychiatric illness: A comparison of schizophrenic and depressed neurotic patients. *British Journal of Psychiatry, 129,* 125–137.

Wallace, C. J., & Liberman, R. P. (1985). Social skills training for patients with schizophrenia: A controlled clinical trial. *Psychiatry Research, 14,* 239–247.

Weinberger, D. R., Wagner, R. L., & Wyatt, R. J. (1983). Neuropathological studies of schizophrenia: A selective review. *Schizophrenia Bulletin, 9,* 193–212.

Wing, J. K., & Brown, G. W. (1970). *Institutionalization and schizophrenia.* London: Cambridge University Press.

Wong, S. E., Terranova, M. D., Bowen, L., Zarete, T., Massel, H. K., & Liberman, R. P. (1987). Providing independent recreational activities to reduce stereotypic vocalizations in chronic schizophrenics. *Journal of Applied Behavior Analysis, 20,* 77–81.

Yolles, S. F. (1977). A critical appraisal of community health services. In G. Serban & B. Astrachan (Eds.), *New trends of psychiatry in the community.* Cambridge, MA: Ballinger.

Zubin, J., & Spring, B. (1977). Vulnerability—A new view of schizophrenia. *Journal of Abnormal Psychology, 86,* 103–126.

2

Pharmacological Management of Schizophrenia

PHILIP T. NINAN

INTRODUCTION

A number of different pharmacological agents have been shown to be effective in the management of schizophrenia. These pharmacological agents have been variously named antischizophrenic, antipsychotic, neuroleptic, and major tranquilizers. Though these medications do significantly ameliorate the symptoms of schizophrenia, they are not specifically antischizophrenic because they are effective against a number of psychotic illnesses. The term *neuroleptic* is a Greek derivative that literally means to take hold of the nerves. It was first used by Delay and Deniker in 1955 in reference to both chlorpromazine and reserpine (Deniker, 1983) because their extrapyramidal effects resembled central nervous system diseases. By common usage, neuroleptics came to be used interchangeably with the term *antipsychotic medications*. Novel antipsychotic agents exist that do not have prominent extrapyramidal side effects (e.g., clozapine). These have been called atypical neuroleptics, though a consensus is lacking on a clear definition of the term *atypical*.

Because antipsychotic agents had the effect of sedating and calming agitated behavior, they came to be called major tranquilizers (differentiating them from minor tranquilizers, which had similar capacities but no antipsychotic effects). However, antipsychotic medications can have an activat-

PHILIP T. NINAN • Department of Psychiatry, Emory University Clinic, 1365 Clifton Road, N.E., Atlanta, Georgia 30322.

ing effect in withdrawn schizophrenics, and normal subjects consider their effects unpleasant. One of the side effects of these medications is akathisia, which is a subjective sense of restlessness that is in direct contrast to any feelings of tranquillity. Thus, terms like *major tranquilizers* are highly non-specific and reflect the relatively primitive state of the available pharmacological agents and our knowledge about their effects.

Synthesized in 1950, chlorpromazine was initially evaluated as an adjunct for anesthesia and was reported to produce a detached affect. It was first used in psychiatry for "states of excitement, agitation, mania, confusion and acute psychosis" (Deniker, 1983, p. 166) in 1952, and within that year at least 15 scientific articles related to the use of chlorpromazine were published in the literature. Subsequently, a number of other phenothiazines were released for clinical use, essentially with the same therapeutic effects. Butyrophenones were introduced in the mid-1960s and had the same profile as high-potency phenothiazines.

With the use of chlorpromazine, the pharmacological management of schizophrenia began a new era. At about the same time, reserpine was also being evaluated for its efficacy in treating psychotic states. It is important to remember that before the discovery of neuroleptic agents, the treatments that were available for the management of schizophrenia were limited to sedatives like barbiturates, insulin-induced coma, and ECT. Such treatments were largely ineffective, resulting in patients' being essentially warehoused in large state institutions for custodial care.

Once the effectiveness of neuroleptic agents was clearly established, the search for its mechanism of action ensued. This also spawned hypotheses about the pathophysiology of the illness, based on the premise that a pharmacological treatment that was effective must be correcting the underlying pathological state. This assumption is only partially true, especially in situations in which one is controlling rather than curing the illness. Thus, understanding how aspirin controls fever provides little information about the infectious agent. Similarly, it seems that, at least in some patients with schizophrenia, the positive symptoms that are the hallmarks of the illness and are most responsive to neuroleptics are probably secondary phenomena to an underlying primary illness marked by negative symptoms and the defect state.

PREDICTING RESPONSES TO PHARMACOLOGICAL TREATMENT IN SCHIZOPHRENIA

The management of an illness should be based on studies of the diagnosis and clinical manifestations, responsiveness to the treatment under question, maintenance and prophylaxis, and risks of the treatment. There are a number of factors that make it difficult to study pharmacological responses in schizophrenia. These include *diagnostic, clinical, and pharmacological* issues. There are limitations in what hard science can provide in terms of specific guidelines for the pharmacological treatment of individual patients with schizophrenia. The treatment of an individual patient is guided by the numberous clinical factors to be considered, balanced by the trade-offs of various treatment options. This emphasizes the critical importance of clinical judgment, the relationship with the patient, the ability to elicit and observe symptoms, and the ability to tease out the different possibilities that might explain the observed presentation. Compliance and issues around self-reporting of symptoms do not make the task any easier.

The most basic of all the issues is that of *diagnosis*. Since there is no pathognomonic sign or test that can be used to categorically diagnose the illness and separate people without the illness from those with the illness, we are limited in validating the diagnosis. The term *schizophrenia* does not seem to signify a single disease with a specific etiology or pathophysiology that results in the manifestations of the illness and provides some basis for the response to treatment. Schizophrenia is a simple clustering of symptoms and signs that denote a clinical syndrome or disorder. Thus, current psychiatric nomenclature uses cross-sectional symptomatology and longitudinal outcome in the diagnosis of the illness to increase reliability. A lack, or a partial lack, of response to treatment is necessary for the diagnosis of schizophrenia (i.e., 6 months of symptomatology, including prodromal and residual symptoms). Thus, predicting response to treatment in patients that are at least partially nonresponsive is daunting. If schizophrenia is the result of damage to brain tissue or a developmental dysplasia that is irreversible, treatment response takes on a whole different connotation.

The boundaries of schizophrenia are poorly defined, and illnesses that straddle or lie just outside the boundary may have different responses to treatment. The illness is probably multifactorial in its etiology, with genetic vulnerabilities and environmental triggers or protection; thus, until we are able to tease out the actual vulnerability and the other etiological agents involved, it would be appropriate to take a variety of factors into consideration in the diagnosis. However, this is not easily done because these variables are not absolute. Thus, while schizophrenia tends to aggregate in families, this fact cannot be used for diagnostic purposes since the vast majority of patients with the illness do not seem to have an immediate family history of the illness.

One of the boundary issues for the diagnosis of schizophrenia is deciding what to do about subclinical versions of the disorder. For example, the prodromal symptoms of schizophrenia are remarkably similar to schizotypal personality disorder (SPD). However, the criteria for diagnosing SPD are far from ideal. Part of the problem arises because the social-interpersonal items (as against the cognitive-perceptual ones) in the diagnosis of SPD were derived from familial studies that looked for symptoms in the biological relatives of schizophrenics (Widiger, Frances, & Trull, 1987). This is in contrast to the purely descriptive approach that attempts to separate a cluster of symptoms signifying SPD from other personality disorders, such as borderline personality disorder.

There are also questions about the boundaries between schizophrenia and affective disorders. Thus, schizoaffective disorder has been described broadly, partly to increase the diagnostic stringency of schizophrenia. Similarly, the boundary between depressive disorders with psychotic features (especially with mood-incongruent symptoms) and schizophrenia is operationally based on the temporal association of the psychotic and the affective symptoms, rather than on objective biological measures.

There is a growing consensus that the symptomatic presentations of the illness can be grossly divided into positive and negative symptoms. Positive symptoms are those behaviors that are added to the premorbid functioning of the patient, including such symptoms as delusions, hallucinations, and incoherence. Negative symptoms are those relating to the absence of functions that might have been present premorbidly or should be present, given the developmental progress. Emotional blunting, social withdrawal, and poverty of speech content are considered negative symptoms. Debate still continues on whether some symptoms should be considered positive or negative. Thus, social withdrawal could be an independent domain or the result of impairment from positive symptoms.

The *nature of the illness* also makes it difficult to evaluate treatment response. Because of the effect of the illness on the cognitive, emotional, and behavioral capacities of the patient, he or she is not always the best observer or reporter of the intrapsychic experiences that are a critical element of the illness. Yet many rating scales used to measure change are often dependent on self-report. Denial of symptoms is a common phenomenon that further complicates the picture. Such issues might become more problematic as the symptoms increase in severity.

An illness as complex in its presentation as schizophrenia cannot easily be quantified. The criteria used to measure response (i.e., rating scales) are imprecise measures. For example, some symtpoms might be all-or-none phenomena while others, like social functioning, might be graduated. Graduated items might not be linear, although rating scales often seem to make that assumption. In treatments that are geared to controlling the symptoms of the illness rather than curing it, the mechanism of response induced by the medication might be different from the pathophysiology of the disorder.

Such control of symptoms might move the patient not in the direction of normality but toward another state that has to be fitted into the scale that presumes a linear direction between the pathological symptom and normality. For example, activation of a withdrawn schizophrenic is attenuated by the akinesia of neuroleptics.

Neuroleptics have tremendous differences in their steady-state levels in the plasma of different individuals. It would seem logical that some of the variance in treatment response would be the result of these differences in plasma levels in patients. However, a clear-cut association between plasma levels of neuroleptics and clinical response has yet to be convincingly demonstrated. Some of the problems have been related to technical issues, such as the measurement of active metabolites, while others have been methodological ones. Flexible dose strategies, which are commonly used in clinical management, result in nonresponders' getting higher doses of medication. Higher doses are also associated with greater side effects, which can be difficult to differentiate from the symptoms of the illness. For example, akathisia is often mistaken for agitation. Thus, to find a dose–response relationship, fixed-dose studies, in which all patients regardless of response get the same regimen of medication, are required. The presence of spontaneous responders also makes it difficult to find an association between plasma levels and clinical response. It is not surprising that it took many years from the clinical discovery of the effectiveness of neuroleptics to studies that clearly documented the diagnostic groups that responsded and the nature of the response (NIMH-PSC Collaborative Study, 1964).

There are some data to suggest that, at least for haloperidol, there is a curvilinear relationship between plasma levels and clinical response, such that at higher plasma levels clinical response deteriorates. However, for such a relationship to be convincingly demonstrated, an adequate number of both responders and nonresponders have to be in the sample studied, and nonresponders with high plasma levels should have their neuroleptic dose reduced to see if lowering the plasma level will result in clinical response (Kane, 1987).

DOPAMINE AND SCHIZOPHRENIA

The purpose of this section is not to review the literature on the pathophysiology of schizophrenia but to address an area that has specific relevance to the understanding of the pharmacological management of schizophrenia. Dopamine is not the sole neurotransmitter of relevance in the current understanding of schizophrenia, but having an understanding of its function is critical in developing at least some guidelines for the rational therapy of schizophrenia with neuroleptic agents. There are a number of dopamine systems in the brain. The ones of relevance to this chapter include the mesolimbic and mesocortical, which are thought to be integrally related to the illness, and the nigrostriatal and tuberoinfundibular, which are more related to side effects.

The dopamine hypothesis has provided the major thrust in the search for a biological understanding of schizophrenia. As originally proposed, it stated that the symptoms of the illness were the result of functional overactivity of the dopamine system. Until recently, there was only indirect evidence to support this hypothesis. Dopamine agonists could induce schizophreniclike states, while antagonism of the dopamine receptor in time resulted in clinical improvement. The affinity that various neuroleptic agents had for the dopamine receptor correlated highly with the average therapeutic dose used for antipsychotic effect, strongly suggesting that neuroleptic actions at the dopamine receptor were pharmacologically relevant for their therapeutic effects. More recently, PET scan studies have shown an increase in the density of D2 dopamine receptors in the brains of schizophrenics, some of whom were never treated with neuroleptics (Wong et al., 1986). However, adequate replication of this finding is lacking and might have to await clarification of methodological issues.

The nature of the symptomatology of the illness and the functional organization of the brain makes the likely structural areas of the brain involved in schizophrenia to be the prefrontal lobes and the limbic brain. Damage to the prefrontal areas results in an amotivated, withdrawn state with lack of initiative thought and emotion (Fuster, 1980). These effects closely parallel the negative symptoms of schizophrenia. The positive symptoms, such as hallucinations and delusions, on the other hand, seem to be the result of pathology in the limbic system (Seidman, 1983). Since it is easier to measure positive symptoms than negative symptoms (there is an inherent difficulty in measuring a symptom that is defined as an absence of function), and the positive symptoms are more striking, they have been given greater weight in the diagnostic criteria of schizophrenia. Hence, they have also received more focus in the dopamine hypothesis of the illness.

There is an intriguing confluence of the possible anatomical localization of pathology in schizophrenia and the mesocortical and mesolimbic dopamine pathways. There are important differences between these cortical and limbic dopamine pathways. The mesocortical system does not have autoreceptors on the cell bodies and nerve terminals (Bannon & Roth, 1983). Possibly related to this, the mesocortical dopamine neurons have a higher rate of physiological activity, are less responsive to dopamine agonists and antagonists, and do not develop tolerance to chronic neuroleptic treatment. It is possible that at low doses, neuroleptics have a predominent effect on the nigrostriatal and mesolimbic dopamine system, and higher doses result in effects on the mesocotrical dopamine system. Blockade of the mesocortical dopamine pathway could theoretically result in a worsening of negative symptoms.

Lesioning of the mesocortical dopamine system in rats (Pycock, Kervin, & Carter, 1980) results in the functional overactivity of the mesolimbic dopamine system, with increased dopamine turnover and upregulation of the dopamine receptors. Such effects in the limbic system are reported in postmortem studies of schizophrenic brains (Weinberger & Kleinman, 1986), although differentiating the effects of the illness from its treatment are difficult with this methodology. A model can be proposed in which an underactivity of the mesocortical dopamine system and an overactivity of the mesolimbic system can possibly explain the symptomatology in schizophrenia. Thus, a number of different lines of information from the clinical, structural, physiological, biochemical, and pharmacological areas come together to aid in understanding the complex illness of schizophrenia. These advances in our understanding of dopamine and schizophrenia are important because of their implications for the rational use of neuroleptics in the treatment of patients with schizophrenia.

CLASSIFICATION OF ANTIPSYCHOTIC AGENTS

Neuroleptics can be classified on the basis of structure and effects, including clinical and biochemical.

The basic skeleton of the antipsychotic agents belonging to the phenothiazines and the thioxanthenes are a tricyclic ring structure formed by two benzene rings connected by sulfur at position 5 and nitrogen (carbon for thioxanthenes) at position 10. Various substitutions at positions 10 and 2 provide the compounds with antipsychotic activity. Chlorpromazine, the first phenothiazine demonstrated to have antipsychotic activity, belongs to the phenothiazines that have an aliphatic side chain at position 10. A piperidine side chain at position 10 results in thioridazine and mesoridazine. A piperazine side chain results in compounds like fluphenazine, which have greater potency. Esterification with long-chain fatty acids of piperazine derivatives results in long-acting phenothiazines that are slowly absorbed when given as an injection. Other antipsychotic agents like haloperidol (a butyrophenone), loxapine (a dibenzoxazepine), and molindone (a dihydroindolone) also have heterocyclic ring structures but are chemically unrelated to the phenothiazines and thioxanthenes.

The therapeutic effects of the currently available neuroleptics are comparable. What differentiates them are issues of milligram potency and side-effect profiles. The high-potency neuroleptics (e.g., haloperidol) are used in low-milligram doses (2–75 mg), while the low-potency neuroleptics (e.g., chlorpromazine) are used in doses of hundreds of milligrams. The former tend to have greater propensity toward the development of extrapyramidal side effects, while the latter have more anticholinergic, sedative, and hypotensive side effects.

PHARMACOLOGICAL EFFECTS OF NEUROLEPTICS

In animal studies, neuroleptics reduce both conditioned and unconditioned (spontaneous) motor responses, in a dose-dependent manner. In fact, neuroleptics seem to modulate the control of external stimuli on overall behavior (Iversen & Iversen, 1981). The effect is particularly true for operant conditioning, where the response is tied to reinforcement (positive) and punishment (negative). Neuroleptics reduce behaviors that are maintained by positive reinforcement but have less of an effect on responses that are suppressed by punishing stimuli. Self-stimulation of electrodes placed in the median forebrain bundle by animals is a model for positive reinforcement. Neuroleptics block such self-stimulatory behavior.

The antipsychotic effect of neuroleptics is directly correlated with their capacity to suppress conditioned avoidance behavior. The antipsychotic activity is also highly correlated with the ability of neuroleptic agents to antagonize the behavioral, physiological, and biochemical effects of dopamine agonists. Thus, such effects became screening tools in the search for newer antipsychotic agents. However, these strategies have their limitations. For example, the conditioned avoidance effect develops tolerance and is blocked by anticholinergic agents. Such a screening test predicts the development of extrapyramidal symptoms better than antipsychotic effects. Similarly, clozapine, a new antipsychotic agent that does not have prominent extrapyramidal side effects, also does not block conditioned avoidance behavior.

Since spontaneous motor behavior is reduced by neuroleptics, behavioral pharmacologists have been unable to identify a specific action of neuroleptics in animals that can predict antipsychotic action. This lack of a true animal model for the neuroleptic and antipsychotic effects has been a major stumbling block. The inability to overcome this problem can reflect the greater phylogenetic evolution of the human brain (i.e., a truly representative animal model for human psychosis is impossible), or because the effect of neuroleptics in a nonpsychotic brain is different from that seen in a psychotic one—and unless one can come up with a model that replicates the pathophysiology of psychosis in animals, a screening system to detect antipsychotic activity in pharmacological agents is simply not feasible.

Other effects of neuroleptics include a calming of normally aggressive animals, including sham rage in decorticated animals. Neuroleptics also have a generalized slowing and synchronizing effect on EEG. There also is a reduction in the arousing effects of sensory stimuli. However, there is a danger of seizure induction at high doses of neuroleptics, particularly with aliphatic phenothiazines like chlorpromazine, which reduce the threshold for the development of seizures.

Dopamine inhibits prolactin release in the anterior pituitary and, therefore, neuroleptics cause prolactin levels in the serum to rise. Tolerance does not seem to develop over time, and prolactin levels revert to normal when the neuroleptic is discontinued. Neuroleptics also have effects on gonadotrophins, although the effects are not consistent. The result of these endocrine effects can be impotence, gynecomastia, and galactorrhea.

Neuroleptics accelerate the turnover of dopamine following acute administration, as evidenced by an acute increase in plasma and CSF homovanillic acid, a metabolite of dopamine. This increased turnover is the result of increased firing of the dopamine neurones when the dopamine receptors are blocked acutely (Bunney & Aghajanian, 1974). Chronic neuroleptic treatment eventually results in a depolarization block of the dopamine neurones. This reduction of firing of the dopamine neurons is temporally related to clinical improvement.

Chlorpromazine is a potent alpha-adrenergic antagonist, while drugs like haloperidol and fluphenazine are relatively weak in this action. The hypotensive effect of neuroleptics is thought to be mediated through this mechanism. Other pharmacological effects of neuroleptics include anticholinergic ones that are a source of distressing side effects (see below).

TREATMENT OF SCHIZOPHRENIA WITH NEUROLEPTIC AGENTS

Neuroleptic agents in the treatment of schizophrenia are clearly superior to antianxiety agents, antidepressant agents, antimanic agents, and psychostimulants, none of which is significantly better than placebo.

Neuroleptic agents have two prominent indications in the treatment of schizophrenia: control of the symptoms of the illness, and a prophylactic effect in preventing relapse. Thus, one is geared to the control of an episode of illness while the other is primarily involved in maintenance management. Quite often, since the symptomatic control of the illness is only partial, these two components of the treatment are combined. However, for the purposes of this chapter, we will address these two issues separately.

Studies from the beginning of the neuroleptic era to more recent ones have clearly shown the efficacy of neuroleptics in controling manifestations of psychotic behavior (Baldessarini, Cohen, & Teicher, 1988). This is predominantly true for the positive symptoms of the illness. It is generally believed that negative symptoms do not, or only partially, respond to neuroleptics, although this is still being debated (Goldberg, 1985). The defect state is believed to be irreversible and not responsive to neuroleptics. The control of symptoms is complete in some patients and partial in others, while neuroleptics are almost totally ineffective in some patients with schizophrenia. The capacity to predict response to treatment is limited (Lydiard & Laird, 1988) and depends primarily on clinical judgment. Patients who have responded well in the past are likely to respond again. In general, predictors of good outcome in schizophrenia are also predictors of good response to pharmacological treatment. Initial clinical and subjective responses when exposed to neuroleptics also are thought to predict later response (Hogan, Awad, & Eastwood, 1985; Van Putten, May, & Marder, 1980).

A number of studies have shown clearly that neuroleptic medications are effective in controlling the symptoms of schizophrenia acutely when compared to placebo (Davis, 1975). The therapeutic benefit generally takes a couple of weeks to manifest, although it can occasionally be seen within a few days. Such early responses are thought to be the result of nonspecific effects, such as sedation and calming of agitation, which can secondarily have an impact on psychotic symptoms. Antipsychotic benefits can continue to accrue for a considerable period of time.

Studies seem to suggest a range of 400 to 600 mg of chlorpromazine or equivalent to be necessary for the successful treatment of an acute psychotic episode for most patients (Kane, 1987). There is possibly a dose–response curve for neuroleptics, but the range seems to happen at a very low dose. Haloperidol has been reported to have a curvilinear dose–response relationship, where blood levels between roughly 5 and 15 ng/ml are associated with clinical benefit while levels below and above that are not. Tremendous individual differences in neuroleptic blood levels and other factors may have obscured a dose–response relationship in studies of other neuroleptics. High doses (2000 mg and over of chlorpromazine or 50 mg of haloperidol or equivalent) do not result in greater or faster improvement (Baldessarini et al., 1988; Kane, 1987).

In light of the studies that look at therapeutic response, it would be advisable to treat a patient needing control of the acute symptoms of schizophrenia with roughly 600 mg of chlorpromazine or 15 mg of haloperidol or equivalent. Because some patients are extremely sensitive to the side effects of neuroleptics, it would be advisable, especially in someone receiving neuroleptics for the first time, to give an initial test dose before the institution of a regular dose. Intolerable side effects that cannot be adequately managed require a reduction in neuroleptic dose. Failure to see any response in psychotic symptoms within a couple of weeks is indication to increase the dose of neuroleptic within tolerable limits to see if higher doses will result in any improvement. It should be recognized that a clinical response associated with an increased dose could also be the result of the passage of time, rather than the increase in dosage.

A common reason for the early use of high doses of neuroleptic is agitation and threatening behavior. Such behaviors, if not responsive to initial doses of neuroleptic, might be responsive to sedative-hypnotic agents, such as benzodiazepines. The advantage of using targeted benzodiazepines to control agitated behavior is that the dose of neuroleptic used can still be relatively low. The disadvantages include the possibility of disinhibiting behavior. Use of benzodiazepines should be for only a few days at a time, to prevent the development of tolerance and dependence.

The neuroleptic agents in use today are all equally efficacious in treating psychosis. No neuroleptic has been consistently shown to be superior to another (Davis & Garver, 1978). Even neuroleptics that have a greater sedative effect are effective in psychomotor retardation associated with psychosis, and the less sedating neuroleptics calm agitated patients. Thus, neuroleptics across the spectrum have a normalizing effect on patient behavior. It is possible that a subgroup of schizophrenics exist who will specifically respond to one neuroleptic rather than another, and that a failure to find this is related to a type II statistical error (false negative). Although the remarkable similarity of results in studies comparing neuroleptics would make this unlikely, there are clinical examples in which patients do seem to respond to one neuroleptic agent and relapse when switched to another (Gardos, 1974).

What should be done with patients who do not respond to a neuroleptic within a specified period of time? Since the response to neuroleptics can vary from a few days to many weeks, it is difficult to know whether any benefit obtained from switching medications is from the switch or from the passage of time. The logical recommendation would be that if a patient is nonresponsive to a neuroleptic for a number of weeks (adequate trial of an adequate dose), a trial of another neuroleptic might be indicated. Since the differences in structure are greater between chemical classes of neuroleptics than within a class, it would make sense to choose a neuroleptic from another class (e.g., switching from a phenothiazine to a butyrophenone). Failure to respond to an adequate trial of different classes of neuroleptics would be considered to constitute a nonresponsive condition.

The combination of different neuroleptics simultaneously is rarely indicated. There are no therapeutic advantages to these combinations, while the likelihood of negative reactions is increased. For example, the risk of neuroleptic malignant syndrome is reported to be greater when a combination of neuroleptic agents is used (although this might be explained on the basis of a higher dose, which by itself is a risk factor for neuroleptic malignant syndrome).

Another question is whether nonresponders to the standard dose of neuroleptic agents will respond to high or megadose strategies (e.g., over 2000 mg of chlorpromazine or 50 mg of haloperidol or equivalent). High-dose strategies are based on the premise that if a standard dose of neuroleptic resulted in partial benefit, then more medication might provide even greater benefit. High-dose strategies could be necessary because of pharmacokinetic factors resulting in lower blood levels at standard doses, or because a subgroup of schizophrenic patients require higher blood levels for pharmacodynamic reasons. However, such strategies do not provide any greater therapeutic benefits and are marked by greater side effects (Quitkin, Rifkin, & Klein, 1975). This is particularly true for negative symptoms, which can be worsened by high doses of neuroleptics.

Would rapid delivery of high doses of neuroleptic result in a quicker response? Methodologically stringent studies fail to support this possibility (Neborsky, Janowsky, Munson, & Debry, 1981). Methodological issues in addressing these questions are numerous. A failure to find an improvement in these strategies does not mean that individual patients will not be helped by them, but that a group of patients treated along these lines fail to show statistically greater improvement over the control condition. It is possible that a type II error has occurred because the numbers of patients studied are inadequate to rule out the possibility that a small subgroup of patients will be aided by these strategies.

MAINTENANCE STRATEGIES IN THE MANAGEMENT OF SCHIZOPHRENIA

The value of maintenance neuroleptics in preventing relapse is clear (Davis, 1975; Davis, Schaffer, Killian, Kinard, & Chen, 1980). These have focused on reducing relapse and hospitalization. More recently, psychosocial functioning and the risk for the development of tardive dyskinesia have also been addressed (Kane, 1987).

Patients whose acute psychotic symptoms have been controlled for a few months are eligible for maintenance therapy strategies. What should the maintenance dose of a patient be relative to dose for acute control? In a review of the studies that have tried to answer this question (Baldessarini & Davis, 1980), there was no correlation between the maintenance dose and the capacity to prevent relapse. Clinical experience would suggest that unless side effects require a reduction in dose, it is generally advisable to maintain the patient on the same dose of neuroleptic that was required to obtain control of the acute episode if standard dosage strategies were used (i.e., 600 mg of chlorpromazine or 15 mg of haloperidol or equivalent daily). If higher doses were needed to control the acute symptomatology, consideration should be given to a slow and gradual decrease in dose (i.e., 100 mg of chlorpromazine or 2.5 mg of haloperidol or equivalent roughly every month) for maintenance treatment. Such a decrease should be coupled with education of the patient and significant others, and attempts to monitor the development of early warning signs of an impending relapse. Such a decision should also take into consideration the stability of the environment around the patient, and the extent of emotional hostility or intrusiveness the patient has to endure.

There is a dearth of information about maintenance strategies for patients who have had a first psychotic break that was brought under control quickly, because of the current inability to predict possible relapse. Patients with predictors of good outcome are probably better off being placed on maintenance neuroleptics at least for some time, with the understanding that a trial off medication will be tried in the future when psychosocial stressors are minimal. Clinical judgment is critical in making these decisions.

The rate of relapse in treated schizophrenics at the end of a year is in the area of 30%, even if compliance is monitored through the use of long-acting injectable neuroleptics (Schooler et al., 1980). The risk for relapse is greatest in the first year following discontinuation of medication, and the risk seems to partially level off in the second year (Hogarty & Goldberg, 1973). Thus, neuroleptics have a definite advantage in the prevention of relapse, although the control again is not absolute.

There are no clear predictors of relapse following successful control of psychotic symptoms in schizophrenia. The predictors of relapse are probably the same as the predictors for a poor outcome in the illness. Poor control of an acute episode of psychosis suggests the liklihood of relapse. Dose of medication needed to control an acute episode may also predict the likelihood of relapse (Prien, Lewine, & Switalski, 1971). The higher the dose needed for the control of the acute episode, the greater the likelihood of relapse. Presumably, the higher dose reflected either greater severity of symptoms, chronicity, or nonresponsiveness to treatment. Thus, the factors to consider in deciding on maintenance strategies (compliance being assumed) should include issues such as chronicity, medication responsiveness, and previous experiences of relapse at certain doses (Davis, 1975).

Relapse rates with neuroleptic medications have been reduced even further with the addition of various psychosocial treatment strategies. This is particularly important because neuroleptics often do not result in complete symptomatic control, and residual symptoms can prevent a return to premorbid functioning.

EXTRAPYRAMIDAL EFFECTS OF NEUROLEPTICS AND THEIR MANAGEMENT

Although neuroleptics have many side effects, for the purposes of this chapter only extrapyramidal side effects of the CNS will be addressed. The extrapyramidal systems are involved in the nonconscious control of voluntary musculature. Neuroleptics have complex effects on parts of the extrapyramidal systems, and since these effects are clinically undesirable, they are considered to be side effects. Extrapyramidal side effects are exaggerated by anxiety, disappear in sleep, and can be consciously controlled for a limited time with effort. Extrapyramidal side effects can be classified into those that happen early or late in treatment.

Acute dystonic reactions (*dystonia* literally means "abnormal tone") are involuntary spasms of voluntary muscle groups that are often painful and frightening to patients. They most commonly involve the orofacial and head and neck areas, although any part of the body with voluntary muscles can be involved. Young patients and males taking high-potency neuroleptics are at greatest risk for the development of acute dystonic reactions. All neuroleptic medications have the capacity to cause acute dystonic reactions, although low-potency neuroleptics that also have significant anticholinergic effects (e.g., thioridazine) have them less frequently. Acute dystonic reactions tend to happen early in treatment, and although some level of tolerance develops, they can also happen late in treatment (Rifkin, Quitkin, Kane, Struve, & Klein, 1978). When it involves the laryngeal muscles, it can be life-threatening and require emergency action. Parenteral anticholinergic agents are indicated in these rare situations.

The prophylactic use of anti-Parkinsonian agents (anticholinergic agents and dopamine agonists) for acute dystonic reactions is still debated. Prophylactic use of these agents would mean that they are prescribed simultaneously with neuroleptics even before the development of extrapyramidal side effects. Anticholinergic agents (e.g., benztropine mesylate, diphenhydramine hydrochloride) have been reported to be more effective in the acute treatment of dystonic reactions than in a prophylactic role (Sramek, Simpson, Morrison, & Heiser, 1986), although others disagree (Gelenberg, 1987). The clinical trend appears to favor prophylactic use of anti-Parkinsonian agents because the development of acute dystonic reactions can lead to noncompliance with neuroleptic treatment (Van Putten, 1974). Such a practice results in significant anticholinergic side effects and, especially in the elderly and in brain-damaged patients, the risk of developing a central toxic state has to be considered. In patients who have been on a constant dose of neuroleptic and are compliant and responsible, and can recognize extrapyramidal side effects, the possibility of changing the anti-Parkinsonian agent to a PRN schedule could be considered.

In idiopathic Parkinson's disease there is a degeneration of dopamine cells in the substantia nigra, resulting in an imbalance between the dopamine and cholinergic systems. Neuroleptics, by blocking dopamine receptors, produce a condition that has functional similarity to idiopathic Parkinson's disease. *Parkinsonian side effects* include tremor, rigidity, and akinesia. The tremor seen most often with neuroleptic treatment is a fine tremor of the fingers. It may occasionally involve the lips and jaw and resemble the chewing movements of a rabbit. The rigidity is generally of the cog-wheeling type, often best felt in the upper arm during passive flexion of the elbow. Pharmacological treatment of Parkinson's disease is to use dopamine agonists or anticholinergic agents to correct this imbalance.

Akinesia was described by Rifkin, Quitkin, and Klein (1975) as a "behavioral state of diminished spontaneity characterized by few gestures, unspontaneous speech and, particularly, apathy and difficulty with initiating usual activities." Akinesia can have effects on complex social behavior and, as a side effect, can have an impact on the social functioning of a patient making efforts at rehabilitation. Akinesia can also be difficult to differentiate from depression and the apathy and blunting of negative symptoms. Improvement of the symptoms on reducing the neuroleptic dose or adding anti-Parkinsonian agents would suggest akinesia. Terms like *akinetic depression, pharmacologic depression,* and *postpsychotic depression* are imprecise terms that need further elaboration. Clinically, at least some of the patients who seem to have postpsychotic depression respond to anti-Parkinsonian agents.

Anticholinergic agents are effective in treating early features of Parkinson's disease and for neuroleptic-induced Parkinsonian side effects. Benztropine mesylate, an anticholinergic agent, also has an effect in blocking the reuptake of dopamine, an effect that is possibly related to its mildly activating effect. Dopamine agonists like amantadine are also used in the treatment of neuroleptic-induced Parkinsonian side effects. Amantadine, which is a predominantly indirect dopamine agonist, has the advantage of not causing the tachycardia and other autonomic side effects of anticholinergic agents. Amantadine also lowers prolactin through its effects on the pituitary.

Akathisia is a subjective sense of restlessness that is often manifested by patients' being motorically restless (e.g., rocking from one foot to the other while standing, or walking on the same spot). It is often associated with a dysphoric mood. Generally considered a late complication of neuroleptic treatment, akathisia has also been reported to be present relatively early in treatment with high-potency neuroleptics in the majority of patients (Van

Putten, May, & Marder, 1984). Akathisia is difficult to differentiate clinically from anxiety and psychotic agitation. One of the disconcerting possibilities is that akathisia is misdiagnosed as agitation, resulting in patients' getting more neuroleptics in a spiraling manner when less neuroleptics or treatment for akathisia is indicated. Anticholinergic agents and dopamine agonists are only partially effective in the treatment of akathisia. Propranalol also has been shown to be partially effective. The best treatment, of course, is reducing the dose of the neuroleptic.

Tardive dyskinesia (TD) is "a syndrome consisting of abnormal, stereotyped involuntary movements, usually of choreoathetoid type, principally affecting the mouth, face, limbs and trunk, which occurs relatively late in the course of drug treatment and in the etiology of which the drug treatment is a necessary factor" (Jeste & Wyatt, 1982). Like other dyskinesias, it is exacerbated by anxiety and focusing on unaffected parts, and is temporarily controlled by volition. Like all movements that involve the extrapyramidal system, they disappear during sleep. It appears in approximately one-third of the individuals treated with neuroleptics on a chronic basis, although some populations of patients might be more susceptible than others. Risk factors for the development of tardive dyskinesia are total amount of neuroleptic exposure, age, being female, a history of extrapyramidal side effects, and affective disorder. There is an annual cumulative incidence of about 3 to 4% in chronically treated patients. Early diagnosis is critical. It seems that even with continued neuroleptic exposure, the condition is mild and not progressive in the majority of patients (Casey, 1983). Continuation of the neuroleptic results in the symptoms' becoming irreversible (Kane, 1987). Discontinuation of the neuroleptic results in either remission or improvement in half the patients. The improvement can happen over a period of 2 years. The difficult question is in the patients in whom discontinuation of neuroleptics is not an affordable luxury, or the risk–benefit ratio is weighed heavily in favor of continuation of neuroleptic treatment. In these individuals, the neuroleptic treatment should be with the lowest dose necessary for therapeutic effects.

At a simple level, TD is thought to result from supersensitive dopamine receptors that result in a functional hyperdopaminergic-hypocholinergic state. The data supporting this hypothesis are that transient improvement results from the use of a higher dose of neuroleptics and of cholinomimetic agents like physostigmine (a choline esterase inhibitor), while the symptoms are exacerbated by dopaminergic agents (e.g., L-dopa) and anticholinergic agents. No cure exists for this condition, and symptomatic treatment for it leaves much to be desired.

Tardive dystonia is a more malignant form of tardive dyskinesia, characterized by "sustained, involuntary, twisting movements, generally slow, which may affect the limbs, trunk, neck or face" (Burke et al., 1982). The clinical manifestations can be retrocollis, torticollis, and abnormal posture and gait. It seems to be more common in younger patients, associated with brain damage, and less reversible, and it could respond to anticholinergic agents. It tends to cause greater functional impairment than tardive dyskinesia.

Neuroleptic malignant syndrome (NMS) has been reported to have an annual prevalence rate of 1.4% in an inpatient setting (Pope, Keck, & McElroy, 1986). The clinical manifestations of neuroleptic malignant syndrome include hyperthermia, muscle rigidity, and associated mental status changes, including delirium. Other symptoms include tachycardia, labile blood pressure, excessive perspiration, sialorrhea, resting tremor, dystonia, dysphagia, and akinetic mutism. Pulmonary difficulties are thought to be secondary manifestations of the illness due to general cachexia. Laboratory findings include a leukocytosis, abnormal liver function tests, and abnormalities in blood gases and electrolytes. Other laboratory tests do not show a pathognomonic pattern. Postmortem studies fail to demonstrate lesions that can be used retrospectively to confirm the diagnosis. On the basis of the case report literature, the mortality from NMS appears to be about 20%.

The nature of NMS makes it particularly difficult to study. Its relative infrequency, presence in patients often with a number of other complicating circumstances, varied presentation, responses to treatment that might be nonspecific, and lack of an adequate animal model make the literature in this area suspect because it is based only on clinical case reports.

Multiple neuroleptics prescribed simultaneously are reported to have been used in 40% of patients with NMS. NMS appears to occur more in younger patients. NMS also has been associated more often with high-potency neuroleptics than with low-potency ones. This might be a factor based on the prescription practices of the physicians, because high-potency neuroleptics are used more often and are also used in higher chlorpromazine-equivalent doses. Thus, if the amount of neuroleptic prescribed were a critical issue in the generation of NMS, it would explain the reports of high-potency neuroleptics and the combination of neuroleptics as more likely to result in NMS.

NMS by definition requires the use of neuroleptic agents. However, there are similar conditions in neurologic patients (Parkinson's disease, Huntington's chorea) who have not received neuroleptics. Further, the symptoms of NMS closely resemble malignant hyperthermia, which is a disorder affecting skeletal muscles. It follows exposure to halogenated inhalant anesthetics in susceptible individuals, possibly with an abnormal phospholipase activity. Dantrolene is effective in the treatment of malignant hyperthermia if instituted in the early stages of its development.

In general, the pathophysiology of NMS might be an abnormal thermal regulation that is aggravated by compounds that have an effect on dopamine. Thus, heat loading can result in a susceptibility to NMS. The treatment should include discontinuing the neuroleptic, supportive measures, dopamine agonists, and possibly dantrolene sodium.

CONCLUSION

The discovery of the effectiveness of neuroleptic agents had a tremendous effect in the treatment of psychotically ill patients. However, we are still learning today how to use these agents to their best advantage, and to balance the various trade-offs that are involved with their usage. Future research may well identify entirely new compounds, as well as refine use of those currently available. Despite the imitations and negative side effects associated with current neuroleptics, they serve an indespensible role in the treatment of schizophrenia.

ACKNOWLEDGMENTS

This work was supported, in part, by U.S. Public Health Service (NIMH) grants MH 40597 and MH 42298.

REFERENCES

Baldessarini, R. J., Cohen, B. M., & Teicher, M. M. (1988). Significance of neuroleptic dose and plasma level in the pharmacological treatment of psychosis. *Archives of General Psychiatry, 45*, 79–91.

Baldessarini, R. J., & Davis, J. M. (1980). What is the best maintenance dose of neuroleptics in schizophrenia? *Psychiatry Research, 3*, 115–122.

Bannon, M. J., & Roth, R. H. (1983). Pharmacology of mesocortical dopamine neurons. *Pharmacological Review, 35*, 53–68.

Bunney B. S., & Aghajanian, G. (1974). In E. Usdin & S. H. Snyder (Eds.), *Frontiers in catecholamine research*. Oxford: Pergammon Press.

Burke, R. E., Fahn, S., Jankovic, J., Marsden, C. D., Lang, A. E., Gollomps, S., & Ilson, J. (1982). Tardive dystonia: Late-onset and persistent dystonia caused by antipsychotic drugs. *Neurology, 32*, 1335–1346.

Casey, D. E. (1983). Tardive dyskinesia: What is the natural history? *International Drug Therapy Newsletter, 18*, 13–16.

Davis, J. M. (1975). Overview: Maintenance therapy in psychiatry I. Schizophrenia. *American Journal of Psychiatry, 132*, 1237–1245.

Davis, J. M., & Garver, D. L. (1978). Neuroleptics: Clinical use in psychiatry. In L. L. Iverson, S. D. Iverson, & S. H. Snyder (Eds.), *Handbook of psychopharmacology* (Vol. 10, pp. 129–164). New York: Plenum Press.

Davis, J. M., Schaffer, C. B., Killian, G. A., Kinard, C., & Chan, C. (1980). Important issues in the drug treatment of schizophrenia. *Schizophrenia Bulletin, 6*, 70–87.

Deniker, P. (1983). Discovery of the clinical uses of neuroleptics. In M. J. Parnham & J. Bruinvels (Eds.), *Discoveries in Pharmacology, Volume 1: Psycho- and Neuropharmacology* (pp. 163–180). New York: Elsevier Science.

Fuster, J. (1980). *The prefrontal cortex*. New York: Raven Press.

Gardos, G. (1974). Are antipsychotic drugs interchangeable? *Journal of Nervous and Mental Disease, 159,* 343–348.

Gelenberg, A. J. (1987). Treating extrapyramidal reactions: Some current issues. *Journal of Clinical Psychiatry, 48*(9) (Suppl.), 24–27.

Goldberg, S. C. (1985). Negative and deficit symptoms in schizophrenia do respond to neuroleptics. *Schizophrenia Bulletin, 11,* 453–456.

Hogan, T. P., Awad, A. G., & Eastwood, M. R. (1985). Early subjective response and prediction of outcome to neuroleptic therapy in schizophrenia. *Canadian Journal of Psychiatry, 30,* 246–248.

Hogarty, G. E., & Goldberg, S. C. (1973). Drugs and sociotherapy in the aftercare of schizophrenic patients: One year-relapse rates. *Archives of General Psychiatry, 28,* 54–64.

Hogarty, G. E., Schooler, N. R., Ulrich, R., Mussare F., Ferro, P., & Herron, E. (1979). Fluphenazine and social therapy in the aftercare of schizophrenic patients. Relapse analyses of a two-year controlled study of fluphenazine decanoate and fluphenazine hydrochloride. *Archives of General Psychiatry 36,* 1283–1294.

Iversen, S. E., & Iversen, L. L. (1981). *Behavioral pharmacology* (2nd ed.). New York: Oxford University Press.

Jeste, D. V., & Wyatt, R. J. (1982). *Understanding and treating tardive dyskinesia* (p. 84). New York: Guilford Press.

Kane, J. M. (1987). Treatment of schizophrenia. *Schizophrenia Bulletin, 13,* 133–156.

Lydiard, B. R., & Laird, L. K. (1988). Prediction of response to antipsychotics. *Journal of Clinical Psychopharmacology, 8,* 3–13.

National Institute of Mental Health Psychopharmacology Service, Collaborative Study Group. (1964). Phenothiazine treatment in acute schizophrenia: Effectiveness. *Archives of General Psychiatry, 10,* 246–261.

Neborsky, R., Janowsky, D., Munson, E., & Depry, D. (1981). Rapid treatment of acute psychotic symptoms with high- and low-dose haloperidol: Behavioral considerations. *Archives of General Psychiatry, 38,* 195–199.

Pope, H. G., Keck, P. E., & McElroy, S. L. (1986). Frequency and presentation of neuroleptic malignant syndrome in a large psychiatric hospital. *American Journal of Psychiatry, 143,* 1227–1232.

Prien, R. F., Lewine, J., & Switalski, R. W. (1971). Discontinuation of chemotherapy for chronic schizophrenics. *Hospital and Community Psychiatry, 22,* 4–7.

Pycock, C. J., Kerwin, R. W., & Carter, C. J. (1980). Effect of lession of cortical dopamine terminals on subcortical dopamine receptors in rats. *Nature, 286,* 74–76.

Quitkin, F., Rifkin, A., & Klein, D. (1975). Very high dosage vs. standard dosage fluphenazine in schizophrenia: A double-blind study of non-chronic treatment-refractory patients. *Archives of General Psychiatry, 32,* 1276–1281.

Rifkin A., Quitkin, F., Kane, J. M., Struve, F., & Klein, D. F. (1978). Are prophylactic antiparkinson drugs necessary? A controlled study of procyclidine withdrawal. *Archives of General Psychiatry, 35,* 483–489.

Rifkin A., Quitkin, F., & Klein, D. F. (1975). Akinesia: A poorly recognized drug-induced extrapyramidal behavioral disorder. *Archives of General Psychiatry, 32,* 672–674.

Schooler, N. R., Levine, J., Severe, J. B., Brauzer, B., DiMascio A., Klerman G. L., & Tuason, V. B. (1980). Prevention of relapse in schizophrenia: An evaluation of fluphenazine decanoate. *Archives of General Psychiatry, 37,* 16–24.

Seidman, L. J. (1983). Schizophrenia and brain dysfunction: An integration of recent diagnostic findings. *Psychology Bulletin, 94,* 195.

Sramek, J. J., Simpson, G. M., Morrison, R. L., & Heiser, J. F. (1986). Anticholinergic agents for prophylaxis of neuroleptic-induced dystonic reactions: A prospective study. *Journal of Clinical Psychiatry, 47,* 305–309.

Van Putten, T. (1974). Why do schizophrenic patients refuse to take their drugs. *Archives of General Psychiatry, 31,* 67–72.

Van Putten, T., May, P. R., & Marder, S. R. (1980). Subjective response to thiothixene and chlorpromazine. *Psychopharmacology Bulletin, 16,* 36–38.

Van Putten, T., May, P. R. A., & Marder, S. R. (1984). Akathisia with haloperidol and thiothixene. *Archives of General Psychiatry, 41,* 1036–1039.

Weinberger, D. R., & Kleinman, J. E. (1986) Observations on the brain in schizophrenia. In R. E. Hales & J. A. Frances (Eds.), *Psychiatry update: American Psychiatric Association annual review* (Vol. 5, pp. 42–67). Washington DC: American Psychiatric Association Press.

Widiger, T. A., Frances, A., & Trull, T. J. (1987). A psychometric analysis of the social-interpersonal and cognitive-perceptual items for the schizotypal personality disorder. *Archives of General Psychiatry, 44,* 741–745.

Wong, D. F., Wagner, H. N., Tune, L. E., Dannals, R. F., Pearlson, G. D., Links, J. M., Tamminga, C. A., Broussolle, E. P., Ravert, M. T., Wilson, A. A., [Thomas Toung, J. K., Malat, J., Williams, J. A., O'Tuane, L. A., Snyder, S. M., Kuhar, M. J., Gjedde, A.]. (1986). Positron emission tomography reveals elevated D2 dopamine receptors in drug-naive schizophrenics. *Science, 234,* 1558–1563.

3

Innovations in the Psychopharmacologic Treatment of Schizophrenia

JOHN M. KANE

INTRODUCTION

The treatment of schizophrenia represents a major challenge to clinicians. The role of pharmacologic and somatic treatments in this disorder is an important one; however, clinicians must appreciate both the complexity and the potential heterogeneity of the disorder in order to provide optimal management within a particular modality.

Antipsychotic medication remains a mainstay in both the acute and long-term treatment of schizophrenia as it has for approximately three decades. The emphasis in the recent past has focused on several concerns: to improve response rates by attempting to understand factors that might influence drug response, either positively or negatively; to improve the benefit-to-risk ratio by reducing or eliminating adverse effects; to identify minimum effective dosage requirements; to establish alternative treatments for patients who fail to respond to standard pharmacologic approaches; to develop

JOHN M. KANE • Department of Psychiatry, Hillside Hospital, Division of Long Island Jewish Medical Center, 75-59 263rd Street, Glen Oaks, New York 11004, and School of Medicine, Health Sciences Center, State University of New York at Stony Brook, Stony Brook, New York 11794.

drugs with greater specificity of therapeutic activity as well as treatments that might be useful in alleviating some of those signs and symptoms that may not respond adequately to antipsychotic drugs (i.e., so-called deficit symptoms). In addition, considerable attention has been given to developing strategies for identifying patients who may be taken off neuroleptic drugs for substantial intervals of time. Further advances have been made in exploring the impact of psychological and psychosocial treatments administered in conjunction with various antipsychotic drug strategies.

In this chapter we will review some of the developments in these areas, focusing on their clinical relevance as well as their implications for improving our overall understanding of the disorder we label as schizophrenia.

ACUTE TREATMENT

This phase of treatment refers usually to a period of exacerbation of psychotic signs and symptoms frequently, though not always, requiring hospitalization. The goal of this treatment phase is to control the "florid" psychotic signs and symptoms and enable the patient to return to the community and, to the extent possible, to previous levels of psychosocial and vocational adaptation. Although we usually associate acute exacerbation with so-called positive symptoms, such as delusions, hallucinations, thought disorder, or agitation, some patients may experience an increase in negative symptoms, such as withdrawal, lack of motivation, or diminished attention to personal hygiene. A psychotic episode may be rapid in onset or insidious; it may represent a worsening of preexisting symptomatology, the emergence of new symptoms, or the reemergence of symptoms that occurred during the prior episode. Clinically, it is important to recognize that we rely very heavily on the subjective reporting of perceptual experiences and feeling states that cannot necessarily be subjected to external validation; however, behavioral observation and information derived from significant others can also be critical in establishing a diagnosis and assessing the severity of the symptomatology.

Considerable advances have been made in recent years in improving the reliability of psychiatric diagnosis, and the first step in treatment planning for patients with psychosis is a careful delineation of the differential diagnosis in order to assure appropriate pharmacologic treatment. In a situation where a major affective component is present, the use of alternative treatments such as lithium or electroconvulsive therapy should be considered. Any pharmacologic treatment, even in a patient who clearly meets criteria for schizophrenia, should be viewed as a therapeutic trial and evaluated in that context with a statement of clear goals and objectives, target symptoms, and other factors by which clinicians can evaluate the efficacy of the treatment provided.

Antipsychotic (neuroleptic) drugs remain the primary modality in the treatment of an acute episode or an acute exacerbation of the schizophrenic illness. The value of medication in this context has been established in numerous double-blind, placebo-controlled trials. Variability in drug responsiveness, however, remains a major clinical problem, given the fact that a substantial subgroup of patients derives little, if any, benefit from drug treatment.

It is possible that variability in drug response is influenced by pharmacologic (e.g., drug type, dosage, blood levels) and biological (e.g., genetic, neurochemical, neuroanatomical) factors as well as psychological, psychosocial, and environmental influences. Subsequent advances in any of these areas may ultimately lead to improvements in treatment efficacy or specificity.

There are several pharmacologic factors that should be considered in planning the treatment of an acute episode although we are far from having developed definitive guidelines in all of these areas.

DRUG TYPE

At the present time there are five different classes of antipsychotic drugs available in the United States; however, there are no convincing data that among medications currently marketed in this country any one is more effective, either in schizophrenia in general or in specific subtypes of the disorder (although an experimental drug, clozapine, may be an exception to this, as we shall discuss subsequently). It is possible, however, that there are differences between available medications but that appropriately designed studies have not been carried out in order to establish this. Very few studies provide data on differential treatment response to particular pharmacologic agents, and most of the available data are based on comparisons of overall response rates in group data contrasting one drug with another.

A major question grows out of this in terms of an acute episode of schizophrenia when an individual fails to respond to an adequate dose and adequate time period of administration with a particular antipsychotic drug. Should the clinician switch to another class of antipsychotic, and what is the likelihood that this will produce the desired response? Although these are questions that arise daily in clinical practice, there are remarkably few data that address these issues. One methodological problem that would require consideration is the fact that the time course of response to antipsychotic drugs in schizophrenia is somewhat unpredictable. Many patients will experience substantial therapeutic response within the first 2 to 3 weeks, whereas other patients may take substantially longer to derive full therapeutic benefit from this treatment. As a result, if a clinician switches from one antipsychotic drug to another after a lack of response to 3 weeks of initial therapy, it may be difficult to attribute subsequent improvement to the change in pharmacologic agents rather than the passage of additional time. Obviously, appropriately controlled studies would be necessary to answer this question.

The preclinical observations that antipsychotic drugs differ enormously in their relative affinities for specific brain receptors, including the dopamine receptors felt to mediate therapeutic response, also support the possibility that all classes of antipsychotic medication do not have the same spectrum of therapeutic activity. At the same time, however, it has been suggested that the potency of various antipsychotic drugs on a milligram per milligram basis does correlate with receptor affinity in theoretically relevant binding assays. It is clear that antipsychotic drugs do differ in their adverse effects profile, and these differences may be attributable to variability in affinity for specific receptors. In addition, these differences may be important clinically in choosing a particular drug for those individuals with known sensitivity to specific adverse affects. Obviously, knowledge of a patient's previous therapeutic response to a particular antipsychotic drug or drugs should be heavily weighted in choosing a particular treatment approach. One belief that continues to be prevalent in some clinical settings is that highly sedating drugs (e.g., chlorpromazine) are more effective in controlling the extremely excited or agitated patient than are nonsedating drugs (e.g., haloperidol, trifluoperazine), with the latter being more appropriate for withdrawn or psychomotorically retarded patients. This relationship has never been systemically established, and numerous studies suggest that high-potency and low-potency drugs are equally effective in both types of patients.

In terms of treating the agitated or excited patients, many clinicians have reported the benefits of anxiolytics as adjunctive agents in combination with antipsychotic drugs. In our view, the potential added benefit of these compounds has not been sufficiently studied, and the degree to which these agents are exerting an antipsychotic as opposed to anxiolytic effect has not been clearly established.

DOSAGE

We continue to have insufficient information regarding dose response curves for antipsychotic drugs. (The issue of blood levels will be discussed separately.) Many investigations of drug efficacy have not employed fixed doses. When flexible dose strategies are employed, this means that the clinician is adjusting the dosage on the basis of clinical response. The problem with drawing conclusions regarding dose–response relationships in this context is that if a patient receiving a given dose of an antipsychotic shows little improvement after 10 days and the clinician decides to increase the dose, the subsequent improvement may be due to the passage of additional time rather than to the increase in dosage. Controlled trials are necessary to establish a putative cause-and-effect relationship. In those investigations comparing high doses (arbitrarily defined as in excess of 2000 mg chlorpromazine equivalents) with "standard" dose treatment, there is no evidence of a statistically significant advantage for the high-dose approach. This does not preclude, however, the possibility that some individuals may benefit from higher doses, but it would suggest that such individuals may represent a small subgroup. Clearly, better means of identifying those patients who would be appropriate candidates for relatively high-dose treatment should be established, but in general, our reading of the literature would suggest that doses of 400 to 600 mg/day of chlorpromazine or equivalents should be sufficient for the average patient.

It is also our impression that strategies employing rapid neuroleptization with very high doses of parenteral medication offer no advantage over more traditional approaches. This is not to say that vigorous pharmacotherapy should not be employed in the highly agitated or violent patient, but that further therapeutic gains may not result from increasing the dosages.

DOSE EQUIVALENCE

As indicated in the introduction, there has been increasing attention in recent years focused on establishing minimum effective dosage requirements for both acute and long-term treatment. In this context a clear understanding of the dose equivalence among antipsychotic drugs would be highly desirable. Chlorpromazine has usually been the standard against which equivalent doses are established; however, we should recognize the fact that dosage equivalencies that have been published should serve as mere guidelines and may be crude and unsystematic. The most frequent method for establishing dose equivalency has involved a double-blind clinical trial comparing two antipsychotic drugs, with the clinician adjusting the dosage as he sees fit. When the trial is completed, statistical comparisons are made of the doses employed and a conversion ratio is suggested. In addition, in some cases results from drug–placebo comparisons may be employed to attempt to identify the clinically "effective" dosage range of a particular drug or drugs. There are a variety of problems in assuming the validity of these results. In addition, it is also important to recognize that the conversion ratios possibly appropriate at the lower end of the dosage spectrum may not apply at higher dosage levels.

It certainly does appear that many clinicians are using dissimilar dosing practices when they employ high-potency drugs as compared with low-potency drugs. Baldessarini, Katz, and Cotton (1984) compared the findings of a survey of 110 private hospital inpatients with the dosing practice as reported in surveys of nearly 16,000 Veterans Administration patients. Doses of high-potency drugs above the daily equivalent of 1 gram of chlorpromazine accounted for more than 40% of all prescriptions. The mean chlorpromazine equivalent dose of the two most potent antipsychotic agents (haloperidol and fluphenazine) was 3.54 times as high as the mean dose prescribed of chlorpromazine or thioridazine. As these authors suggested, the sedative and autonomic effects of low-potency drugs may limit their use in the higher dosage range, whereas it is feasible for clinicians to increase doses of high-potency antipsychotics without a substantial increase in immediate adverse affects.

One additional factor that may have led to the use of higher doses is the apparent increasing pressure on clinicians to shorten the length of inpatient hospital stays. The difficulty, however, is that the use of "rapid neuroleptization" or high-dose treatment has not been shown to shorten the time required for these drugs to exert their therapeutic effect or to improve overall clinical outcome. Though the time course of response may be unpredictable, with some patients improving rapidly and others more slowly, in our general experience and as suggested by the literature, 4 to 6 weeks is usually the minimum necessary to begin to see the full therapeutic benefit, and in some cases it is quite likely that even longer intervals are necessary.

DRUG PLASMA LEVELS

Since it was recognized that antipsychotic medications are subject to enormous individual variability in absorption and metabolism, the availability of assays to measure neuroleptic blood levels appeared to be a major step forward in potentially explaining heterogeneity of clinical response to antipsychotic agents. To a great extent this promise has not been fulfilled, but blood levels may have some utility in specific clinical situations. Over the past 10 years we have seen considerable advances in the laboratory techniques available for measuring minute quantities of antipsychotic and other drugs in clinical specimens (e.g., plasma, cerebrospinal fluid, and even red blood cells). It is ironic, however, that despite this degree of sophisticated technology, it is usually the flaws in the design and methodology employed in clinical trials utilizing blood levels that have, in most cases, limited the potential to draw meaningful and generalizable conclusions. One factor that complicates studies in this area is diagnostic heterogeneity. If patients with a variety of diagnoses or those who have proved nonresponsive to antipsychotic treatments are included in studies, then the ability to find meaningful clinical chemical correlations can be severely limited. (This concern would include, therefore, both diagnostic and prognostic heterogeneity.)

Another concern is that the development of steady-state blood levels following fixed-dose treatment is essential in attempting to relate blood levels to clinical response. If, as mentioned previously, dosage adjustment is based purely on clinical response, then those patients who are intrinsically poor responders to antipsychotic medications (regardless of dose or blood level involved) may end up with the highest blood levels in that particular patient sample. This could then be interpreted as negating the value of blood levels or even suggesting that high blood levels are countertherapeutic.

It is also extremely important to consider the length of the clinical trial since many patients with schizophrenia can require several weeks to achieve full benefit from pharmacotherapy. Those investigations that have examined blood level clinical response relationships after relatively brief periods of time (e.g., 14 days) may be focusing on only one aspect of clinical effect, such as the alleviation of psychomotor agitation or excitement, whereas other aspects of psychopathology (delusions, hallucinations, thought disorder) may not have improved to the same degree within that particular time frame. It is also important to consider the influence of other psychotropic drugs that the patient may be receiving in influencing the metabolism or absorption of the antipsychotic drug or influencing the clinical state more directly (e.g., sedative, hypnotic or anti-Parkinsonian drugs). Table 1 summarizes 18 studies involving some type of fixed-dose design. In reviewing reports, we excluded those that focused on treatment-resistant patients. Almost all these studies have some methodological flaws, but it is extremely difficult to carry out such investigations in the types of clinical settings where appropriate patients can be found.

The drug that has been most frequently studied is haloperidol, and several of these investigations have suggested a curvilinear relationship between blood levels and clinical response, or what is sometimes called a "therapeutic window." Although these results are intriguing, considerable further work would be necessary to firmly establish and define a therapeutic window. Most studies suggesting this phenomenon have had relatively few patients above the suggested upper limit to the therapeutic window, and, more important, hardly any attempts have been made to conduct trials involving random assignment of patients whose blood levels are out of the therapeutic range to a dosage necessary to manipulate the blood level into a

Table 1. Neuroleptic Blood Levels and Clinical Response

Author	N	Dose	Duration	Method	Blood level	Results	Window
Smith et al. (1984)	26	Thioridazine fixed-random	24 days	GLC	195–1685 ng/ml (thiorid and mesorid)	No significant correlation	No
Wode-Helgodt et al. (1978)	38	Chlorpromazine fixed-random	28 days	GC/MS	0–150 ng/ml	Significant correlation at 2 weeks but not 4 weeks	No
Dysken et al. (1981)	29	Fluphenazine fixed	15 days	GLC	0.1–4.4 ng/ml	Significant correlation	Yes 0.2–2.8 ng/ml
Cohen, Lipinski, Pope, et al. (1980)	11	Thioridazine fixed	14 days	RRA	1100–6200	Significant correlation	No
Bergling et al. (1975)	40	Thioidazine or thiothixene	56 days	Fluorometric	Thiorid 1000–6000 ng/ml thiothixene 0–160 ng/ml	No significant correlation	No
Neborsky et al. (1984)	20	Haloperidol fixed-random	7 days	RIA	Low X = 8.2 High X = 34.0	Plasma: RBC correlation with response	No
Garver et al. (1977)	10	Butaperazine flexible-fixed	12 days	Fluorometric	2.3–321 ng/ml	Plasma and RBC curvilinear relationship	30–80 ng/dl RBC
Garver et al. (1984)	14	Haloperidol fixed-random	17 days	GLC	0.7–87 ng/ml	Significant correlation for plasma but not RBC	Window for plasma but not RBC
Smith et al. (1985)	33	Haldoperidol fixed-random	4 days	GLC	2–23 ng/ml	Significant correlation	6.5–16.5 ng/ml plasma; 2.2–6.8 ng/ml RBC

Study	N	Drug (design)	Duration	Method	Range	Correlation	Plasma levels
Mavroidis et al. (1983)	14	Haloperidol fixed-random	14 days	GLC	2–19 ng/ml	Significant correlation	Plasma—4.2–11.0 ng/ml
Mavroidis et al. (1984)	19	Fluphenazine fixed-random	14 days	GC	0.1–2.4 ng/ml	Significant correlation	Plasma—0.1–0.7 ng/ml; RBC—0.2–0.6 ng/ml
Cohen, Lipinski, Harris, et al. (1980)	58	Various drugs flexible-partial fixed	?	RRA	—	Significant correlation	No
Casper et al. (1980)	24	Butaperazine random-fixed	14 days	Fluorometric	23–250 ng/ml	Significant correlation with RBC, but not plasma	RBC only 30–60 ng/ml
Potkin et al. (1985)	73	Haloperidol flexible-fixed	42 days	RIA	0–75 ng/ml	Trend	Curvilinear (trend) 4–26 ng/ml
Van Putten et al. (1985)	47	Haloperidol random-fixed	28 days	RIA	?	Significant at 1 week but not at 2 or 4 weeks	Curvilinear at 1 week (5–16 ng) but no relationship at 2 or 4 weeks
Magliozzi et al. (1981)	17	Haloperidol flexible-fixed	21–84 days	GLC	0–96 ng/ml	Significant correlation	8–17.7 ng/ml
Bolvig-Hansen et al. (1981)	14	Perphenazine flexible-fixed	56 days	GC	.6–10.1 ng/ml	No significant correlation	No
May et al. (1981)	48	Chlorpromazine fixed	28 days	GC/MS	?	No significant correlation (plasma or saliva)	No

putative therapeutic range or to remain at their current blood level (the latter being necessary to control for the effects of continued time on drug). Until such studies are accomplished and results are replicated, any conclusions regarding a therapeutic window must remain cautious.

This concern is also important in considering the role of high-dose or very high (megadose) treatment. If patients were specifically selected owing to their having low blood levels on standard doses of antipsychotics, then it is possible that a substantial dose increase might have a likelihood of providing some added benefit. On the other hand, if those studies employing substantial dosage increase involve a heterogeneous group of drug nonresponders, the likelihood of seeing a desired clinical effect may be reduced considerably since there may be various other factors responsible for drug refractoriness besides those pharmacokinetic factors that may lead to a low drug blood level.

Another important issue in considering the possibility of a therapeutic window is the concern that some of those patients showing a poor or minimal clinical response at the higher blood level may in fact be experiencing behaviorally manifest adverse effects that might alter or impede the therapeutic response. Although some investigators have suggested that an increase in side effects does not account for the lack of beneficial effects at higher blood levels, this question continues to require further study. Behaviorally manifest adverse effects may be difficult to distinguish from psychopathology, and a patient in the midst of a psychotic episode may not be able to articulate subjective feelings and sensations in a way that would contribute to a differential diagnosis. The overall value of measuring blood levels of antipsychotic drugs, therefore, remains far from clear, but the available data should encourage clinicians and investigators to recognize the potential problems of using dosages that are very high as well as the importance of appropriate clinical evaluation and research methodology in using or studying high-dose treatment in specific subgroups of schizophrenic patients.

There has also been some renewed interest in attempting to use the neurologic side effects of neuroleptics as a guide to identifying appropriate therapeutic dose. This concept was first suggested and explored by Haase (1961; Haase & Janssen, 1965), who suggested that the first appearance of hypokinesia-rigidity, as reflected by changes in handwriting, indicated that a sufficient dosage for antipsychotic effect had been reached. This suggestion has been either largely ignored or misinterpreted to imply that there is a linear relationship between extrapyramidal side effects in clinical response, or that more clinically obvious extrapyramidal side effects are necessary to indicate adequate dosage. McEvoy, Stiller, and Farr (1986) have pointed out the potential importance of this suggestion and have begun to test the neuroleptic threshold hypothesis in a systematic fashion. Their initial open pilot study found that the mean daily dose of haloperidol at which the neuroleptic threshold (the emergence of subtle extrapyramidal side effects) was crossed was 4.2 ± 2.4 ng/day. The plasma haloperidol levels obtained at these neuroleptic threshold doses averaged 4.9 ± 2.9 ng/ml, which is very close to the lower end of the therapeutic range reported in several studies (Mavroidis, Kanter, Hirschowitz, & Garver, 1983; Potkin et al., 1985; Van Putten, Marder, May, Poland, & O'Brien, 1985). Sixty-seven percent of the patients in McEvoy's study had at least moderate therapeutic response at the neuroleptic threshold dose. This is an extremely interesting finding, and further double-blind, random-assignment studies should prove of great interest.

PREDICTORS OF RESPONSE AND THE ROLE OF ALTERNATIVE SOMATIC TREATMENTS

It is clear to clinicians who have worked with antipsychotic drugs in the treatment of schizophrenia that there is considerable variability in clinical response. Repeated attempts have been made to identify predictors of response. Although there are suggestions in the literature involving a broad range of variables, there are no well-established predictors of antipsychotic drug response during an acute episode or exacerbation. At the same time, there have been some suggestions that subgroups of patients with schizophrenia may respond to lithium (Delva & Letemendia, 1982; Hirschowitz, Casper, Garver, & Chang, 1980; Small, Kellams, Millstein, & Moore, 1975) or electroconvulsive therapy (ECT) (Brandon et al., 1985; May, 1968; Salzman, 1980; Taylor & Fleminger, 1980), or may at times improve without somatic treatment.

These two lines of evidence may at some point produce data on which to base recommendations for a particular alternative somatic therapy in the acute treatment of specific individuals. However, at our present level of knowledge, antipsychotic drugs are clearly the most effective treatment for the largest proportion of patients with this illness; therefore, currently there is no basis on which to select alternative somatic treatments for an initial therapeutic trial for patients with schizophrenia.

STRATEGIES FOR MANAGING NONRESPONSIVE PATIENTS

Although, as indicated, antipsychotic medications have a dramatic effect on the majority of individuals with schizophrenia, we continue to be faced with a substantial number of patients who derive little if any benefit from these compounds. The treatment of such individuals remains a major clinical dilemma. It is frequently in this context that clinicians consider or employ therapeutic trials of all antipsychotic drug classes, megadoses, high doses of long-acting injectable medication, concomitant lithium, propranolol, carbamazepine, high doses of benzodiazepines, ECT, and experimental compounds under development. Although there are some anecdotal reports describing patients who benefit from such strategies, few systematic well-controlled studies have been carried out suggesting any more than occasional benefit. It is probably reasonable for the clinician to conduct a "therapeutic trial" of some alternative treatment strategy in patients who fail to respond to an adequate course (or courses) of antipsychotics, but there is also a point where we may have to recognize and accept our relative inability to help some patients, given our current level of knowledge. Fortunately, many patients who fail to respond adequately to antipsychotic drugs do derive some clinical benefit, and many of these patients are even more ill when they receive no treatment at all.

If such therapeutic trials are conducted, a clear process of identifying and documenting target symptoms as well as response over a reasonable time should be employed to avoid either an inadequate trial or the lack of follow-up and evaluation necessary to justify continuation of a specific treatment. In our experience, in reviewing numerous medical records in such patients, it is not unusual to see nonstandard or experimental treatment continued for months in a given patient without any clear evidence of a beneficial effect.

Other than the potential value of identifying patients who are rapid or idiosyncratic metabolizers through assays showing unusually low or unusually high blood levels, we are not aware of any logical basis for determining the next treatment to be tried. To our knowledge, no comparisons have been made of ECT, lithium, and other alternatives in this context. Even the determination of blood levels requires caution in interpretation since laboratories may vary in their methods. Values published by one laboratory should not be assumed to be relevant to results produced by a laboratory using different methodology. Therapeutic levels have not been well established, and for some drugs there are hardly any data. Unless blood levels are obtained and interpreted in collaboration with experts in this area, they can be used only as a guide in identifying relative extremes in drug absorption and metabolism.

A particularly important emphasis in evaluating apparently nonresponsive patients should be the adequacy of the length of the initial trial before a failure to respond is assumed. Four weeks may not be adequate in this context, but clinicians may find it difficult to continue a treatment beyond 4 weeks when it does not appear to be working. At the same time, abandoning a treatment before 4 weeks may very well be premature.

It is informative to look at a series of studies that included treatment-resistant schizophrenic patients who were randomly assigned to a standard-dose treatment or a high-dose treatment (see Table 2). None of these studies found a significant advantage for the very high-dose treatment, but it is of considerable interest to note the overall improvement rate among these apparent neuroleptic nonresponsive patients. This could suggest that additional time on medication may lead to improvement in some patients. It is also possible that nonpharmacological aspects of the research contributed to improvement, but in either case these findings argue for the avoidance of premature closure and the need for systematic research with appropriate controls. Considering a patient as treatment-resistant does not automatically eliminate the need for appropriate controls, as evidenced by the improvements seen on standard treatment.

We are also particularly concerned about the premature application of treatment for this patient population on the basis of single-case or anecdotal reports. There is a particular responsibility to do carefully controlled clinical trials in refractory patients, not only because of the potential to improve their treatments but also because we are dealing with an area of considerable desperation where the application of premature conclusions or preliminary data to large numbers of patients is extremely common and potentially unfortunate.

Our own recommendation is that two or three different classes of antipsychotic drugs be employed for at least 4 weeks each in doses in excess of 400 to 600 mg per day of chlorpromazine equivalence before the initiation of more unproven or experimental approaches. Obviously, this requires a relatively lengthy period of ongoing observation and evaluation; however, there is no shortcut in providing appropriate therapeutic trials in this particular patient population.

Table 2. Therapeutic Response in Neuroleptic Resistant Schizophrenia

Investigator	Drug(s)	Dosage	Overall improvement (combined groups)	
Itil et al. (1970)	Fluphenazine	30 mg		
	Fluphenazine	300 mg	9/17	53%
McCreadie and McDonald (1977)	Haloperidol	100 mg		
	Chlorpromazine	600 mg	7/20	35%
Quitkin et al. (1975)	Fluphenazine	30 mg		
	Fluphenazine	1200 mg	13/31	42%
Bjorndal et al. (1980)	Haloperidol	15 mg (mean)		
	Haloperidol	103 mg (mean)	10/23	43%

CLOZAPINE

Clozapine is an experimental antipsychotic drug that belongs to the chemical class of dibenzodiazepines, related chemically to the antipsychotic dibenzoxazepine drug, loxapine. Clozapine's pharmacologic characteristics, however, are strikingly different from those of loxapine.

Clozapine has several novel preclinical effects that have stimulated considerable research in light of its potential for novel activities in the clinic. Specifically, clozapine has produced only slight, transient elevations in serum prolactin levels in patients even on moderate to high daily doses. Its profile of extrapyramidal effects is substantially different from that of typical neuroleptics. Clozapine produces relatively few extrapyramidal side effects and does not appear to produce dystonia or tardive dyskinesia.

Several controlled clinical trials had been conducted with clozapine, establishing its efficacy as an antipsychotic agent (Claghorn et al., 1987; Gerlach et al., 1974). In addition, Honigfeld, Patin, and Singer (1984), in a review of the major controlled trials involving clozapine versus typical neuroleptics (e.g., chlorpromazine and haloperidol), suggested that this drug might have superiority in some treatment-refractory schizophrenic patients. In 1975, however, 16 patients in Finland developed granulocytopenia, and 13 of these developed agranulocytosis (with 8 fatalities resulting from secondary infection). Worldwide evidence now reveals over 100 cases of agranulocytosis in patients receiving clozapine. Because of this, use of the drug was curtailed in many countries and withdrawn for a time from controlled clinical research by the United States sponsor. For humanitarian purposes, some countries, including the United States, continue to allow use of the drug for carefully selected treatment-refractory patients, with intensive monitoring of white blood cell and differential counts. Since the introduction of restrictions in the use of the compound and the intensive monitoring for hematologic adverse effects, the overall worldwide incidence of agranulocytosis, as well as the lethal risk in patients developing this condition, has declined. At the present time in the United States, there have been 10 cases of agranulocytosis among the approximately 850 patients who have received the drug. All of these individuals have recovered without any apparent sequelae. Using the life-table method of calculating risk, the available data on those individuals receiving the drug in the United States indicates a 2% incidence after 52 weeks of clozapine treatment (95% confidence limits of 0.2% to 4%). Given both the potential risk of agranulocytosis and clozapine's possible benefit for treatment of refractory patients, a multicenter collaborative study was initiated in 1984 with the hope of determining whether or not this compound had any clinical advantage for the treatment of resistant patients.

The results of this study suggest that clozapine may have some utility in treatment-refractory patients (Kane, Honigfeld, Singer, & Meltzer, 1988). In a carefully selected sample of patients who had failed to respond to at least three periods of treatment in the preceding 5 years with neuroleptic agents from at least two different chemical classes at doses equivalent to 1000 mg/day of chlorpromazine or higher for a period of 6 weeks, and who then failed to respond to a prospective trial of haloperidol up to 60 mg/day for 6 weeks, clozapine proved to be significantly superior to chlorpromazine in a double-blind 6-week comparison. A total of 268 patients participated in the clozapine versus chlorpromazine double-blind comparison. Clozapine proved to be significantly superior on all of the clinical efficacy measures (BPRS, CGI, Nosie-30). In addition, patients were classified as having "improved" to a clinically significant extent if they experienced over a 20% reduction from baseline on the BPRS total score, and either a posttreatment CGI-scale score of 3 (mild) or less, or a posttreatment BPRS total score of 35 or lower. When these criteria were applied across all patients who completed at least 3 weeks of the double-blind chlorpromazine–clozapine comparison, it was found that only 4% of the chlorpromazine-treated patients improved, as compared with 30% of the clozapine patients ($p < .0001$). The results of these studies suggest that clozapine may be an alternative treatment strategy available for carefully selected treatment-refractory patients; however, the potential risk of agranulocytosis is a serious one, and patients must be monitored with extreme care in order to minimize the potential consequences of this adverse effect. Fortunately, the period of maximum risk for agranulocytosis does not begin until 4 to 6 weeks of clozapine treatment; therefore, it is possible for the clinician to have some sense that the patient will benefit from clozapine before continuing the drug through the period of maximum risk for the development of agranulocytosis. Further work is under way to identify risk factors and mechanisms for the development of this particular adverse effect. At the present time, however, despite this drug's unusual clinical profile, it should be reserved for the treatment of refractory patients, or possibly patients with severe involuntary movement disorders, if more data become available to support its utility in that context. It is hoped that the apparent advantages of this particular compound will also stimulate investigators to identify those features that are responsible for its novel effects as well as to identify other potential compounds that may have a superior benefit-to-risk ratio.

MAINTENANCE NEUROLEPTIC TREATMENT

The "acute" phase of the treatment of schizophrenia involves an attempt to alleviate the signs and symptoms associated with an acute psychotic episode or an acute exacerbation. Antipsychotic medications generally have a substantial effect on the symptoms of schizophrenia (e.g., delusions, hallucinations, thought disorder) within 4 to 6 weeks, although improvement may continue well beyond that. The clinical response achieved during this treatment phase does, to some extent, determine the rationale and expectations of subsequent continuation or maintenance treatment. In an illness that is subject to remission and exacerbations, the pharmacologic treatment can be divided into three sequential phases: acute, continuation, and maintenance (or prophylactic). In those individuals who achieve full or substantial recovery from an acute psychotic episode, the continuation phase would begin at that point when maximal improvement is reached. Its intent is to continue the treatment long enough to be sure that the episode for which the original treatment was administered is, in fact, over. Once this period has passed, then further pharmacologic treatment would be intended to prevent the occurrence of a new episode rather than the reemergency of the original episode. This model has been applied more readily to affective illness where episodes of psychopathology may be more discrete, but, in our view, this conceptualization may be useful in schizophrenia as well. Clearly, the actual delineation of these different phases in the treatment of schizophrenia may be difficult since, for example, some patients do not necessarily achieve complete remission of psychopathology even with continuous drug treatment. At the same time, however, the results of antipsychotic drug discontinuation studies suggest that many of these patients would experience even more symptomatology without medication. In this instance, however, pharmacotherapy may be viewed as controlling or suppressing the ongoing manifestations of the illness rather than actually preventing the new episode. These individuals, therefore, may be considered relatively poor candidates for drug discontinuation or substantial dosage reduction.

Maintenance antipsychotic medication has proved to be of enormous value in reducing the risk of psychotic relapse and rehospitalization. Numerous double-blind placebo-controlled studies support this conclusion and have been the subject of several review articles (Davis, 1975; Davis, Schaffer, Killian, Kinard, & Chan, 1980; Kane & Lieberman, 1987). In the last 10 years we have seen the initiation of a second generation of clinical trials that have been much more sophisticated in focusing not only on relapse and rehospitalization but also on various other factors relevant to assessing the overall benefits and risks of maintenance medication. Several different concerns have determined the types of studies carried out in the recent past: high rates of noncompliance in taking medication for long periods of time; the frequent occurrence of adverse effects, particularly tardive dyskinesia; the relative lack of substantial improvement in various areas of functioning, leading to continued impairment in psychosocial and vocational adjustment in many patients; considerable variability in clinical course, and the potential importance of other therapeutic modalities, environmental and personality factors; and increasingly sophisticated methodologic and data-analytic strategies being available to assist in the design and interpretation of long-term clinical trials. Table 3 summarizes the results of double-blind comparisons of active drug versus placebo; two different active drugs (or forms of administration, e.g., oral vs. long-acting injectable); or the same drug given in different dosages. We have included only maintenance trials of at least 9 months' duration.

It is clear that there is enormous variability in relapse rates reported in these studies, both on active treatment and on placebo. Meaningful comparisons are complicated by differences in design and methodologies, such as diagnostic criteria, level and length of clinical remission, criteria for patient selection and recruitment methods, as well as the definition of relapse. In addition, not all of these reports have presented cumulative relapse rates or "life-table" analyses that would allow for appropriate handling of patients with incomplete data (e.g., those who drop out or are discontinued from the trial owing to adverse effects or other factors). When cumulative relapse curves are presented, then data from different studies can be contrasted, even though investigators may have used different assessment intervals, carried out trials for different periods of time, or encountered substantial differences in dropout rates.

So-called guaranteed medication delivery (i.e., long-acting injectable neuroleptics) has played an important role in many of the major maintenance medication trials in the recent past because this strategy enables the investigator to be certain that a relapse that occurs in the context of long-term pharmacotherapy is not due to noncompliance in oral medication-taking and, therefore, the impact of other patient, treatment, or environmental factors can be considered and explored (Kane & Borenstein, 1985).

In addition, the use of long-acting injectable drugs in clinical trials has also made it quite clear that many patients will continue to experience psychotic relapse or exacerbation despite medication, and this has underscored the potential importance of exploring other factors that might contribute to poor outcome.

COMPLIANCE

As indicated in the previous section, the potential for noncompliance in maintenance treatment of schizophrenia is an important concern in assuring optimal outcome. Compliance to any treatment plan is a major concern in all areas of medicine; however, factors related to compliance are frequently

Table 3. Maintenance Pharmacotherapy in Schizophrenia

Author	N	Age (mean or range)	Sex	Prior episodes	Time since discharge (weeks)	Level of remission	Duration	Outcome Treatment	Outcome Relapse	Dropout rate
Troshinsky et al. (1962)	43	40–50	63% female	2–3	2–4 years	No hallucinations, delusions, or obvious thought disorder; required 300 mg CPZ	1 year	Drug[a]	4%	?
Engelhardt et al. (1963, 1964, 1967)	446	18–44	?	?	?	?	48 months	CPZ	1 year 15% 4 years 20%	36% in 18 months
								PBO	1 year 30% 4 years 31%	
Leff and Wing (1971)	35	16–55	?	?	6–12	Preadmission level	12 months	Drug PBO	35% 80%	14%
Hirsch et al. (1973)	81	43	36% female	70%	50%	?	9 months	FD PBO	8% 66%	9%
Crawford and Forrest (1974)	31	20–65 X̄ = 40s	71% female	≥4	52	?	10 months	Trifl TD	40% 14.3%	7%
Hogarty et al. (1974)	347	34	58% female	60% ≥2	?	?	24 months	Drug	12 months 31% 24 months 48%	8%
								PBO	12 months 68% 24 months 80%	
Cheung (1981)	30	40	60% female	1.6	3–5 years	Fully remitted 3–5 years	18 months	Antipsychotic Benzodiazepine	13% 62%	7%
Kane et al. (1982)	28	22	50% female	1	X̄ = 17	Remitted	1 year	Drug PBO	0% 41%	35%
McCreadie et al. (1982)	28	55	All male	?	Inpatients	"Well controlled"	10 months	Pimozide FD	15% 7%	25%
Odejide and Aderounmu (1982)	70	?	?	≥2	?	Well for ≥12 months	12 months	FD PBO	19% 56%	25%

Study	N	Age	Sex			Criterion	Duration	Drug/Dose		
Kane, Rifkin, et al. (1983, 1986)	163	29	37% female	3.2	X̄ = 64	Remitted or stable plateau	12 months	FD dose Low / Intermediate / Standard	56% / 24% / 14%	10%
Marder et al. (1984, 1986)	50	36	All male	?	X̄ = 23 months	Stable	1 year	FD dose Low / Standard	1 year 22% / 2 years 44% / 1 year 20% / 2 years 31%	14%
Crow et al. (1986)	120	26	38% female	1	1 month	Able to be discharged	2 years	Drug / PBO	58% / 70%	11%
Chien (1975)	47	43	57% female	Former long-term inpatients	?	?	12 months	FE[b] / FE[c] / PBO	12% / 37% / 86%	?
Rifkin et al. (1977)	73	23	32% female	1.9	X̄ = 26	Remitted or stable plateau	12 months	FD + oral / PBO	5% / 75%	11%
Kelly et al. (1977)	60	42	66% female	?	?	?	9 months	FD / Flupen D	10% / 10%	2%
Falloon et al. (1978)	44	17–60	55% female	80% ≥2	0	?	12 months	Pimozide / TD	24% / 40%	12%
Quitkin et al. (1978)	56	X̄ = 39	44% female	2.7	X̄ = 64	Remitted or stable plateau	12 months	Pen / FD	7% / 10%	20%
Hogarty, Goldberg, et al. (1979); Hogarty, Schooler, et al. (1979)	105	34	54% female	4.6	0	?	24 months	Oral / FD	2 years 65% 12–24 months 42% / 2 years 40% 12–24 months 8%	13%
McCreadie et al. (1980)	35	50	All male	?	?	"Well controlled"	9 months	Pimoide / FD	19% / 17%	3%
Schooler et al. (1980)	214	29	41% female	≥2	0	?	12 months	FHCL / FD	38% / 46%	25%

aPBO = placebo, CPZ = chlorpromazine, FD = fluphenazine decanoate, Trifl = trifluoperazine, FE = fluphenazine enanthate, Flupen D = flupenthizol decanoate, Pen = penfluridol, FHCL = fluphenazine hydrochloride.
bDoctor-regulated interval.
cPatient-regulated interval.

given inadequate attention, compared with the effort and sophistication that goes into diagnosis and treatment planning in general. In the clinical management of psychiatric disorders, the problem of compliance is even more difficult and complex because of the nature of the illnesses, and their potential impact on the judgment and insight that patients can apply to their own health care. In addition, psychiatric illnesses continue to evoke more of a stigma, and patients may be embarrassed by the mere fact of taking antipsychotic medication.

The methods employed by clinicians to detect noncompliance have varied considerably. By far the simplest but potentially most misleading strategy is to ask the patient directly. It is important that during any medical work-up and history-taking, individuals should be asked about past as well as present levels of compliance. It may be more informative to phrase the question, for example, "What did you do when you found the medication was not helping?" or "How many times did you forget to take your medication?" rather than a more confrontational inquiry. Many patients, however, regardless of how the question is posed, will deny noncompliance when questioned. Counting pills in returned medication bottles is another method employed, but this technique is very frequently misleading since there is no assurance that the medication removed from the bottle has actually been taken by the patient, and many patients will forget to bring in unused medication even when asked. In some studies, markers such as riboflavin have been used. More recently, sensitive assays have been developed to measure psychotropic drug blood levels, as discussed previously. However, these measures, when applied in the context of noncompliance, are really qualitative rather than quantitative. In order for clinicians to interpret a blood level in this context, they would have to know what the appropriate steady-state level would be under controlled (compliance-assured) conditions before they could make a judgment as to any ongoing levels of compliance. In addition, this procedure is extremely cumbersome and costly to carry out in any routine fashion.

Rates of noncompliance among psychiatric patients in the range of 40 to 50% have frequently been reported and are not dissimilar to those seen in a variety of medical conditions. Even in medical illnesses in which noncompliance has potentially serious physical consequences (e.g., hypertension), compliance rates have been found to be much lower than many clinicians assume.

FACTORS IN NONCOMPLIANCE

The nature of the treatment regimen has been suggested as an important factor in compliance. Patients are much more likely to adhere to a simple regimen, and when multiple medications are prescribed simultaneously where doses are to be taken several times a day, compliance is reduced. The single daily dosage has increased in popularity and is certainly feasible in most patients receiving antipsychotic drugs.

The clinical recognition of adverse effects is an extremely important factor in reducing rates of noncompliance. Many patients feel that their treating clinicians are unresponsive to their complaints regarding side effects, and this belief may frequently lead to reduced compliance. At times, physicians may be uncertain as to the association between a specific problem and the medication being administered and may dismiss it as unrelated, while the patient continues to attribute the difficulty to the drug. In a severe illness like schizophrenia, some complaints that may be drug-related have the potential to be viewed by the clinician as much less serious than the underlying disorder, and therefore minimized. In the patient's mind, however, this attitude may be misinterpreted as a lack of concern. It is important that even for those adverse effects that may appear relatively trivial to the clinician, some discussion take place to put them in the proper perspective. In the case of neuroleptic drugs, the physician must remain particularly sensitive to the possibility of extrapyramidal side effects, which may be subtle and may continue even during the maintenance phase of treatment. There may be debate among psychopharmacologists as to the appropriate use of prophylactic anti-Parkinsonian medication, but whatever strategy is employed, the fundamental necessity is the recognition of this potential problem and careful examination of the patient.

Van Putten (1974) investigated the medication-taking behavior of 85 mostly chronic schizophrenic patients, both in and out of hospital. Of these individuals, 39 (46%) were believed to have taken less antipsychotic medication than had been prescribed. The author found a statistically significant association between noncompliance and extrapyramidal side effects, particularly akathisia. Van Putten emphasized that many of the extrapyramidal side effects associated with noncompliance were "mild," or subclinical, and might be apparent only to a careful observer who knows how the patient behaves both off and on medication.

It is also important to consider the individual patients' own conception of their illness, and their understanding of the need for continued treatment, particularly during the long-term maintenance or prophylactic phase. It is apparent that even in more common and less emotionally laden medical illnesses, individuals who are feeling well will tend to discontinue medication. The concept of prevention, or prophylaxis, is difficult for people to fully accept. It requires the continued recognition and acceptance of the risk of becoming ill again, something that most of us would prefer to deny. In the case of schizophrenia, some individuals may attribute the acute illness to life circumstances or stresses, emotional concerns, or other environmental factors that they feel will not occur again, and may therefore conclude that preventive treatment is not necessary. In addition, as previously mentioned, the stigma associated with mental illness may also contribute substantially to the denial seen among patients suffering from schizophrenia.

Although we should not dismiss the avoidance or reduction of stress as an important goal in potentially reducing the risk of relapse, this aspect of ongoing treatment does not negate or minimize the need for continued pharmacologic treatment. Psychologically, acceptance of a biologic factor in the illness also removes a potential element of control and can be extremely frightening, both to patients and to their families. It is therefore important to discuss these issues fully in order to help overcome these potential contributing factors in noncompliance.

Another important aspect of the course of schizophrenia needs to be considered in promoting medication compliance. Specifically, the time-course of schizophrenic relapse is such that the discontinuation of antipsychotic medication does not usually lead to an immediate relapse or recurrence of psychotic symptoms. In fact, patients may remain well for many months before the full consequence of medication discontinuation becomes apparent. This delay may blur the cause-and-effect relationship in the mind of the patient, and sometimes even in the mind of the mental health professional. The modal time period for psychotic relapse following drug discontinuation in remitted or stable schizophrenic patients appears to be from 3 to 7 months. Therefore, in the case of those individuals who may experiment with medication discontinuation for several weeks, it is important to educate them to the fact that the lack of recurrence of psychotic signs and symptoms is in no way evidence that they no longer continue to require antipsychotic medication.

It is obviously important to assure close follow-up and supervision of patients in long-term treatment in order to reduce potential noncompliance. If problems do arise in any of the areas referred to, it is much more likely to be recognized and successfully dealt with if the patient has an ongoing therapeutic relationship with a health care professional. In addition, the importance of family and social support systems cannot be overemphasized. Not only is a great deal of patient and family psychoeducation required, but mental health professionals must also be adequately sensitized to the issue of noncompliance, its frequency, its causes, and strategies that may help to reduce it.

As indicated previously, the use of long-acting injectable antipsychotic medication may be very helpful in reducing the risk of relapse in patients who are, or have a potential to become, noncompliant in the taking of oral medication. It is our impression that these particular forms of medication are underutilized in this country, and that many patients might avoid the risk of noncompliance and subsequent psychotic relapse if more consideration were given to the use of long-acting injectable drugs. We are not impressed with any available data in the literature that suggest that these compounds are more likely to produce adverse effects than other routes of administration, given the same dosage and degree of neuroleptic exposure.

DRUG DOSAGE IN LONG-TERM TREATMENT

The wish to reduce adverse effects, particularly tardive dyskinesia, but also behaviorally manifest Parkinsonian side effects, has led to an increasing emphasis on identifying minimal effective dosage requirements for the long-term pharmacotherapy of schizophrenia. Attempts to identify minimum dosage requirements have taken three major paths: (1) exploring the relationship between dosage and relapse in those clinical trials that have been reported and can allow for such analyses; (2) carrying out prospective studies that compare patients undergoing gradual dosage reduction with those individuals maintained on stable doses of medication; and (3) assigning patients randomly to different fixed dosage levels for comparison.

The first type of analysis may be complicated by the fact that the dosage employed could have been influenced by other factors and cannot be assumed to be random. In the second type of study, dosage reduction and time may be confounded. As discussed previously, even if patients discontinue medication completely, a psychotic relapse may not occur for several weeks or several months, and we are unable at this time to accurately predict the time frame involved. In a gradual reduction strategy, it is difficult to determine minimal dosage requirements, again given the unpredictable time frame in which patients relapse. If dosage is reduced below the "therapeutic threshold," the relapse that results may not occur immediately, and therefore it becomes difficult to identify the point at which the threshold was passed. Although the fixed-dose strategy eliminates some of these concerns, an arbitrary fixed dose or dose range must be set, and this design does not necessarily allow for the identification of the lowest effective dose for a given individual, although it may provide some general guidelines as to where to begin.

FIXED DOSE COMPARISONS

Caffey et al. (1964) conducted the first controlled dosage reduction study in hospitalized inpatients and demonstrated that those individuals whose dosage was reduced to 3/7ths of their original dosage experienced a 15% relapse rate within 4 months as compared with 45% relapse rate for those patients receiving placebo and a 5% rate for those continuing on their original dose. The mean daily dosage of either chlorpromazine or thioridazine, which the patients had been receiving for at least 3 months before the study began, was 350 to 400 mg/day.

Goldstein, Rodnick, Evans, May, and Steinberg (1978) studied the efficacy of two dose levels of fluphenazine enanthate, with and without crisis-oriented family therapy, in 104 recently discharged schizophrenic patients. These predominantly first-episode patients were randomly assigned to fluphenazine enanthate, 25 mg, or 6.25 mg IM every 2 weeks and were studied for 6 weeks following discharge from hospital. Only 10% relapsed within the 6 weeks following discharge, but 24% of those in the low-dose/no therapy condition relapsed as compared with none of the high-dose/therapy patients. The low-dose/therapy and the high-dose/no-therapy group had relapse rates of 9 and 10%, respectively. Although this study involved a relatively brief period of control and treatment, it is a classic investigation suggesting the potential additive effects of medication and such psychotherapeutic strategies as crisis-oriented family therapy.

We have reported (Kane, Rifkin, Woerner, Sarantakos, et al., 1983, 1985, 1986) results from a 1-year, random-assignment study of different dosage ranges of fluphenazine decanoate (12.5 to 50 mg every 2 weeks as compared with 1.25 to 5.0 mg every 2 weeks) involving stable outpatient schizophrenics. At the end of 1 year, the cumulative relapse rate (determined by the psychotic items of the Brief Psychiatric Rating Scale) on the low dose was 56%, as compared with 14% for the standard dose. An intermediate dose (2.5–10.0 mg every other week) was also studied and produced a cumulative relapse rate of 24%. Despite the significantly higher relapse rate among patients receiving the low-dose treatment, most of the patients who did relapse were restabilized with temporary dosage increase and without requiring rehospitalization. On average, patients were back to their baseline state within 9 weeks. In addition, significantly fewer early signs of tardive dyskinesia were observed in the patients receiving the very low dose, and they were performing better on some measures of psychosocial adjustment than the patients treated with the standard dose. Interestingly, patients receiving the very low dose also manifested less evidence of emotional withdrawal, blunted affect, tension, and psychomotor retardation. These differences were statistically significant in group comparisons of rating scale data but were not of such significant magnitude as to be obvious in individual patients. These findings do, however, emphasize the potential importance of persistent Parkinsonian side effects even during the maintenance phase of treatment, and highlight the complexity of assessing so-called negative symptoms.

Marder et al. (1984, 1986) studied 66 male veteran outpatients who were randomly assigned double-blind to 5 mg or 25 mg of fluphenazine deconoate administered every 2 weeks. Patients were followed for 2 years and were maintained on the assigned fixed dose of 5 or 25 mg as long as they did well. The investigators defined three levels of unfavorable outcome that could lead to a dosage change. When patients had an increase of three or more points on the BPRS cluster scores for thought disturbance or paranoia, they were considered to have had a "psychotic exacerbation." These exacerbations were relatively mild and seldom led to rehospitalization, but the clinician was allowed to increase the dose up to 10 or 50 mg for the respective groups. When patients' symptoms could not be adequately controlled within this range, they were considered to have a relapse. The third level of outcome was rehospitalization. The results from this study highlight the importance of a long-term perspective. At the end of 1 year, the "exacerbation rate" was almost identical in the two treatment groups (35% on the 5 mg treatment, and 43% on the 25 mg treatment). During the second year, however, the two doses produced significantly different rates of exacerbation. Sixty-nine percent experienced an exacerbation on 5 mg, as compared with only 36% on the 25-mg treatment. However, when the outcome of relapse is considered (indicating those patients who could not be controlled on the allowed dosage increase), the two treatments did produce similar results after 2 years: 44% relapsing on the lower dose and 31% relapsing on the higher dose (a nonsignificant difference).

Both of these studies emphasized the potential of substantial dosage reduction in the context of careful clinical observation, allowing for an increase in dosage at early signs of relapse. Clearly, there are potential risks of increasing the likelihood of psychotic relapse when substantial dosage reduction is entertained; however, the potential benefits of reduced adverse effects (including tardive dyskinesia) need to be taken into consideration as well. Clinically, it is most important to emphasize that the benefit-to-risk ratio of these alternative treatment strategies will be greatly influenced by the carefulness of clinical observation and follow-up made available to the patients involved. In addition, there may be patients for whom dosage reduction is not feasible, given past attempts to do this, or potential dire consequences of psychotic relapse (e.g., history of serious suicide attempts or dangerousness).

The underlying assumption behind maintenance pharmacotherapy is that a continued administration of medication is necessary to prevent increase or reemergence of psychotic signs and symptoms. The relative benefits and risks of maintenance treatment in general, or particular alternative maintenance strategies, undoubtedly vary from one patient to another. It is also important to keep in mind that the relative desirability of specific strategies may also vary, depending upon the stage of illness that a given patient is experiencing. Results from long-term naturalistic follow-up studies (Bleuler, 1978; Ciompi, 1980a, 1980b; Harding, Brooks, Askihaga, Strauss, & Breier, 1987; Huber, Gross, & Schuttler, 1979; Huber, Gross, Schuttler, & Linz, 1980) emphasize the heterogeneity of outcome in this illness. Some patients appear to experience a more chronic and deteriorating course, while others may experience a much more benign outcome after one or two decades. Unfortunately, we have relatively little information on the very long-term impact of drug treatment on the course of schizophrenia, despite the dramatic benefits of antipsychotic drugs during a period of several years, as evidenced by the data resulting from the controlled clinical trials.

The variability in symptom pattern as well as in drug responsiveness (even among patients presenting with similar phenomenology) also makes our attempts to identify true drug effects more difficult. The extent to which maintenance treatment is, in fact, prophylactic may vary from individual to individual. If this distinction could be made with any reliability, it would clearly be useful in establishing the most appropriate treatment strategy for a given patient.

The possibility that some patients may not require continuous medication has fostered a series of investigations of "intermittent" or "targeted" strategies that go well beyond earlier suggestions of "drug holidays" in supporting the possibility that some individuals may do well without antipsychotic medications for substantial periods of time, and that a full-blown psychotic relapse might be prevented by identifying early or prodromal signs of exacerbation and then reinstituting medication rapidly.

The targeted or intermittent treatment strategy is a partial outgrowth of observations by Herz and Melville (1980) that many patients experience characteristic signs or symptoms, during the early stages of relapse, and that the clinician's knowledge of this pattern (obtained from the patient, family, and previous treatment sources) may facilitate early recognition and re-institution of drug treatment. Implicit in the strategy is the assumption that lengthy interruptions in drug administration may minimize the risks of adverse effects. Although this is clearly the case for many adverse effects (e.g., Parkinsonian, cognitive, and neuroendocrine), the impact of the strategy on the incidence of tardive dyskinesia has yet to be clearly established.

Herz, Szymanski, and Simon (1982) and Carpenter and colleagues (Carpenter & Heinrichs, 1984; Carpenter, Stephens, Rey, Hanlon, & Heinricks, 1982) have demonstrated the feasibility of targeted or intermittent treatment, but direct comparisons of continuous low-dose versus targeted or intermittent strategies have yet to be completed. The National Institute of Mental Health has been carrying out a multicenter study under the direction of Schooler and Keith (1983) that will provide extremely valuable data on this question.

It would be ideal to have methods that would allow us to identify specific patients who are best suited for a particular strategy on the basis of their propensity to relapse within a relatively short time following antipsychotic drug discontinuation. The work of Lieberman et al. (1987), using response to methylphenidate infusions as a potential predictor of relapse, is a logical extension of earlier work by Janowsky, El-Yousef, Davis, and Sekerke (1973), Janowsky and Davis (1976), Angrist, Rotrosen, and Gershon (1980), and Angrist, Pesselow, Rubenstein, Wolkin, and Rotrosen (1985). Lieberman's results suggest that those patients experiencing a transient exacerbation of psychotic signs and symptoms following 0.5 mg/kg of intravenous methylphenidate will relapse sooner (following antipsychotic drug discontinuation) than will patients not responding to methylphenidate in this manner. This strategy does not necessarily identify patients who can be maintained off medication on an indefinite basis, but in our experience this remains a very small subgroup.

Even among patients who have been in remission for a considerable length of time on antipsychotic drugs, the risk of relapse following drug discontinuation appears to be considerable. In reviewing a series of neuroleptic discontinuation studies among patients who had been in remission for intervals ranging from 6 months to as long as 5 years, on average 75% relapsed within follow-up intervals ranging from 6 to 24 months (Cheung, 1981; Dencker, Lepp, & Malm, 1980; Hogarty, Ulrich, Mussare, & Aristigueta, 1976; Johnson, 1976, 1979; Wistedt, 1981).

Even among those individuals recovering from an acute-onset first episode of schizophrenia, a statistically significant drug effect is apparent in preventing relapse. There are two published double-blind, random-assignment trials that focused exclusively on first-episode patients. In a 1-year double-blind study comparing fluphenazine and placebo, we (Kane, Rifkin, Quitkin, Nayak, & Ramos-Lorenzi, 1982) found a 40% relapse rate on placebo compared with none on drug. Crow, McMillan, Johnson, and Johnstone (1986) reported a less striking drug effect after 2 years in a population of first-episode patients, many of whom were not acute onset. Fifty-eight (58%) relapsed on active medication, as compared with 70% on placebo. The lack of a more dramatic drug effect is surprising but may be due to the fact that many patients in the latter study had been ill for substantial periods of time prior to the initiation of antipsychotic drug treatment. The investigators found a statistically significant relationship between the length of time ill before initiation of medication and poor outcome.

An important question has also been raised concerning the possibility that the long-term administration of antipsychotic drugs may have a negative impact on the course of schizophrenia. Chouinard and Jones (1980) have proposed a concept of "supersensitivity psychosis," which implies that following long-term drug treatment, the risk of relapse is actually increased by an increase in the sensitivity of dopamine receptors in relevant brain areas. This phenomenon could be manifested clinically by a more rapid relapse following drug discontinuation than would have occurred without ongoing maintenance drug treatment, or by the need for continually increasing dosages of medication to maintain the same degree of remission. There are, however, insufficient data to allow meaningful conclusions, and enormous methodological problems exist in adequately testing this hypothesis. It is also relevant to consider the well-known fact that some individuals with schizophrenia do have a chronic, deteriorating course despite or without antipsychotic drug treatment, rather than as a potential consequence of such treatment.

CONCLUSION

Although we may feel that no major breakthrough has occurred, considerable progress has been made in recent years in the pharmacologic treatment of schizophrenia. Our ability to use available medications in the most judicious way and our understanding of potential benefits and risks has clearly improved. As further research progresses along a variety of fronts, it is likely that our treatment strategies will also improve.

Though this chapter has focused on pharmacologic treatment, such treatment interacts in a variety of ways with other treatment modalities as well as patient and environmental characteristics. As clinicians we must maintain an eclectic view of therapeutic strategies while at the same time being self-critical as to efficacy and cost-effectiveness.

REFERENCES

Angrist, B., Pesselow, E., Rubenstein, M., Wolkin, A., & Rotrosen, J. (1985). Amphetamine response and relapse risk after depot neuroleptic discontinuation. *Psychopharmacology, 85*, 277–283.

Angrist, B., Rotrosen, J., & Gershon, S. L. (1980). Responses to apomorphine, amphetamine and neuroleptics in schizophrenic subjects. *Psychopharmacology, 67*, 31–38.

Baldessarini, R., Katz, B., & Cotton, P. (1984). Dissimilar dosing with high-potency and low-potency neuroleptics. *American Journal of Psychiatry, 141*, 748–752.

Bergling, R., Mjorndal, T., Oreland, L., Rapp, W., & Wold, S. (1975). Plasma levels and clinical effects of thioridazine and thiothixene. *Journal of Clinical Pharmacology, 15*, 178–186.

Bjorndal, N., Bjerre, M., Gerlach, J., Kristjansen, P., Magelund, G., Oestrich, I. H., & Wachrems, J. (1980). High dosage haloperidol therapy in chronic schizophrenic patients: A double-blind study of clinical response, side effects, serum haloperidol and serum prolactin. *Psychopharmcology, 67*, 17–23.

Bleuler, M. (1978). *The schizophrenic disorder: Long-term patients and family studies* (S. M. Clemens, Trans.). New Haven: Yale University Press.

Bolvig-Hansen, L. B., Larsen, N. E., & Vestergaard, P. (1981). Plasma levels of perphenazine (Trilafon) related to development of extrapyramidal side effects. *Psychopharmacology, 74*, 306–309.

Brandon, S., Cowley, P., McDonald, C., Neville, P., Palmer, R., Wellstood-Eason, S., & Leicester, R. (1985). ECT trial: Results in schizophrenia. *British Journal of Psychiatry, 146*, 177–183.

Caffey, E. M., Jr., Diamond, L. S., Frank, T. V., Grasberger, J. C., Herman, L., Klett, C. J., & Rothstein, C. (1964). Discontinuation or reduction of chemotherapy in chronic schizophrenics. *Journal of Chronic Diseases, 17*, 347–358.

Carpenter, W. T., & Heinrichs, D. W. (1984). Intermittent pharmacotherapy of schizophrenia. In J. Kane (Ed.), *Drug maintenance strategies in schizophrenia* (pp. 69–82). Washington, DC: American Psychiatric Press.

Carpenter, W. T., Stephens, J. H., Rey, A. C., Hanlon, T. E., & Heinrichs, D. W. (1982). Early intervention vs. continued pharmacotherapy of schizophrenia. *Psychopharmacology Bulletin, 18*, 21–23.

Casper, R., Garver, D. L., Dekirmenjian, H., Chang, S., & Davis, J. M. (1980). Phenothiazine levels in plasma and red blood cells: Their relationship to clinical improvement in schizophrenia. *Archives of General Psychiatry, 37*, 301–305.

Cheung, H. K. (1981). Schizophrenics fully remitted on neuroleptics for 3–5 years: To stop or continue drugs? *British Journal of Psychiatry, 138*, 490–494.

Chien, C. P. (1975). Drugs and rehabilitation in schizophrenia. In M. Greenblatt (Ed.), *Drugs in combination with other therapies* (pp. 13–34). New York: Grune & Stratton.

Chouinard, G., & Jones, B. (1980). Neuroleptic induced supersensitivity psychosis: Clinical and pharmacologic characteristics. *American Journal of Psychiatry, 137*, 16–21.

Ciompi, L. (1980a). Three lectures on schizophrenia: The natural history of schizophrenia in the long-term. *British Journal of Psychiatry, 136*, 413–420.

Ciompi, L. (1980b). Catamnestic long-term study on the course of life and aging of schizophrenics. *Schizophrenia Bulletin, 6*, 606–618.

Claghorn, J., Honigfeld, G., Abuzzahab, F. S., Wang, R., Steinbook, R., Tuason, V., & Klerman, G. (1987). The risks and benefits of clozapine vs. chlorpromazine. *Journal of Clinical Psychopharmacology, 7*, 377–384.

Cohen, B. M., Lipinski, J. F., Harris, P. O., Pope, H. G., & Friedman, M. (1980). Clinical use of the radioreceptor assay for neuroleptics. *Psychiatry Research, 2*, 173–178.

Cohen, B. M., Lipinski, J. F., Pope, H. G., Harris, P. O., & Altesman, R. I. (1980). Neuroleptic blood level and therapeutic effect. *Psychopharmocology, 70*, 191–193.

Crawford, R., & Forrest, A. (1974). Control trial of depot fluphenazine in outpatient schizophrenics. *British Journal of Psychiatry, 124*, 385–391.

Crow, T. J., McMillan, J. F., Johnson, A. L., & Johnstone, E. C. (1986). The Northwick Park study of first episodes of schizophrenia: II. A randomized controlled trial of prophylactic neuroleptic treatment. *British Journal of Psychiatry, 148*, 120–127.

Davis, J. M. (1975). Overview: Maintenance therapy in psychiatry—I. Schizophrenia. *American Journal of Psychiatry, 132*, 1237–1245.

Davis, J. M., Schaffer, C. B., Killian, G. A., Kinard, C., & Chan, C. (1980). Important issues in the drug treatment of schizophrenia. *Schizophrenia Bulletin, 6*, 70–87.

Delva, N. J., & Letemendia, F. J. J. (1982). Lithium treatment in schizophrenia and schizo-affective disorders. *British Journal of Psychiatry, 141*, 387–400.

Dencker, S. J., Lepp, M, & Malm, U. (1980). Do schizophrenics well adapted in the community need neuroleptics? A depot neuroleptic withdrawal study. *Acta Psychiatrica Scandinavica (Suppl.), 279*, 64–76.

Dysken, M. W., Javaid, J. I., Chang, S. S., Schaffer, C., Shaid, A., & Davis, J. M. (1981). Fluphenazine pharmacokinetics and therapeutic response. *Psychopharmacology, 73*, 205–210.

Engelhardt, D. M., Freedman, M., Rosen, B., Mann, D., & Margolis, R. (1964). Phenothiazines in the prevention of psychiatric hospitalization: III. Delay or prevention of hospitalization. *Archives of General Psychiatry, 11*, 162–169.

Engelhardt, D. M., Rosen, B., Freedman, N., Mann, D., & Margolis, R. (1963). Phenothiazines in the prevention of psychiatric hospitalization: II Duration of treatment exposure. *Journal of the American Medical Association, 186*, 981–983.

Engelhardt, D. M., Rosen, B., Freedman, N., & Margolis, R. (1967). Phenothiazines in prevention of psychiatric hospitalization: IV. Delay or prevention of hospitalization—A reevaluation. *Archives of General Psychiatry, 16*, 98–101.

Falloon, I. R. H., Watts, D. C., & Shepherd, M. (1978). A comparative controlled trial of pimozide and fluphenazine decanoate in continuation therapy of schizophrenia. *Psychological Medicine, 8*, 59–70.

Garver, D. L., Dekirmenjian, H., Davis, J. M., Casper, R., & Ericksen, S. (1977). Neuroleptic drug levels and therapeutic response: Preliminary observations with red blood cell bound butaperazine. *American Journal of Psychiatry, 134*, 304–307.

Garver, D. L., Hirschowitz, J., Glicksteen, G. A., Kanter, D. R., & Mavroidis, M. L. (1984). Haloperidol plasma and red blood cell levels and clinical antipsychotic response. *Journal of Psychopharmacology, 4*, 133–137.

Gerlach, J., Koppelhus, E., Helweg, E., & Monrad, A. (1974). Clozapine and haloperidol in a single-blind cross-over trial: Therapeutic and biochemical aspects in the treatment of schizophrenia. *Acta Psychiatrica Scandinavica, 50*, 410–424.

Goldstein, M. J., Rodnick, E. H., Evans, J. R., May, P. R. A., & Steinberg, M. R. (1978). Drug and family therapy in the aftercare of acute schizophrenics. *Archives of General Psychiatry, 35*, 1169–1177.

Haase, H. J. (1961). Extrapyramidal modification of fine movements—A "conditio sine qua non" of the fundamental therapeutic action of neuroleptic drugs. In J. M. Bordeleau (Ed.), *Extrapyramidal system and neuroleptics* (pp. 329–353). Montreal: Montreal Editions Psychiatriques.

Haase, H. J., & Janssen, A. P. J. (1965). *The action of neuroleptic drugs.* Chicago: Yearbook Medical Publishers.

Harding, C. M., Brooks, G. W., Askihaga, T., Strauss, J. S., & Breier, A. (1987). The Vermont longitudinal study: II. Long-term outcome of subjects who retrospectively met DSM-III criteria for schizophrenia. *American Journal of Psychiatry, 144*, 727–735.

Herz, M. I., & Melville, C. (1980). Relapse in schizophrenia. *American Journal of Psychiatry, 137*, 801–805.

Herz, M. I., Szymanski, H. B., & Simon, J. C. (1982). Intermittent medication for stable schizophrenic outpatients: An alternative to maintenance medication. *American Journal of Psychiatry, 139*, 918–922.

Hirsch, S. R., Gaind, R., Rohde, P. D., Stevens, B. C., & Wing, J. K. (1973). Outpatient maintenance of chronic schizophrenic patients with long-acting fluphenazine: Double-blind placebo trial. *British Medical Journal, 1*, 633–637.

Hirschowitz, J., Casper, R., Garver, D. L., & Chang, S. (1980). Lithium response in good prognosis schizophrenia. *American Journal of Psychiatry, 137*, 916–920.

Hogarty, G. E., Goldberg, S. C., & the Collaborative Study Group. (1974). Drug and sociotherapy in the aftercare of schizophrenic patients: One year relapse rates. *Archives of General Psychiatry, 28*, 54–64.

Hogarty, G. E., Goldberg, S. C., Schooler, N. R., Ulrich, R. F., & the Collaborative Study Group. (1979). Drug and sociotherapy in the aftercare of schizophrenic patients: II. Two year relapse rate. *Archives of General Psychiatry, 31*, 603–608.

Hogarty, G. E., Schooler, N. R., Ulrich, R. F., Mussare, F., Ferro, P., & Herron, E. (1979). Fluphenazine and social therapy in the aftercare of schizophrenic patients: Relapse analyses of a two-year controlled study of fluphenazine decanoate and fluphenazine hydrochloride. *Archives of General Psychiatry, 36*, 1283–1294.

Hogarty, G. E., Ulrich, R. F., Mussare, F., & Aristigueta, N. (1976). Drug discontinuation among long-term successfully maintained schizophrenic outpatients. *Diseases of the Nervous System, 37*, 494–500.

Honigfeld, G., Patin, J., & Singer, J. (1984). Antipsychotic activity in treatment resistance schizophrenics. *Advances in Therapy, 1*, 77–97.

Huber, G., Gross, G., & Schüttler, R. (1979). Verlaufs-und Sozialpsychiatriche langzeituntersuchunder an den 1945–1959 in Benn Hospitalizierten Schizophren Kranken Monogr. Gesantgeb Psychiatr. (Berline). *English Abstract, 21*, 1–3999.

Huber, G., Gross, G., Schüttler, R., & Linz, M. (1980). Longitudinal studies of schizophrenic patients. *Schizophrenia Bulletin, 6*, 592–605.

Itil, T. M., Keskiner, A., Heinemann, L., Han, T., Gannen, P., & Hsu, W. (1970). Treatment of resistant schizophrenics with extreme high dosage fluphenazine hydrochloride. *Psychosomatics, 11*, 456–463.

Janowsky, D. S., & Davis, J. M. (1976). Methylphenidate, dextroamphetamine and levamfetamine: Effects on schizophrenic symptoms. *Archives of General Psychiatry, 33*, 304–308.

Janowsky, D. S., El-Yousef, K., Davis, J. M., & Sekerke, J. (1973). Provocations of schizophrenic symptoms by intravenous administration of methylphenidate. *Archives of General Psychiatry, 28*, 185–191.

Johnson, D. A. W. (1976). The duration of maintenance therapy in chronic schizophrenia. *Acta Psychiatrica Scandinavica, 53*, 298–301.

Johnson, D. A. W. (1979). Further observations on the duration of depot neuroleptic maintenance therapy in schizophrenia. *British Journal of Psychiatry, 135*, 524–530.

Kane, J. M., & Borenstein, M. (1985). Compliance in the long-term treatment of schizophrenia. *Psychopharmacology Bulletin, 21*, 23–27.

Kane, J., Honigfeld, G., Singer, J., & Meltzer, H. (1988). Clozapine for the treatment-resistance schizophrenic: A double-blind comparison versus chlorpromazine/benztropine. *Archives of General Psychiatry, 45*, 789–796.

Kane, J. M., & Lieberman, J. A. (1987). Maintenance pharmacotherapy in schizophrenia. In H. Y. Meltzer (Ed.), *Psychopharmacology, the third generation of progress: The emergency of molecular biology and biological psychiatry* (pp. 1103–1109). New York: Raven Press.

Kane, J. M., Rifkin, A., Quitkin, F., Nayak, D. V., & Ramos-Lorenzi, J. R. (1982). Fluphenazine versus placebo in patients with remitted, acute first episodes of schizophrenia. *Archives of General Psychiatry, 39*, 70–73.

Kane, J. M., Rifkin, A., Woerner, M., Reardon, G., Kreisman, L., Blumenthal, R., & Borenstein, M. (1985). High-dose versus low-dose strategies in the treatment of schizophrenia. *Psychopharmacology Bulletin, 21*, 533–537.

Kane, J. M., Rifkin, A., Woerner, M., Reardon, G., Sarantakos, S., Schiebel, D., & Ramos-Lorenzi, J. R. (1983). Low dose neuroleptic treatment of outpatient schizophrenics. I. Preliminary results for relapse rates. *Archives of General Psychiatry, 40*, 893–896.

Kane, J. M., Rifkin, A., Woerner, M., & Sarantakos, S. (1986). Dose response relationships in maintenance drug treatment for schizophrenia. *Psychopharmacology Bulletin, 6*, 205–235.

Kane, J. M., Woerner, M., Borenstein, M., Wegner, J., & Lieberman, J. (1986). Integrating incidence and prevalence of tardive dyskinesia. *Psychopharmacology Bulletin, 22*, 254–258.

Kelly, H. B., Freeman, H. L., Banning, B., & Schiff, A. (1977). A clinical and social comparison of fluphenazine decanoate and flupenthixol decanoate in the community maintenance therapy of schizophrenia. *International Pharmacopsychology, 12*, 54–64.

Leff, J. P., & Wing, J. K. (1971). Trial of maintenance therapy in schizophrenia. *British Medical Journal, 3*, 559–605.

Lieberman, J., Kane, J., Sarantakos, S., Gadaleta, D., & Woerner, M. (1987). Prediction of relapse in schizophrenia. *Archives of General Psychiatry, 44*, 597–603.

Magliozzi, J. R., Hollister, L. E., Arnold, K. V., & Earlie, G. M. (1981). Relationship of serum haloperidol levels to clinical response in schizophrenic patients. *American Journal of Psychiatry, 138*, 365–367.

Marder, S. R., Van Putten, T., Mintz, J., Lebelle, M., Faltico, G., & May, P. R. A. (1984). Costs and benefits of two doses of fluphenazine. *Archives of General Psychiatry, 41*, 1025–1029.

Marder, S. R., Van Putten, T., Mintz, J., Lebelle, M., McKenzie, J., & May, P. R. A. (1987). Low and conventional dose maintenance therapy with fluphenazine decanoate: Two year outcome. *Archives of General Psychiatry, 44*, 518–521.

Mavroidis, M. L., Kanter, D. R., Hirschowitz, J., & Garver, D. L. (1983). Clinical response and plasma in haloperidol levels in schizophrenia. *Psychopharmacology, 81*, 354–356.

Mavroidis, M. L., Kanter, D. R., Hirschowitz, J., & Garver, D. L. (1984). Therapeutic blood levels of fluphenazine: Plasma or RBC determinations? *Psychopharmacology Bulletin, 20*, 168–170.

May, P. R. A. (1968). *Treatment of schizophrenia: A Comparative study of five treatment methods.* New York: Science House.

May, P. R. A., Van Putten, T., Jenden, D. J., Yale, C., & Dixon, W. J. (1981). Chlorpromazine levels and the outcome of treatment in schizophrenic patients. *Archives of General Psychiatry, 38*, 202–207.

McCreadie, R. G., Dingwall, J. M., Wiles, D. H., & Heykants, J. J. P. (1980). Intermittent pimozide versus fluphenazine decanoate as maintenance therapy in chronic schizophrenia. *British Journal of Psychiatry, 137*, 510–517.

McCreadie, R. G., Mackie, M., Morrison, D., & Kidd, J. (1982). Once weekly pimozide versus fluphenazine decanoate as maintenance therapy in chronic schizophrenia. *British Journal of Psychiatry, 140*, 280–286.

McCreadie, R. G., & McDonald, I. M. (1977). High dosage haloperidol in chronic schizophrenia. *British Journal of Psychiatry, 131*, 210–316.

McEvoy, J., Stiller, R. L., & Farr, R. (1986). Plasma haloperidol levels drawn on neuroleptic threshold doses: A pilot study. *Journal of Clinical Psychopharmacology, 6*, 133–138.

Neborsky, R. J., Janowsky, D. S., Perel, J. M., Munson, E., & Depry, D. (1984). Plasma/RBC haloperidol ratios and improvement in acute psychotic symptoms. *Journal of Clinical Psychiatry, 45*, 10–13.

Odejide, O. A., & Aderounmu, A. F. (1982). Double-blind placebo substitution: Withdrawal of fluphenazine decanoate in schizophrenic patients. *Journal of Clinical Psychiatry, 43*, 195–196.

Potkin, S. G., Shen, Y., Zhou, D., Pardes, H., Shu, L., Phelps, B., & Poland, R. (1985). Does a therapeutic window for plasma haloperidol exist? Preliminary Chinese data. *Psychopharmacology Bulletin, 21*, 59–61.

Quitkin, F., Rifkin, A., Kane, J. M., Ramos-Lorenzi, J. R., & Klein, D. F. (1978). Long-acting oral versus injectable antipsychotic drugs in schizophrenics: A one-year double-blind comparison in multiple episode schizophrenics. *Archives of General Psychiatry, 35*, 889–892.

Quitkin, F., Rifkin, A., & Klein, D. F. (1975). Very high dosage versus standard dosage fluphenazine in schizophrenia: A double-blind study of non-chronic treatment refractory patients. *Archives of General Psychiatry, 32*, 1276–1281.

Rifkin, A., Quitkin, F., Rabiner, C. J., & Klein, D. F. (1977). Fluphenazine decanoate, fluphenazine hydrochloride given orally, and placebo in remitted schizophrenics. *Archives of General Psychiatry, 34*, 43–47.

Salzman, C. (1980). The use of ECT in the treatment of schizophrenia. *American Journal of Psychiatry, 137*, 1032–1041.

Schooler, N. R., & Keith, S. J. (1983). *Treatment strategies in schizophrenia study protocol.* Rockville, MD: National Institute of Mental Health.

Schooler, N. R., Levine, J., Severe, J. B., Brauzer, B., DiMascio, A., Klerman, G. L., & Tauson, V. B. (1980). Prevention of relapse in schizophrenia: An evaluation of fluphenazine decanoate. *Archives of General Psychiatry, 37*, 16–24.

Small, J. G., Kellams, J. J., Millstein, V., & Moore, J. (1975). A placebo controlled study of lithium combined with neuroleptics in chronic schizophrenic patients. *American Journal of Psychiatry, 132*, 1315–1317.

Smith, R. C., Baumgartner, R., Ravichandran, G. K., Shvartsburd, A., Schooler, J. C., Allen, P., & Johnson, R. (1984). Plasma and cell levels of thioridazine and clinical response in schizophrenia. *Psychiatry Research, 12*, 287–296.

Smith, R. C., Baumgartner, R., Shvartsburd, A., Ravichandran, G. K., Vroulis, G., & Mauldin, M. (1985). Comparative efficacy of red cell and plasma haloperidol as predictors of clinical response in schizophrenia. *Psychopharmacology, 85*, 449–455.

Taylor, P. J., & Fleminger, J. J. (1980). ECT for schizophrenia. *Lancet, 1*, 1380–1382.

Troshinsky, C. H., Aaronson, H. G., & Stone, R. K. (1962). Maintenance phenothiazine in the aftercare of schizophrenic patients. *Pennsylvania Psychiatric Quarterly, 2*, 11–15.

Van Putten, T. (1974). Why do schizophrenic patients refuse to take their drugs? *Archives of General Psychiatry, 31*, 67–72.

Van Putten, T., Marder, S. R., May, P. R. A., Poland, R. E., & O'Brien, R. (1985). Plasma levels of haloperidol and clinical response. *Psychopharmacology Bulletin, 21*, 69–72.

Wistedt, B. (1981). A depot neuroleptic withdrawal study: A controlled study of the clinical effects of the withdrawal of depot fluphenazine decanoate and depot flupenthioxol decanoate in chronic schizophrenic patients. *Acta Psychiatrica Scandinavica, 64*, 65–84.

Wode-Helgodt, B., Borg, S., Fyro, B., & Sedvall, G. (1978). Clinical effects and drug concentrations in plasma and cerebrospinal fluid in psychotic patients treated with fixed doses of chlorpromazine. *Acta Psychiatrica Scandinavica, 58*, 149–173.

4

Case Management

CHRISTINE W. MCGILL AND ROBERT W. SURBER

INTRODUCTION

Case management is a concept that has gained much credence and popularity in human services. Case management is viewed as a necessary component to the care of a variety of populations that are perceived as disabled and/or as having multiple service needs. These populations include the developmentally disabled, dependent children, the frail elderly, the homeless, and the severely mentally ill. Because of the diverse populations served, a broad array of models of practice, the diverse backgrounds and training of individuals providing this service, and multiple organizational approaches, there is no consistent definition or understanding of this term.

Despite this lack of clarity, case management programs have proliferated in mental health services in recent years and are seen as a critical aspect in the care of the severely mentally ill. The community support initiative (Turner & Shifren, 1979) developed by the National Institute of Mental Health includes case management as a central component in the system of care necessary to support severely mentally ill individuals living in the community. Indeed, several states have mandated case management for their public mental health services. For instance, in California, state law requires that each county mental health service submit a plan to provide case management services for the following adult target population:

1. All clients who have been admitted to local acute or state psychiatric

CHRISTINE W. MCGILL • University of California San Francisco, Department of Psychiatry, San Francisco General Hospital, 1001 Potrero Avenue, San Francisco, California 94110. • ROBERT W. SURBER • Department of Psychiatry, San Francisco General Hospital, 1001 Potrero Avenue, San Francisco, California 94110.

hospitals two or more times within the past 12 months and requiring 14 days or more of treatment on each occasion.

2. All clients whose mental or emotional condition has been diagnosed chronic, *or* who have had a continuous mental disorder for the previous 5 years.

3. Any persons who have been diagnosed as having a mental illness that makes them incapable of appropriately utilizing available mental health resources, or grossly interferes with their ability to live independently in the community (California Department of Mental Health, 1985).

With this wide acceptance of the need for case management there is an equally wide disparity within mental health as to what the term means, how it should be provided, and by whom. This disparity is most dramatic in the variety of people who are described in the literature as providing this care. Not only are case management programs staffed with professionals of all mental health disciplines and paraprofessionals as well, but the functions of case management have also been reported as being provided by indigenous community members, by volunteers, and even by family members (Levine & Fleming, 1984).

Additionally, case management is provided through numerous organizational structures. Some case management programs assign individual case managers to individual clients, while others provide a team of staff, all of whom serve the clients of the program (Reinke & Greenly, 1986). Comprehensive model programs, such as the Training in Community Living program (TCL) in Dane County, Wisconsin, provide total service provision to clients with schizophrenia (Stein & Test, 1985). Case management services are also provided within a variety of traditional mental health modalities, including outpatient clinics, day treatment services, psychosocial rehabilitation centers, residential treatment services, and private practitioners.

One important debate in the field centers on whether case management is a clinical activity that requires that staff have clinical training and provide psychotherapeutic interventions, or whether case managers provide an adjunct to clinical services and act as coordinators and brokers of services, rather than as providers of direct service.

Our purpose in this chapter is not to provide a single definition of case management or to suggest an optimal organizational structure for this service. The diversity of approaches suggests the vitality of the concept and provides an opportunity to compare the effectiveness of varying approaches with different populations and within different contexts. Our purpose is rather to provide a framework for conceptualizing case management services for clients with schizophrenia, and to discuss the particular issues involved in case management with this illness. In doing this, we will present a comprehensive model for the treatment of schizophrenia, and then describe how the generally accepted functions of case management are molded to respond to this model. We will then suggest several requirements necessary to establish effective case management services.

We admit to a bias, based on our own experience, that a case manager's effectiveness increases with increasing knowledge of the illness and its practical and psychological effects on the lives of its victims, and with knowledge of its treatment from both biological and psychosocial perspectives. We are particularly concerned with those programs that report that their case managers are not aware of their clientele's psychopathology (Baker & Weiss, 1984). In our view, effectiveness also increases with the ability of the case manager to establish, maintain, and utilize a therapeutic alliance, particularly around specific aspects of schizophrenic illness. Nevertheless, we intend that this discussion will be useful to any individual providing case management or therapeutic services to clients with schizophrenia.

We are aware that family members of individuals with schizophrenia often provide many of the functions of case managers because appropriate services are not available. Since this is done by default rather than by design (Levine & Fleming, 1984), we do not define the efforts of families as case management; nor do we think it is appropriate to ask families to assume the role of a case manager. However, because families can be extremely helpful, we will pay particular attention to discussing the role of the case manager when family is available to take an active role in the life of the client.

THE CONCEPTUAL MODEL OF SCHIZOPHRENIA AND ITS TREATMENT

We define schizophrenia as a complex and heterogenous biopsychosocial disorder that is diagnosed on the basis of the presence of certain characteristic disturbances of thinking and perception. Effective treatment of this disorder requires a combination of biological and psychosocial interventions (Schooler & Hogarty, 1987). Although the course and severity of the illness is highly variable, case management will usually be offered to those individuals whose schizophrenia is likely to be both chronic and severe, and whose prognosis is less than optimal.

Several authors have developed conceptual models of schizophrenia which go beyond disease- or symptom-based diagnosis, and which take into account the marked social impairment often associated with the illness (Strauss & Carpenter, 1981; Wing, 1978). John Wing distinguishes between the acute and chronic impairments of schizophrenia, secondary handicaps associated with the illness, and extrinsic factors presumably unrelated to the illness. Wing suggests that effective intervention for the disorder must address all of these dimensions.

The acute condition, or period of florid psychosis, is characterized by such symptoms as thought insertion, thought broadcast, thought withdrawal, hallucinations, and delusions. Wing describes these phenomena as highly discriminating for schizophrenia.

The chronic symptoms suggest the presence of intrinsic impairments of schizophrenia, such as the commonly held "negative symptoms," including apathy, slowed thought and movement, lack of activity, amotivation, poverty of speech, and social withdrawal. According to Wing, presence of one negative symptom usually signals others, and they are a good measure of the overall severity of illness-related impairment. The negative symptoms are highly correlated with social performance and are characteristic of the chronic condition. Other intrinsic impairments are the residual disturbances of thinking characterized by vagueness, confusion, looseness or incoherence, unremitting delusions and hallucinations, and behavioral disturbances that may persist as severely disabling.

Wing outlines a number of secondary impairments or handicaps that are often likely to be associated with chronic schizophrenia. These encompass both personal and societal reactions to the circumstances of the illness. An example of this is the effect of long-term institutionalization. Much of the loss of social and living skills and resultant dependency was related to the impact of the limited role expectations on chronic back wards. Similarly, low self-esteem and lack of social activity may be linked to the stigma associated with being a mental patient in our society. Problems such as poverty, homelessness, and poor housing, as well as social attitudes toward mental illness, are likewise associated with patient adjustment to schizophrenia.

The last dimension that Wing stresses are the extrinsic factors that, although seemingly unrelated to the illness, nevertheless have a substantial impact on lifetime course and outcome. Premorbid characteristics such as social adjustment, basic intelligence and intellectual development, physical appearance, and health status are major areas that must be taken into consideration in planning treatment. Environmental stress may also play an important role in the course of schizophrenia. The stress-diathesis model assumes that schizophrenia is a broad spectrum disorder with a biological component. A core genetic predisposition, or vulnerability, may be exacerbated by stressors in the environment. That is to say that stressors may have a deleterious effect on the course of the patient's illness. The role of stress on the course of the illness has been documented in the study of life events and familial expressed emotion, with both factors associated with relapse (Leff & Vaughn, 1985).

The stress-diathesis model hypothesizes that: (1) life events will add stress to the ongoing ambient stress of living; (2) stress is associated with psychological symptoms; (3) stress may lead to exacerbation of psychotic symptoms; (4) if stress persists, a cycle of chronicity may be established or perpetuated; (5) individual and family coping efforts may modify stress; and (6) stress may be moderated by neuroleptic drugs, even in small doses (Falloon, Boyd, & McGill, 1984).

Strauss and Carpenter (1981) have suggested the importance of a multi-axial assessment process in schizophrenia. These authors maintain that the longitudinal course of the disorder is highly variable and that the best predictors of future functioning may be determined from the history of prior performance. They note that an individual's functioning in terms of social relationship and work or vocational capacity may be quite independent of severity of the symptoms experienced. They suggest a system of diagnosis with three independent axes in addition to symptoms and life events: (1) course of disorder, (2) social functioning and relationships, and (3) work or vocational functioning (Strauss & Carpenter, 1981).

We are suggesting a model of treatment that incorporates all of these approaches to the illness. This model incorporates biological, social, and psychological interventions that are individualized to each client's symptoms, level of disability, needs, and strengths.

Neuroleptic medication is a necessary component of treatment for control of acute symptoms and is usually required on an ongoing basis to maintain symptomatic relief and prevent relapse. During acute episodes it may also be necessary to provide care and protection in secure settings.

It is also necessary to respond to long-term disabilities and symptoms that are not ameliorated with medications. This may include support, rehabilitation, and training over a protracted period of time. During this long-term effort, it is necessary to continuously balance the desire to encourage clients to meet their fullest potential with the real and often severe limitations imposed by the illness.

The long-term effort must also respond to difficulties clients have in meeting survival needs and obtaining other needed services. This includes an active effort at helping clients obtain and maintain housing, income, medical care, legal aid, and any other required services. In addition to concrete services, this long-term effort needs to respond to less tangible problems such as stigma, unrealistic expectations of family and friends, and the depression that often accompanies a long-term disabling illness. A combination of education and psychotherapeutic interventions is helpful with these issues.

Treatment must also address the client's social and vocational functioning by offering social skills training and vocational rehabilitation. However, we would define vocational efforts very broadly to include any activity that helps clients to use their time constructively.

Finally, treatment is to be provided in the context of the client's capacities and the client's environment. Treatment must be individualized to respond to the client's particular strengths, weaknesses, aspirations, and limitations. Equally important is the potential support available from family, community resources, and culture. Effective treatment will utilize the strengths in the client's environment to the best advantage.

CASE MANAGEMENT IN SCHIZOPHRENIA

It follows from this model that the treatment of schizophrenia must necessarily be broad and that treatment and supportive services must be available over time. Historically, mental health services have often failed the client with schizophrenia and other severe mental disabilities because of their limited scope and fragmentation. The difficulties of the design of traditional services have been compounded by the fact that no one person or agency has been assigned responsibility for continuously coordinating and integrating all of the care for individual clients.

Case management is a construct that has developed to respond to this need for comprehensive and continuous care, and it is particularly useful in the treatment of schizophrenia. We believe that the goal of case management, as in all treatment of schizophrenia, is to help clients achieve their life goals to the maximum extent possible, notwithstanding the limitations imposed by the illness.

There is considerable consensus as to the important components of case management. To our knowledge, most authors include the five basic elements of assessment, planning, linkage, monitoring, and advocacy in describing the service (Intagliata, 1982). Levine and Fleming (1984) add the component of client identification and outreach, while Ballew and Mink (1986) have suggested that engagement is an additional function. We will discuss the five basic functions as they relate to the treatment of schizophrenia. It is necessary to first note that although these functions are described as discrete entities, in practice there is much overlap between them. Also, they do not occur in succession. That is, a case manager does not assess, then plan, then link, and so on. Rather, one performs all of these functions continuously. Describing these functions successively is primarily to conceptualize a role in the care and treatment of the mentally ill.

ASSESSMENT

A comprehensive assessment is, of course, the beginning of any treatment or social service intervention. The psychiatric diagnosis is a necessary early step in this assessment. However, it is also necessary to know the particular symptoms, both positive and negative, that a client suffers from, under what circumstances these symptoms occur, and how they interfere with the client's functioning. For example, one middle-aged Jewish man who had a very strict moral upbringing heard voices that uniformly told him to do what he felt like doing rather than what he thought he should do. This client believed that he had to do what his voices told him, or he would lose control of his thinking. Once this was understood, his case manager had a tool to understand the client's behavior and motivations.

In terms of symptoms, a case manager must note the particular disturbances of thinking, delusions, hallucinations, and affective disturbance that a client experiences, and the distress that these symptoms engender. In addition, the negative symptoms of apathy, slowed thought and movement, lack of activity, amotivation, poverty of speech, and social withdrawal need to be reviewed. The behavioral disturbances associated with schizophrenia, such as lack of impulse control, impaired judgment, assaultiveness, suicidality, tendencies for violence, and idiosyncratic mannerisms and behaviors, must also be addressed.

Case managers need to obtain as thorough a history of the illness as possible from all available sources, including the client, family and others in the client's support system, and other treatment providers. Factors to consider include age of onset and whether the illness appeared insidiously versus suddenly, previous periods of hospitalization, and patterns of symptom exacerbation. It is also useful to look at symptoms and behaviors longitudinally, particularly in response to treatment and environmental stressors. Finally, the presence of significant life events, such as deaths, losses, illnesses or ongoing stressors (e.g., lack of resources or incarceration), that may have contributed to the course of the disorder need investigation.

Another important consideration for assessment is substance abuse. Since the use of alcohol and/or drugs is endemic in our culture, and since these substances often temporarily ameliorate some of the painful symptoms of mental illness, those with schizophrenia are at high risk for becoming dependent on them. Unfortunately, the long-term use of drugs and/or alcohol is likely to make the symptoms of the illness much worse and to add significant additional problems. Assessment in this area can be particularly difficult and must be done carefully because of the interaction of the two disorders.

Most psychiatric inpatient staff know that one of the greatest impediments to the severely mentally ill receiving voluntary outpatient treatment is their tendency to deny the illness. Understanding the subjective meaning of the illness to the client can be a key to breaking through this denial. For instance, one young black woman told her hospital social worker that for several years she refused to accept her diagnosis of schizophrenia because she was afraid that if she admitted that she had schizophrenia, she would be locked up in a state hospital for the rest of her life.

A case manager is also responsible for assessing a broad spectrum of service needs in addition to those related to the illness of schizophrenia. These include, but are not limited to, income, housing, medical problems, legal problems, the degree of substance use or abuse, educational needs, and vocational history and capacity.

To be an effective case manager one must assess much more than problems. One must look at the entire person. Clients' strengths, assets, goals, and aspirations are as important as their limitations. One also needs to look at clients' functioning in terms of education, work, and social relationships, both prior to and after the onset of the illness. In terms of social relationships, one would want to know the extent of peer relationships: specifically, with whom the client socializes, whether the client has a primary relationship, and whether the client has or is interested in sexual relationships. One of the best ways to evaluate social functioning is to ask clients how they spend their time on a typical day, or, more concretely, to ask them to recount what they did yesterday from the time they got up until they went to bed in the evening.

Social supports in the community may play a crucial role in the course of treatment. For many clients with schizophrenia, the family will provide a major source of such support. Most mental health professionals understand that the family can be a useful source of information to assess the client. However, historically families have been treated poorly by mental health professionals and remain an untapped resource in effective case management activities such as monitoring and acquisition of resources (Intagliata, Willer, & Egri, 1986). Equally important is the need for family assessment, especially in regard to their understanding of the illness, the extent of their resources for the client, and their goals and aspirations, both for themselves and for the client. It is also useful to assess the amount of burden that the family experiences as a result of the patient's illness. Dimensions of family burden may include financial hardship, emotional distress, health problems, and curtailment of leisure activities leading to social isolation. Family members need support to resume former activities independent of the patient, which will ameliorate their sense of burden. When we speak of family, we include any individuals who play important supportive roles in the client's life, whether or not there is a blood or marital relationship.

A critical aspect of a case manager's assessment includes resources available in the client's community. The case manager must be knowledgeable of and able to use treatment services and other human services, as well as vocational resources and any other services or supports that may be necessary for a particular client.

In terms of community resources, it is insufficient simply to know that programs exist. One must have a thorough understanding of what they are, what they do, and, in particular, how they respond to the mentally ill. For instance, a referral to an Alcoholics Anonymous group may seem like an obvious choice for a client who has become addicted to alcohol after years of self-medication. However, an Alcoholics Anonymous group that accepts psychotropic medications as necessary for the mentally ill, and supports compliance, is likely to have a dramatically different impact on the client than one that defines all psychotropic substances as bad and repeatedly discourages clients from staying on their medication regimen.

Finally, the client's cultural background and religious affiliation, as well as community norms, and especially the community's attitudes towards mental illness are all factors that will have impact on recovery. Case managers will be more effective if they can understand and capitalize on these factors on behalf of their clients. As an example, one case manager learned that the church of a young black male client had a pastor who was particularly knowledgeable about and sympathetic to the needs of the mentally ill. Through this connection, the client was encouraged to continue on his medication and also did volunteer work for the church, which enhanced his sense of self-esteem.

One might say at this point that it would take an exceedingly long time for case managers to obtain this much information about their clients and their communities, and that if they had to have all of this information in order to intervene, they could never begin. This is exactly right. Assessment is an ongoing process. In the example given earlier of the client's voices that expressed what the client wanted to do, the case manager did not discover the egosyntonic aspect of the auditory hallucinations until after a year of involvement with the client. This is also a good argument as to why case management needs to be available continuously and indefinitely. A case manager must proceed with the other functions of case management on the basis of only a beginning assessment, and with less than complete information.

PLANNING

Planning is an activity that is done *with* the client, rather than *for* the client. Even though the degree to which clients with schizophrenia can participate in planning for themselves varies among clients, and varies over time for individual clients, it is essential that clients participate to the maximum extent possible in developing their own service plan. If the case manager and clients share the objective of case management as a means of helping the clients to obtain their own life goals, it is obvious that the clients need to participate in the process.

The plan flows from the assessment. Though this assessment must necessarily be broad to cover a range of the client's possible needs and goals, there are some important priorities for the service plan.

The first priority for the case manager is safety. Since schizophrenia is an illness that can produce behaviors that are potentially dangerous, both for the client and for others, the plan must include a means for protecting the client and the community when clients present any risk of violent or self-destructive behavior. Although some clients can identify those circumstances in which they are likely to lose control and can plan accordingly, many cannot. When clients do lose control, case managers must unambivalently take charge of the situation and obtain involuntary constraint and treatment.

To some, this may seem to be contradictory to the principle of client self-determination, but there are times when the effects of the illness preclude the clients' ability to respond in their own best interests. Nevertheless, we recommend that the case manager explain to the clients at the outset of their involvement those instances under which the case manager will take control of the situation, and what the case manager will do in those instances. This includes explaining the criteria for involuntary treatment and local requirements for reporting threatening or abusive behavior. In our experience, making this explicit at the beginning actually helps build trust between the client and the case manager.

The next priority for the case management plan is survival needs, which include food, clothing, and shelter. These must be dealt with regardless of the client's willingness to accept any other aspect of the plan. We believe it is unethical to withhold housing, or the capability of obtaining food, or any other basic survival service as leverage to get the client to take medication, stop drinking, respond to a court order, keep appointments with the case manager, or anything else that the case manager believes might be in the best interest of the client. If the only parts of the plan the client will accept are those dealing with survival needs, then we believe that it is necessary to provide these services. Our experience indicates that unconditionally providing these basic services, which clients often perceive as meeting their needs, helps provide the basis for a therapeutic relationship. Within this relationship the case manager can suggest that the client accept services that the case manager sees as necessary. In this regard, case management must be cooperative and noncoercive. However, the case manager can voice concern for, and disapproval of, the client's decision.

An important role of the case manager is to assure the provision of psychotropic medication. If the client refuses medications and there is any evidence that the client functions more poorly when not on medications, the plan should include a strategy for encouraging the client to accept this aspect of the treatment.

In the case management plan it is necessary to pay special attention to those problems that are likely to have serious consequences for the client if they are not resolved. These may include medical problems, substance abuse, and legal entanglements.

It is also important that case managers plan for the establishment and maintenance of social relationships for the client and ways for the client to use time constructively. The constructive use of time may include work, volunteer activities, school, or just being a friend to someone else. Since clients with schizophrenia vary substantially in their capacity for social relationships and constructive activities, the plan should be realistic in light of the client's abilities. Nevertheless, in our view, even the most regressed client benefits from some social contact and from the sense of contributing to others.

Family can play a very important role in the planning process. If family are available and the client is willing to have them involved, the case manager should work to include the family in the process. The family can both give input into the development of the plan and provide resources to implement it. In the case of clients with schizophrenia, the family most frequently provides or helps provide for basic survival needs. The family may also have the resources to respond to other needs and/or may be available to provide emotional support. Although the family can be of enormous help, they should not be exploited to their own detriment. When the family is involved, the case management plan should include provisions for supporting the family in their efforts to help the client. This support may include education about the illness, consultation on resources, respite from the client, and any other assistance that will improve the family's capacity to support the client.

Case managers must remember that clients retain their rights to confidentiality and that they may discuss clients with their family members only with explicit consent or as allowed by law. However, if the family is highly involved and knows the details of a client's life, the case manager needs to develop strategies for gaining the necessary permission to talk with the family. For a resistant client, this may include discussing the dilemma posed by the lack of consent, and how it interferes with the development of a workable plan.

LINKAGE

The purpose of linkage is to see that the client receives the services indicated in the case management plan. It is much more than making referrals, in that successful linkage implies that the clients utilize and receive the intended benefit of the services to which they are referred.

Successful linkage is often the most complicated and difficult function that case managers perform, yet one that is the most important to the success of their efforts. The first task of the case manager may be to link the client to the case management service itself. This process of engagement, which some define as a separate function of case management, often entails overcoming considerable fear, mistrust, and resistance to change on the part of the client.

The impediments to linkage can be problems emanating from the client, obstacles created by the services to which the client is being referred, or both interacting to defeat the effort. Even when clients express that they want or need a particular service, a variety of problems can come between the client and the front door of the other agency. The client may be ambivalent about the need for the service, may believe that this agency can't meet that particular need, may have a delusion that this particular agency is conspiring against them, may be fearful of the stress of the intake process, may not feel deserving of the attention, may oversleep on the morning of the appointment, or may take the bus in the wrong direction. The possibilities are limitless.

The reasons for the other agency's not providing the services are equally varied. Some of these include admission criteria that exclude the severely mentally ill, not having the resources to serve the needs of the particular client, having a program that does not address the special needs of the mentally ill, having long waiting lists, having program requirements that the client cannot meet, providing overwhelmed and hostile intake staff that frighten off the clients, being geographically inaccessible, being linguistically inaccessible, and/or having high costs. It is the role of the case manager to work to develop strategies to overcome these obstacles.

Even when the client and the service provider are eager to link, the best-laid plans of case managers often go awry. At the time of discharge from the hospital, one case manager made certain that his young Latino male client had vouchers issued by a social service agency for a hotel room and for obtaining food at a local grocery. However, the client called the next day and complained that he was hungry and couldn't get anything to eat. Upon investigation, the case manager learned that this market, which readily accepted these vouchers and had experience with the mentally ill, could not accept them from this client because he had completed them in such a way that the market could not be reimbursed. In addition, the store manager complained that this client had the habit of opening boxes of food while in the store and shoveling handfuls into his mouth. This resulted in much food spilling on the floor and other customers complaining and leaving the store.

Making a successful linkage in this case involved arrangements for the store to complete the voucher for the client, while at the same time teaching the client the finer points of shopping etiquette.

One of the most important linkages for those with schizophrenia is to a psychiatrist for medications. Since the case manager is rarely a physician, he or she will be responsible for assuring that the client has access to psycho-pharmacological treatment, both on a routine basis and in emergencies.

The case manager can play a crucial role in medication compliance. In addition to seeing that the clients can get to a physician, the case manager is in a position to report objectively on symptomatic changes, side effects, and client response to changes in medication regimen. The case manager can also lend further credence to the physician's rationale for prescribing partic-ular medications or changing an individual's regimen.

For clients who clearly demonstrate a need for medications, but stead-fastly refuse to take them, a case manager and a physician need to work in concert. In these situations, the case manager will need to stay in close contact with the client and repeatedly tie the need for medications to conse-quences the client actually suffers as a result of not being medicated or to goals of the client that are unattainable in an unmedicated state.

The ideal medication regimen for voluntary clients is often achieved through a series of successive approximations. The first step is getting the client to consider taking medications. The next step is getting the client to see a physician for evaluation and then to agree to take some medication for a symptom that the client does acknowledge, even if it is not an ideal choice. Once the client is taking medications, it is possible to revise the prescription to a more effective one as the client becomes more comfortable with the need for medications.

One of the major reasons for medication noncompliance is unpleasant side effects (Diamond, 1984). This is another area in which close collabora-tion between physician and case manager can produce beneficial results. By helping the client articulate the effects of the medication to the physician, and by helping the client negotiate a more satisfactory type of medication or dosage level, improved results can often be obtained. In this regard, the case manager can also be helpful in educating the client about the purpose and value of the particular medications prescribed.

Family will frequently be available to play a major role in the linkage process because they are often willing and eager to take responsibility for tasks that the case manager would otherwise complete. From the discussion thus far, it is clear that the role of the case manager is to see that whatever needs to be done is done to assure the best possible quality of life for the client. However, it is not appropriate for the case manager to foster unnecessary dependency. Therefore, the case manager should encourage a client and/or anyone in the client's support system to do as much as they can *and* will do on behalf of the client. As stated earlier, however, the case manager should not overly burden the family, but rather should support them so that they can support the client. To this end it is useful to explicitly delineate the areas of responsibility and tasks to be assumed by the family, and those to be assumed by the case manager. The case manager maintains responsibility when the family is unable to follow through in a particular area.

MONITORING

The essence of monitoring is keeping in touch with the client. The purpose of monitoring is to continuously reassess the client's condition and progress as the case management plan is implemented, so that it can be modified as necessary.

Case managers monitor primarily by observing the client's functioning and circumstances. However, a goal of case management is often to help clients monitor themselves in terms of a number of factors. These include symptoms, side effects of medication, mood, social relationships, functioning capacity, and progress toward their own goals. If clients with schizophrenia are to function more autonomously, it is necessary for them to attain mastery over their illnesses by recognizing their own symptoms, and the circumstances in which they arise, as well as the steps they can take to keep them from becoming worse.

One important area for monitoring is response to medications, and particularly the presence of side effects, which may affect compliance. These may include drowsiness, sensitivity to sunburn, shakiness/tremors, muscle tightness or spasms, increased appetite, dizziness, dry mouth, blurred vision, and constipation. In addition, the patient may have sexual complaints that involve impotence, difficulty with ejaculation, or menstrual irregularities. Finally, one must always be on the lookout for early signs of tardive dyskinesia. It is necessary to discuss any possible side effects with the prescribing physician.

A case manager will also use others with whom the client comes in contact to help with the monitoring process. This is in part because the case manager cannot be available all of the time and needs others to report changes in the client's condition and problems as they occur. However, it is also because the case manager needs as many objective views of the client, from as many perspectives as possible, in order to have a complete picture of the client, the client's needs, and the client's progress.

Others who may help monitor the client include the psychiatrist, other treatment providers, support service programs, staff, family, friends, roommates, apartment managers, and anyone else who comes in contact with the client. Again, it is necessary to note the client's right to confidentiality. A case manager can discuss the client only with those for whom the client gives consent or those with whom the case manager is legally permitted to discuss the client.

How closely clients need to be monitored depends on their condition, and will vary over time. If clients represent a danger to themselves or others, they need to be monitored very closely. At one end of the continuum, this may mean one-to-one observation on a locked inpatient unit. However, a client who has not been hospitalized for years, has long been stable on medications, and faithfully reports all changes in circumstances, may need only very infrequent periodic checks. It is the role of the case manager to determine when and how clients are to be monitored to assure that clients and their community are protected, that the clients' needs for basic services are met, and that the case management efforts are proceeding according to plan. Sufficient monitoring does require some degree of cooperation from the client, and case managers will sometimes have to accept that they will not always be able to stay in as close contact with voluntary clients as they would like.

Family will often play a key role in monitoring clients because they will be spending the most time with them. When this is the case, it is most useful for the case manager to be explicit about what the family should be looking for in the client, how to respond to particular problems as they do arise, and when the case manager or other help should be called in. It is also very helpful to teach the family the specific symptoms the client exhibits, and particularly those that are precursors of decompensation, or those that could portend dangerous behavior.

For instance, one case manager worked with a middle-aged black client who had a history of acting on command hallucinations that told him to jump out of windows. The client's auditory hallucinations were accompanied by tactile hallucinations of wires slapping across his face. The client lived with his mother, who would report to the case manager that she suspected that her son was hearing voices. By instructing the mother to ask her son directly if he were hearing voices, or feeling the wires slapping, and more specifically what the voices were saying to him, she was able to continuously assess the client and provide to the case manager very precise information on the client's condition.

ADVOCACY

By advocating for clients, case managers take an active role in supporting their clients and responding to their needs. Case managers advocate for individual clients in implementing case management plans and advocate for groups or classes of clients by encouraging treatment programs, supportive services, or the community at large to be more responsive to their needs.

To ensure the provision of appropriate services for individual clients, the case manager may perform a variety of tasks with anyone in the client's support system. As an example, a case manager may help the client articulate to a psychiatrist the side effects experienced from a particular medication. The case manager may also try to persuade a day treatment program to reconsider a client who has failed in the past by documenting changes in the client's condition, behaviors, or attitudes that might make success more likely at this time. A case manager might accompany a client to the Social Security Administration office to help with the completion of an SSI application, or provide documentation of the client's disability and inability to work to support this application, or testify on behalf of the client at an appeal hearing if the application is turned down.

Assuring an apartment manager that the case manager will be available to provide backup and support when problems arise may be useful in helping the client obtain housing. The case manager may need to advocate with the client's family by educating them about the client's illness so that they can have realistic expectations and be more supportive.

Case managers may have to advocate with their own clients for their benefit. For instance, a client might wish to live in the community, and might have the capacity to do so with adequate treatment and support, but might face long-term hospitalization because of an unwillingness to participate with available services. The client may not even be willing to use case management services because of a denial of any problems or a mistrust of mental health programs. Case managers may need to persistently encourage or entice such clients to utilize services from which they could benefit.

In many instances necessary services will not exist or will not be established to meet the needs of a number of severely mentally ill clients. In advocating to improve the system of services for groups of clients, case managers are also likely to be involved in a diverse array of activities.

To begin with, the case management's own program may be modified to be more responsive to its clients. One case management service that works with inner-city acute-care recidivists determined that extreme isolation was a problem for many of its clients. Other available services either were full, had expectations that were too high for the case management program's low-functioning clients, or were in settings in which the clients did not feel safe. A partial answer to this problem was a socialization group developed and operated by the case management program.

Most unmet needs of clients cannot be met simply by improving case management programs. It is often useful to improve the relationships between programs. The previously noted case management program perceived a number of difficulties with the hospital in which its clients received emergency services and inpatient care. The problems included the emergency service's not admitting clients that case managers believed needed hospitalization and the inpatient units' making referrals to the case management program at the last moment prior to discharge. Regular meetings between the case management staff and the emergency room staff, as well as case management staff attending inpatient rounds weekly, resolved these problems. Hospital staff also expressed that their capacity to treat the case management team's clients improved because they had improved access to clinical data and a better view of the clients' functioning and resources in the community.

Case managers often need to develop strategies to encourage existing services to be more responsive to the needs of severely mentally ill clients. This may include mental health programs as well as nonmental health services. A timely example is that of the severely mentally ill client who also has an equally severe substance abuse problem. Although the magnitude of this problem is now being recognized (Ridgely, Osher, Goldman, & Talbott, 1987), it remains true that many mental health and substance abuse services systematically exclude these individuals from treatment. Many mental health outpatient clinics will not provide medications or therapy to clients who are intoxicated and/or who have not resolved or are not in concurrent treatment for their substance abuse problem. Similarly, many substance abuse services refuse to treat individuals who are being treated with neuroleptic medications on the misguided notion that all psychoactive drugs are substances of abuse. For the alcoholic or cocaine addict with schizophrenia these policies spell disaster.

Case managers who work with these dual-diagnosis clients need to educate their colleagues in other services as to the needs of these clients and provide documentation of these problems to their superiors in the human service hierarchy, as well as organize and/or participate in committees and task forces in their communities to improve services for these clients.

Often, local communities do not provide adequate resources for individuals with schizophrenia. For instance, most communities do not have sufficient safe and decent, permanent, affordable housing for the severely mentally ill. Dramatic evidence of this failing is the rapidly growing problem of homelessness and mounting documentation that large numbers of the homeless suffer from schizophrenia and other disabling mental illnesses.

Improving the low-income housing stock in a particular community is an issue that goes well beyond the scope and capacity of most case managers. However, since housing is a basic survival need upon which the efficacy of the rest of the case management plan depends, it is an issue that case managers cannot afford to ignore. At the least, case managers are responsible for developing strategies for making available to their clients the housing that does exist, and for documenting the unmet need. As representatives of their programs, or as individuals, case managers may also wish to participate in the political and economic processes that could improve community housing options for the severely mentally ill.

Family can work to great advantage as partners with case managers in advocating for clients with schizophrenia. By encouraging the ill family member to utilize available resources, by monitoring progress in various programs, and by encouraging local services to work appropriately with the family member, families can make the difference between a successful outcome and a less successful one. Again, it is most useful if the case manager and the family spell out clearly what they each will do to support the case management plan.

Through the Alliance for the Mentally Ill and other groups of families of the mentally ill, families are actively advocating for improved services to clients with schizophrenia, and they have begun to have considerable positive impact. For instance, the San Francisco Alliance for the Mentally Ill chapter cosponsors an educational series on mental illness with the University of California, San Francisco Department of Psychiatry at San Francisco General Hospital, for the family members of clients treated in that hospital and for the community at large. Similarly, the California Alliance for the Mentally Ill played a major role in influencing the California state legislature to enhance funding for residential care homes for the mentally ill throughout the state. Recent lobbying efforts by the National Alliance for the Mentally Ill have persuaded Congress to appropriate additional funds for the National Institute of Mental Health to expand biological research in schizophrenia. Similar initiatives need to be launched for service evaluation of case management.

To date there has been a dearth of empirical studies of case management (Intagliata & Baker, 1983). This is in part due to methodological difficulties in defining and measuring case management activity. A reliable method for measuring case management has been proposed by Hargreaves et al. (1984) that involves interviewing of case managers and chart abstraction. However, the validity of such measures remains in question. It is hoped that the record abstraction method can be used for retrospective analysis of case management where adequate clinical documentation exists.

A notable exception to the lack of outcome data on the effectiveness of case management is the community support system model developed by Test and Stein in Madison, Wisconsin. The Training in Community Living Program (TCL) was conceptualized as an intensive psychosocial treatment program, offering an alternative to hospitalization. It delivers a comprehensive range of services from program staff who provide coverage almost around the clock, 7 days a week, with 24-hour crisis care available. TCL staff composition is multidisciplinary, representing all mental health professions as well as paraprofessionals. The established efficacy of TCL has been described previously (Stein & Test, 1980, 1985; Test & Stein, 1980). In controlled outcome studies the model has demonstrated success in the community management of schizophrenia by decreasing hospitalization, psychiatric symptomatology, and noncompliance with medication, while promoting social and occupational functioning and independent living.

The project focused on the needs of individual patients, which included the following:

1. Material resources: food, shelter, clothing, and medical care.
2. Basic coping skills in activities of daily living: public transportation, budgeting money, meal preparation, household cleaning, and personal hygiene.
3. Highly individualized support for community involvement, stress reduction, and problem solving.
4. Vocational and recreational activities, including social skills training.
5. Treatment in the community where the client lives.
6. Assertive staff outreach to prevent dropouts.
7. Community support to caretakers, family, or others involved with patients.
8. Continuity of care through monitoring, review, and liaison activity.
9. Commitment to an ongoing treatment contract.

Thus, although the scope of the program went far beyond most case management efforts, it was consonant with and helped to shape general case management principles. Psychotherapeutic efforts were tailored to improving individual deficits by assisting patients in their daily activities. Patients received help in finding employment or referrals to sheltered workshops where appropriate. Staff provided support for improved social functioning and development of individual strengths. An important ingredient was outreach when patients failed to attend programs or appointments. Medication was prescribed and monitored by the TCL team, and noncompliance was dealt with by the staff.

TCL differs from other case management programs in the depth and breadth of its range of services. In addition, the panoply of services was almost exclusively provided by TCL staff, rather than by linking patients extensively with other agencies. Thus, the demonstrated effectiveness of the TCL model suggests that comprehensive treatment services from a single agency or program should be considered in the future development of case management programs. Finally, efforts to monitor TCL program activity by means of a daily contact log were successful and offer another method of evaluating community support programs (Brekke & Test, 1987).

RECOMMENDATIONS FOR CASE MANAGEMENT IN SCHIZOPHRENIA

As stated earlier, case management services currently use a wide variety of personnel and organizational structures to respond to the needs of their clients. We will enumerate what we consider to be essential ingredients of case management with schizophrenic clients regardless of a case manager's educational background or the design of a case management program.

The first requirement is that the case manager have a thorough knowledge of the illness of schizophrenia and its treatment. This is essential for numerous reasons. An assessment cannot be complete without an understanding of the impact of the illness on the client. Similarly, one cannot adequately monitor a client if one is not aware as to how the treatment (or lack of treatment) is likely to influence the client's behavior. In addition, a case manager will often need to educate others in the client's support system and in the community at large as to the problems that clients are experiencing, their service needs, and the reasons for their behaviors. Obviously, one cannot educate others about the needs and behaviors of a client with schizophrenia without an understanding of the illness and its effect on that particular individual.

To meet this requirement, case management programs must provide adequate orientation, supervision, and in-service training for their case managers. This educational support is necessary even for programs that hire only a professional staff, since the training of most mental health professionals to date has seldom included experience or course work on the comprehensive care of the severely mentally ill. Ongoing in-service training is necessary to keep a case management staff updated on recent developments in the field, as well as to promote teamwork and to strengthen morale.

A second requirement for case management services is that they be available continuously and indefinitely. Schizophrenia is usually a chronic illness and often has a long-term disabling effect. It is also an illness that is likely to interfere with the client's capacity to form and maintain positive interpersonal relationships. Case management programs must respond to these realities by providing the possibility of a constant supportive relationship or relationships for as long as the client needs them. Although the intensity of the client's service needs will vary greatly over time, it is helpful to provide the constancy of one individual or one program. Even clients who are quite stable and need only intermittent contact find it reassuring to have someone to contact if they do need help, and they are much more likely to get in touch with someone that they know and trust.

It is necessary that case managers have the resources to do their work. A most important resource is sufficient time to attend to the needs of their clients. This means keeping case loads to a reasonable size. The actual number of clients that one full-time case manager can serve well varies with the intensity of the client's service needs, the organization of the case management program, and the degree to which other treatment and supportive resources are available in the comunity. Nevertheless, extending case managers beyond their capacity will lead to putting clients at risk, as well as reducing the job satisfaction of case managers (Reinke & Greenley, 1986).

In addition to sufficient time to do their work, case managers depend on the human service resources of the community. Although one purpose of case management is to assure that existing resources are used as effectively and as efficiently as possible, ultimately case managers can only be as good as the service system in which they work. Case management programs, then, must be part of an administrative structure in the community from which case managers can get support in advocating for their efforts and to which they can document the need for additional services. We agree with those who argue that the administrative structure for case management services must clearly define lines of responsibility and decision making (Mechanic & Aiken, 1987).

Case management programs must be flexible in their approach, and treatment plans must be responsive to the individual needs of particular clients. Individuals with schizophrenia vary dramatically in their service needs and in their potential, from those who require long-term care and protection in structured settings to those who can be self-supporting and maintain meaningful interdependent social relationships. Therefore, all case management plans must be individualized to the needs of specific clients, and a case management program must be organized to allow the flexibility to respond to major needs that a client may have.

One central aspect of this flexibility is the importance for case managers to be mobile and community-based. Many clients are too disorganized or too distrustful to keep appointments or to go to an office or program. For these clients, case managers must be able and willing to go where the clients are. Additionally, one can accurately assess a client's resources, functioning, and social relationships better in the environment in which the client lives. This means that case managers will provide more individualized care if they can observe the client in this environment. Also, advocacy with other agencies is sometimes more powerful, and, therefore, likely to be more effective, if it is done in person. Case managers need the capability to provide this advocacy when necessary.

Evaluation of case management services must be conducted in terms of both client outcomes and the monitoring of service delivery. A number of current hypotheses about the general efficacy of case management remain to be tested empirically. These include its cost-effectiveness, role in prevention of relapse and rehospitalization, and promotion of social functioning. Varied clinical models of case management of schizophrenia warrant further investigation.

Finally, case managers must include the families of their clients in their efforts. For too long, mental health professionals have excluded families to the detriment of the clients and their family members. Therefore, when family is available, we believe that the case manager should work with the family, as described above, in developing and implementing a comprehensive case management plan. In working with families, we believe that they have a right to know about the client's illness, its effects on the client, and its treatment. In our discussion of the role of family in case management we hope to have conveyed the message that with education and support, family members can be extremely helpful partners in the case management of schizophrenia.

REFERENCES

Baker, F., & Weiss, R. (1984). The nature of case manager support. *Hospital and Community Psychiatry, 35,* 925–928.

Ballew, J., & Mink, J. (1986). *Case management in the human services.* Springfield, Ill.: Charles C Thomas.

Brekke, J. S., & Test, M. S. (1987). An empirical analysis of services delivered in a model community support program. *Psychosocial Rehabilitation Journal, 10*(4), 51–61.

California Department of Mental Health. DPH Letter No. 85-23, June 1985.

Diamond, R. J. (1984). Increasing medication compliance in young adult psychiatric patients. *New Directions in Mental Health Services,* No. 21, 59–69.

Falloon, I. R. H., Boyd, J. L., & McGill, C. W. (1984). *Family care of schizophrenia.* New York: Guilford Press.

Hargreaves, W. A., Shaw, R. G., Shadoan, R., Walker, G., Surber, R., & Gaynor, F. (1984). Measuring case management activity. *Journal of Nervous and Mental Disease, 172,* 296–300.

Intagliata, J. (1982). Improving the quality of community care for the chronically mentally disabled: The role of case management. *Schizophrenia Bulletin, 8,* 655–674.

Intagliata, J., & Baker, F. (1983). Factors influencing the delivery of case management services to the chronically mentally ill. *Administration in Mental Health, 11,* 75–91.

Intagliata, J., Willer, B., & Egri, G. L. (1986). Role of the family in case management of the mentally ill. *Schizophrenia Bulletin, 12,* 699–708.

Leff, J. P., & Vaughn, C. E. (1985). *Expressed emotion in families.* New York: Guilford Press.

Levine, I. S., & Fleming, M. (1984). *Human resource development: Issues in case management.* Baltimore: University of Maryland.

Mechanic, D., & Aiken, L. H. (1987). Improving the care of patients with chronic mental illness. *New England Journal of Medicine, 317,* 1634–1638.

Reinke, B., & Greenley, J. F. (1986). Organizational analysis of three community support program models. *Hospital and Community Psychiatry, 37,* 624–629.

Ridgely, M. S., Osher, F. C., Goldman, H. H., & Talbott, J. A. (1987). Chronic mentally ill young adults with substance abuse problems: A review of research, treatment, and training issues. Baltimore: University of Maryland.

Schooler, N. R., & Hogarty, G. E. (1987). Medication and psychosocial strategies in the treatment of schizophrenia. In H. Meltzer (Ed.), *Psychopharmacology, the third generation of progress.* New York: Raven Press.

Stein, L. I., & Test, M. A. (1980). Alternative to mental hospital treatment: I. Conceptual model, treatment program, and clinical evaluation. *Archives of General Psychiatry, 37,* 392–397.

Stein, L. I., & Test, M. A. (Eds.). (1985). *The training in community living model: A decade of experience.* New Directions for Mental Health Services, No. 16. San Francisco: Jossey-Bass.

Strauss, J. S., & Carpenter, W. T., Jr. (1981). *Schizophrenia.* New York: Plenum Medical Book Co.

Test, M. A., & Stein, L. I. (1980). Alternative to mental hospital treatment: III. Social cost. *Archives of General Psychiatry, 37,* 409–412.

Turner, J. C., & Shifren J. (1979). Community support systems: How comprehensive. *New Directions for Mental Health Services,* No. 2, 1–13.

Wing, J. K. (1978). *Reasoning about madness.* London: Oxford University Press.

5

Crisis Intervention

GILBERT K. WEISMAN

During the past 20 years crisis intervention has been developed into a technique for the treatment of acute schizophrenic episodes. Several program models have appeared to provide intensive, crisis-oriented treatment for severely disturbed psychiatric patients in a wide spectrum of settings, including crisis residential programs, crisis day treatment centers, crisis-oriented hospital inpatient units, crisis family treatment centers, mobile crisis units, and crisis clinics. Many of these programs were developed to function as alternatives to hospitalization or continued hospitalization.

Governmental interest in these approaches has been spurred by the public's increasing concern about the lack of services for the chronically mentally ill who have been discharged from state hospitals as part of de-institutionalization. In 1977 NIMH began its Community Support Program (CSP) to help local programs develop service systems needed by mentally disabled persons in the community. CSP has identified crisis-oriented treatment programs as a critical part of a comprehensive set of services for the chronically mentally ill. It advocates a "continuum of crisis services" (Stroul, 1987) to help stabilize the crisis, to assist clients and their natural support systems to restabilize, and then to link clients with services and supports in the community. Such a continuum would include: (1) crisis telephone services, (2) walk-in crisis intervention services, (3) mobile crisis outreach services, and (4) crisis residential services.

How can crisis intervention, a brief treatment model, be applied to the treatment of a possibly lifelong illness such as schizophrenia? The answer to

GILBERT K. WEISMAN • Correspondence should be addressed to: 1107 Park Hills, Berkeley, California 94708.

this question emerges as one considers that schizophrenia is a phasic illness requiring various interventions at different points in its clinical course. There is no single treatment for schizophrenia but rather a series of shifting treatment plans and aproaches that are altered as the patient enters various phases of the disorder. Crisis intervention is effective solely in the acute phases of the schizophrenic process. It is only one component of a treatment plan for the acute illness and must be combined with medication, family intervention, and addressing psychosocial problems. Current methods of treating acute schizophrenic episodes on either an inpatient or an outpatient basis can be enhanced by combining them with techniques utilized in treating other crises, such as multidisciplinary crisis teams, time-limited treatment, the use of paraprofessionals and active patient participation in treatment planning and problem solving.

This chapter examines specific crisis intervention techniques and concepts used in treating schizophrenia and describes five clinical programs that have successfully used these techniques: crisis day treatment, residential crisis treatment (halfway house and foster family), inpatient crisis units, and family crisis intervention programs.

SCHIZOPHRENIA AND THE CHRONIC ILLNESS MODEL

Psychiatry has a long history of limited success in treating schizophrenia with the same type of medical model that is used in treating acute infections or injuries. Psychiatrists who approach the treatment of schizophrenia with the idea of effecting a cure by using a definitive therapy, such as medication, intensive psychotherapy, or hospitalization, have found the results disappointing despite the patients' initially favorable response. While, in a small percentage of cases schizophrenia does not recur following the resolution of an initial episode, this illness is most often characterized by relapses and residual manifestations. To the extent that we ignore this reality, we are able to treat only segments of the illness, thus often leaving the patient ill prepared to deal with the next set of stressors. These eventually overwhelm fragile coping mechanisms and lead to an exacerbation of acute symptoms.

In contrast, using a chronic illness model analogous to the kind used for chronic, remitting diseases such as diabetes avoids many of these pitfalls. A chronic illness model allows for planning tailored to the patient's differing needs at various phases during the illness. In treating schizophrenia one needs to differentiate between: acute exacerbations; periods of low-level, relatively stable functioning; periods when psychotherapy and change can occur; and periods when rehabilitative or resocializing approaches are most effective. Over many years of treatment a schizophrenic patient may need chemotherapy, psychotherapy, crisis intervention, day treatment, residential treatment, inpatient treatment, group therapy, rehabilitative efforts, resocialization, or varying combinations of these and other forms of treatment. Crisis intervention is thus but one approach among many that may be required.

One drawback to using a model that requires shifting techniques as clinical needs change is that fragmentation can occur. Since each treatment setting may be separate from the preceding or following one, two problems occur. First, the transition from one program to another is inherently stressful to the patient and fraught with problems if not carefully handled; there must be a commitment to effective transition work and to coordination with other current and subsequent treatment elements. Second, ongoing treatment coordination and planning is needed in order to provide a viable long-term plan. Using crisis intervention without integrating it into a comprehensive approach results in a Band-Aid therapy.

THE CRISIS MODEL

Crisis intervention had its origins in Lindemann's (1944) work with the survivors of the Coconut Grove fire. He viewed a crisis as a brief, time-limited reaction that follows a predictable course through various stages that arise as a normative attempt to master overwhelming stress. Caplan (1964) further developed these ideas to the point where they had broad clinical implications. Caplan's theory of crisis was based on the concept of emotional homeostasis. He viewed crisis as an imbalance between the individual's experience of a difficult life situation and that person's available coping mechanisms. The individual experiencing a stressful situation such as loss, illness, or disruptions in conflictual areas responds initially with habitual coping mechanisms, including both adaptive and pathologic behaviors. Normally these coping mechanisms lead to successful management of the situation. However, when they prove inadequate, the individual faces stress with which he or she is unable to effectively deal and yet cannot tolerate, an intolerable impass. Patients in such circumstances often describe a desperate sense of having "no way out" or of feeling "checkmated." As the stress becomes increasingly intolerable, the individual feels overwhelmed and enters a state of psychological crisis. This state includes characteristics shared by all crises as well as specific features determined by the patient's underlying personality and the patient's psychopathology. When an individual with a schizophrenic history enters a crisis state, the schizophrenic psychopathology emerges as part of the maladaptive crisis response. Treatment is optimally effective when addressing the crisis as well as the specific illness process. If an acute schizophrenic episode is viewed as a type of crisis, then crisis intervention techniques can be combined with well-established methods of treating acute schizophrenia.

Initially, Caplan divided crises into four phases: (1) impact and habitual response, (2) upset and ineffectuality, (3) emergency problem solving, and (4) major disorganization. Others have refined and modified Caplan's ideas, although most tend to agree on the general nature of these phases.

FOUR-PHASE MODEL OF CRISES

The following sections describe the author's adaptation for crises in schizophrenia of a four-phase model proposed by Baldwin (1977):

Phase 1: Emotionally Hazardous Situation. During this prodromal phase the individual, who had been relatively stable, is impinged on by one or more stressors. These may be nonspecific life stresses, such as housing problems, or stresses that directly relate to the individual's conflicts. Usually, two or three stresses develop over a relatively short period of time. Consequently, if only the precipitating stress is considered, much of what may be occurring will be missed. For example, among 20 patients seen in a crisis service the author found that each had experienced a buildup of stresses over periods ranging from several days to 3 months. These stresses often occurred in different spheres of the individual's life (e.g., interpersonal, financial, familial, work). During this period of mounting stress, individuals bring into play their usual adaptive mechanisms. and prodromal symptoms emerge. For chronic schizophrenic patients this includes withdrawal, irritability, mild confusion, hypersensitivity to stimuli, or other typical signs of disruption short of full-blown psychosis. Whatever residual schizophrenic symptoms are present often worsen during this phase. This is an optimal time for therapeutic intervention because preventing decompensation is often still feasible. A final stressor, even a minor one, can result in a full-blown psychotic episode.

Phase 2: Crisis. As life stresses continue to overwhelm the individual's coping mechanisms, a critical point is exceeded and symptoms of the full-blown crisis emerge. The clinical manifestation of the crisis phase is primarily determined by one or more of the following factors: (1) nonspecific symptoms characteristic of crises in general; (2) crisis symptoms specific to the type of situation precipitating the crisis, such as rape or death of a spouse; and (3) psychological predisposition of the individual.

In the schizophrenic, symptoms of this disorder will usually dominate the clinical picture. An initial or recurrent acute schizophrenic episode includes the symptoms of acute schizophrenia within the framework of a non-specific crisis. If the precipitating stressor is grief, rape, geographic dislocation, or similar crisis, features of these specific types of crises will also be present. A comprehensive approach to acute schizophrenia will include treatment directed at the crisis aspects of the problem as well as the clinical symptoms of schizophrenia.

Phase 3: Crisis Resolution. Crisis resolution as observed in psychiatric patients is a distinct phase lasting a few hours or a few days. This period is characterized by the rapid clearing of the nonspecific crisis symptoms and of the acute symptoms of the psychiatric syndrome. The process usually begins as the patient starts to feel the ability to cope with the stresses that initially felt overwhelming. If the patient is in treatment, this occurs once the treatment is experienced as helpful, often prior to the actual solution of psychologic and environmental problems. During the crisis intervention process, problems are identified and solutions are initiated (e.g., counseling is begun, housing is stabilized, medication is started, affects are controlled or identified and expressed). As these solutions are defined and/or initiated, the individual no longer experiences the problems as insoluble and overwhelming, and the sense of hopelessness begins to lift. The actual resolution of these problems may be long- or short-term, but it occurs well past the time of crisis resolution. Crisis resolution emerges in response to awareness of available adaptive solutions rather than to actually solving problems and resolving conflicts. The crisis state emerges when adaptive mechanisms are overwhelmed and ends when new mechanisms begin to develop.

Phase 4: Postcrisis Transition. Crisis intervention does not end with the resolution of the crisis; it extends for several days from the crisis to the reestablishment of stability. Once the crisis is resolved, the individual has the energy, acuity, and time to focus on restructuring the disrupted elements of his or her life through instituting adaptive solutions initiated in the crisis phase. Patients move into their next living situation in a residential program, back home, or to an apartment. Homeless patients may return to the streets, ideally to be followed by a case manager. Many patients enter the next phase of treatment in day treatment programs or individual therapy. Work, job training, or school will be resumed or initiated. The transition phase ends once a new homeostasis is established. Although this is the usual and hoped-for end point for most patients, others find themselves not adequately prepared to deal with their postdischarge situation and may slip back into a crisis state. In such situations, a new crisis intervention must be initiated to avert hospitalization.

SPECIAL IMPLICATIONS OF CRISIS FOR THERAPY

Three nonspecific features of a crisis have special implications for treatment: (1) the time-limited nature of crises, (2) cognitive and affective features of the individual in crisis, and (3) individual openness to help during a crisis.

Time-Limited Nature of Crises. In schizophrenia, crises are time-limited periods within an extended illness process. Caplan (1964) sees crises as lasting from 1 to 5 weeks. The time-limited nature of crises may well be influenced by psychophysiologic mechanisms that function to reestablish homeostasis and prevent exhaustion. This time limit has important implications for designing maximally effective interventions.

Cognitive and Affective Disruption. The crisis itself usually involves painful affective components as well as disruptions of cognitive functioning. These compound the symptoms of the particular psychiatric disorder. Nonspecific feelings of distress, anxiety, and tension are characteristic of the crisis phase, and their disappearance marks the end of the crisis; for example, Caplan (1964) describes "feelings of helplessness and ineffectuality in the face of the insoluble problem." Cognitively, the individual appears incapable of making decisions or of thinking things through logically. Particularly disruptive is the individual's lack of a cognitive framework with which to understand what is being experienced. Patients do not know how to understand what they are experiencing and why they are unable to think their way out of the situation or defend against painful feelings in their usual manner. Some disruption of functioning ensues. The patient may appear stunned and immobilized or involved in frenetic, ineffectual behavior.

In the schizophrenic patient these nonspecific crisis symptoms are not always distinct because they can combine with, aggravate or add to the symptoms of the illness process, such as fragmentation of cognition or speeding up and impoverishment of thoughts.

Openness to Help. Owing to the disruptive and dysphoric aspects of the crisis, the individual is more amenable than usual to accepting help and to making changes. This creates a unique opportunity for achieving considerable psychological growth relatively quickly. Gains made during crisis intervention can effect core conflicts such as dependency, low self-esteem, and family dynamics. Many schizophrenics will only engage in treatment during crisis, refusing all help or accepting only supportive therapy at other times. Consequently, crisis intervention with schizophrenic patients may be more important than with individuals having other psychological diagnoses. Not all schizophrenics are actively seeking help; some are quite antagonistic to attempts at treatment. When crisis intervention is done on a less than voluntary basis it is usually limited to returning the patient to a precrisis level of functioning. However, there is a subgroup of patients who begin treatment antagonistically, but who shift in a few days to exhibiting a desire for help.

THE EVOLUTION OF CRISIS INTERVENTION IN THE TREATMENT OF SCHIZOPHRENIA

During the 40 years since crisis intervention emerged as a clinical model, its scope and use have dramatically expanded. In the 1970s crisis intervention grew from a model primarily used for prevention and dealing with situational reactions to one of the main psychotherapeutic tools in community mental health. In part this occurred because of the realization that many people requesting treatment were in crisis. Often these patients had been placed on waiting lists for several months and then failed to show up for their appointments. Some had decompensated and were hospitalized, while others had committed suicide. Most struggled through the crisis as best they could. Caplan has pointed out that timely crisis intervention can turn the crisis in a positive direction versus a potentially pathologic resolution if treatment is not available.

Crisis intervention was often used in clinics as a temporary measure for those cases where it appeared urgent that immediate treatment be provided even if longer-term care was not yet available. Many of these patients were able to resolve their problems adequately in a matter of weeks, often to the point where they no longer felt a need for therapy. Soon crisis intervention became a standard service offered by clinics. It also became evident that a significant number of psychiatric patients requiring long-term treatment were, in fact, willing to be in therapy only during crises. Whereas these patients were not considered candidates for psychotherapy before, they now could be considered for crisis-oriented and short-term treatment. With increasingly scarce financial support for mental health services, providing crisis intervention became a high priority.

Crisis Teams. As the crisis model became part of the urban mental health system, techniques were modified to better treat problems previously beyond the scope of crisis intervention. The primary factor enabling this expansion was the development of the crisis team. The use of small, multidisciplinary teams rather than individual therapists made it possible to treat highly complex situations involving patients with severe psychopathology using crisis intervention as an intensive treatment modality. Acutely psychotic patients could now be treated at home or in various treatment facilities by a team for the many hours a day required to deal with acute psychosis or suicidal behavior. Within a few hours a crisis team could provide psychiatric assessment, initiate medication, involve the family, establish a temporary support system, provide one-to-one counseling, companionship, and monitoring, and identify many of the community resources needed to restabilize the patient. Involvement and treatment could be more intense and rapid than than usually provided by most acute inpatient psychiatric facilities.

The first inpatient use of a crisis team was at the Connecticut Mental Health Center in a 72-hour intensive treatment program developed by Claudwell Thomas (Thomas & Weisman, 1970; Weisman, Feirstein, & Thomas, 1969). Intensive treatment was provided by a crisis team that included a psychiatrist, nurses, a psychologist, a social worker, and psychiatric technicians. The crisis team utilized in this program is described in detail by Lieb, Lipsitch, and Slaby in *The Crisis Team* (1973). The program discharged 82% of those hospitalized within 72 hours.

During the ensuing years the average length of hospital stays on a national level has decreased. By the 1980s the median length of stay in state and county mental hospitals was 3 weeks and much less in urban hospitals. If this 20-year trend continues, the length of hospital stays will be reduced to 1 week within the next decade or two. Concepts of short-term hospital treatment increasingly resemble crisis intervention, and the merging of the two seems to be a matter of time.

Crisis Intervention as a Hospital Alternative. While hospital treatment of schizophrenia has been shifting in the direction of crisis intervention, most programs designed specifically as crisis intervention approaches for the treatment of schizophrenia have developed as alternatives to hospitalization or to extended hospitalization. These programs have evolved out of concerns that hospital treatment in general has serious drawbacks in terms of institutionalization and its effect on the patient's identity. Hospital treatment implicitly encourages a dependent "patient identity" associated with expected compliance with the medical model. Such roles usually fail to foster independence, the ability to make decisions, and autonomy. In its more severe form, institutional adaptation leads to behavior patterns that militate against reentry into the normal community (Goffman, 1961; Gruenberg, 1969). In response to these concerns the deinstitutionalization process—shifting psychiatric patients out of the hospital and into the community—began. Belatedly, local and state governments are realizing that their communities lack the resources needed to treat many of these patients. A commitment to dealing with this problem is only now beginning to emerge.

A considerable array of hospital-alternative models have developed over the years (Lamb, 1979; Stein & Test, 1978b). The early works of Pasamanick, Scarpitti, and Dinitz (1967) and Langsley, Pittman, Machotka, and Flomenhaft (1968) provided well-controlled studies showing that home treatment alternatives could be as good as or better than hospitals in providing treatment for the severely disturbed patient. Langsley's work used a crisis model of family therapy as an alternative to hospitalization. Some more recent programs were broader in the range of patients treated, such as the Training in Community Living program developed in Madison, Wisconsin (Stein & Test, 1978a). This program diverted all but 18% of patients from hospital admission into normative community settings (rooms and apartments), where they were treated by a mobile interdisciplinary team. A major factor promoting the development of hospital alternatives is that they have usually proven to be more cost-effective than hospital treatment.

Crisis Intervention in Emergency Rooms and Mobile Crisis Units. Hospital alternatives and crisis intervention followed parallel and, at times, combined development over the past 20 years. An early form of combined evolution occurred in the psychiatric emergency room. In the late 1960s and early 1970s psychiatric emergency services emerged as distinct entities with their own specialized techniques and multidisciplinary teams. This involved a shift in emergency room psychiatric services from an assessment and triage model to one that included treatment. Emergency room teams could see acutely psychotic individuals in the emergency room, begin them on phenothiazines, and then follow them over the next several days until they had improved enough to wait for an outpatient appointment, thus at times avoiding hospitalization.

Once crisis teams demonstrated the ability to intervene in acute psychosis in the emergency room, programs were developed with mobile crisis teams to provide emergency services and crisis intervention in the community. Mobile crisis teams not only worked with the individual but often focused on the resolution of family crises (Bengelsdorf & Alden, 1987; Foxman, 1976). They were able to provide emergency services in virtually any community setting, including homes, hotels, and board-and-care homes, and to the homeless. By providing crisis intervention in the community, the mobile crisis team was able to reduce the use of emergency rooms and outpatient crisis services, and provided an alternative to hospitalization.

Crisis Residential Programs. While treating acute schizophrenia in medical and community settings has worked for many patients, a number of models have developed that employ various types of therapeutic residential environments in the community. These programs provide homelike milieus that have some of the advantages of the presence of a natural family setting combined with the advantages of a trained crisis team. In 1976 the La Posada program was developed to provide crisis intervention in a house in a residential area of San Francisco (Weisman, 1985a,b). La Posada combined the halfwayhouse model with the use of a crisis team. The halfway house orientation gave the program a strong therapeutic community and resocialization component. La Posada treated a predominantly chronic population and was able to avert hosptalizing 92% of those admitted to the program.

Another variant of residential treatment was a "crisis foster homes" model developed by the Southwest Denver Mental Health Center (Polak & Kirby, 1976; Polak, Kirby, & Deitchman, 1979). This program combined foster homes for acutely disturbed patients with the use of a mobile crisis team. The program trained foster families to work with acutely psychotic patients, and these families were supported by a mobile crisis team that provided the direct treatment for the patient and consultation to the foster family in the home.

In November 1986 the Community Support Services Branch of NIMH convened the NIMH Crisis Residential Services Meeting, which brought together people working and interested in this area to facilitate sharing of information. The plan was to formulate recommendations in this area and provide information and speakers to facilities interested in developing similar programs. The final report was issued in 1987 (Stroul, 1987).

Crisis-Oriented Day Treatment. Another area in which crisis intervention can readily be applied is the day treatment center. Although day treatment programs have traditionally been long-term, open-ended settings, increasingly such programs have been designed on a shorter-term model for more acutely disturbed patients. Wilder (1966) described the use of a day treatment program as a hospital alternative. Patients in his program stayed for an average of 8 weeks. In 1970 San Francisco's Mission Mental Health Center Acute Day Treatment program was developed as a 3-week crisis-oriented service. The program combined the major elements of crisis intervention and day treatment.

The programs discussed thus far do not provide methods by which the private practitioner or outpatient clinic can use crisis intervention with acute schizophrenia. If the intensive crisis programs described are available in the community, therapists can refer their patient and continue the individual therapy while the patients are in the program. This works particularly well with day treatment or residential treatment programs. The therapist can often avert hospitalization and maintain continuity of treatment in the process. When such alternative programs are not available, the therapist can use crisis intervention techniques including frequent visits, rapid tranquilization, intervention in the environment, work with the family, the use of contracts, and other techniques elaborated on in the next section. The individual therapist can thus shift to a crisis-oriented approach when the patient becomes acute and can return to the regular treatment mode when the crisis is resolved.

Although these crisis intervention approaches can provide an alternative for hospitalization for many patients, each has its limitations. A solution to this problem, advocated by NIMH, is to construct a "continuum of crisis services." This model (Stroul, 1987) utilizes a comprehensive network of crisis programs, each of which is designed to meet somewhat different needs. For example, the Southwest Denver Community Mental Health Services (Polak & Kirby, 1976; Polak et al., 1979) is based on a continuum model. Services include a mobile crisis team, home treatment, crisis foster homes, and an intensive observation apartment. The crisis team picks up the case initially, evaluates the patient, and then provides whatever services are needed, one member continuing as the therapist and case coordinator throughout the crisis. Any sequence of services may be used as dictated by the evolving clinical picture. This crisis network allows for maximal use of crisis intervention for the treatment of acute schizophrenic episodes and makes hospital services essentially a backup for the most difficult cases. A similar program, the Kent County Mental Health Center (1986) in Warwick, Rhode Island, provides, in addition, a crisis-oriented inpatient program.

TECHNIQUES FOR CRISIS INTERVENTION IN SCHIZOPHRENIA

In its early years, crisis intervention techniques were used in a limited number of situations, such as disasters, and in preventive approaches to treatment. The techniques developed for these types of problems, which most often occurred in healthy individuals, were relatively direct and often easily mastered by people who had little training. These early techniques still form the basis of most crisis intervention programs. They include the use of time limits, a primary focus on current problems, a reality orientation, an active theraputic stance, development of new adaptive mechanisms, and dealing with families and social networks. With the evolution of the crisis team and the various crisis programs described earlier, the complexity and severity of the problems treated increased and new techniques for crisis intervention had to be developed. The following paragraphs describe therapeutic techniques frequently used in the crisis-oriented treatment of acute schizophrenia. Individual crisis programs use some of these techniques and not others. The list of techniques does not attempt to be comprehensive but rather illustrates some of the most effective components of the crisis treatment of schizophrenia, with an emphasis on factors differentiating them from more generic crisis intervention techniques.

ASSESSMENT

Assessment of the acute schizophrenic episode for crisis intervention has several features that differentiate it from inpatient evaluation. Since the duration of the treatment process is short and interventions must be initiated as quickly as possible, it is essential to develop a fairly comprehensive problem list during the first interview so that a treatment plan can be initiated within the first 24 hours. By the end of the intake interview the clinician should be able to identify and discuss with the patient the main problem areas. In a preliminary manner, he or she should also discuss potential solutions, such as the nature of the treatment the patient is going to receive, the possibility of family therapy, alternative answers to financial problems, and solutions to problematic living situations. The process of hearing one's problems articulated along with potential solutions sets the stage for the process of crisis resolution. The intake interview, which may take up to 2 hours, is usually the most potent interview in the treatment process; it introduces the patient to treatment, initiates the treatment, and establishes the basis for a therapeutic alliance.

As part of the initial assessment it is often essential to interview the family or whomever the patient is living with in order to understand the systemic aspects of the current crisis. Frequently there is a crisis in the patient's family that is causally related to his or her decompensation; this may become the primary focus of the crisis intervention.

In the crisis treatment of schizophrenia the initial interview in an emergency room followed by an intake interview in the treatment program is the central forum for assessment. This contrasts with assessment of hospitalized patients, where the assessment process can be extended over a longer time.

MEDICATION

One of the major factors enabling crisis intervention to be effective in treating schizophrenia is the use of antipsychotic medication (Polak, 1978). Phenothiazines must be initiated as early as possible, in order to rapidly control disorganized thought and disruptive behavior. Similarly, it is important to quickly alleviate any sleep problems. Often, lack of sleep exacerbates psychotic disorganization, and attempts to facilitate reorganization are ineffectual until the individual obtains sufficient sleep.

Despite the need for rapid tranquilization, the doses used in crisis intervention are usually 25% to 50% lower than those required for hospitalized patients. The use of lower doses is the result of two factors. Because of the need for high-intensity treatment and the patient's active involvement in the program for many hours a day, the sedative effects of phenothiazines must be minimized. In addition, lower levels of medication are adequate in the homelike residential crisis treatment settings because the settings themselves have a calming, integrative effect in contrast to the often frightening, impersonal ambience of an acute psychiatric ward. Normative, homelike settings often calm the patient shortly after entering, leading to a dramatic lessening of anxiety and clearing of symptoms.

EXPECTATIONS AND CLINICAL CHANGE

The expectations of the clinician, the program, and the therapeutic community all have an important effect on the course of psychiatric illness. By carefully building expectations into the program one can harness this formidable clinical tool. Expectations can be used to alter various aspects of the treatment process, including influencing behavior, control of affects, the quality of social interactions, and the patient's level of functioning. Expectations can emanate from many sources. In residential crisis programs the homelike building and the family-like structure of the milieu generate a set of expected behaviors that, although powerful, are experienced by the patient as noncoercive. In a crisis foster home, patients will automatically begin to behave with house-appropriate rather than hospital-appropriate behavior. They will relate to the home sponsors as hosts rather than as psychiatric nurses and attendants. Usually patients automatically take responsibility for maintaining their own area and try to be as sociable as their problems permit. Analogous changes occur in group residential crisis programs such as La Posada. Such changes often begin soon after the patient enters the program and develop at a pace determined by the individual's capabilities. In general, expectations are high in these programs as compared with other treatment settings.

Although concern has been expressed in the literature about the negative effect of high expectations and high-intensity treatment on schizophrenics, this does not appear to be a problem when expectations are individualized and carefully reassessed on a daily basis.

TIME LIMITS

One of the central tenets of crisis intervention is that the duration of the crisis is relatively short but is influenced by the treatment setting and expectations. Acute schizophrenic episodes that take weeks to resolve in an inpatient setting are usually brought to resolution and the patient discharged within several days in time-limited crisis programs. Burgess and Baldwin (1981) have succinctly described this phenomenon by restating Parkinson's law: "The work of adaptive change expands or contracts to meet the time available for its completion as defined through structure and limits created early in the therapeutic process." In crisis programs the time limit facilitates the necessary work being accomplished within the time frame. In contrast, time limits imposed from sources outside the treatment team, such as by insurance companies or utilization review, can truncate the treatment plan rather than being integral to it.

Time limits also have a therapeutic effect through providing a structure for both patient and therapist. Patients in crisis usually have some degree of confusion about what is happening, how help can be obtained, and how long treatment will take. They are actively seeking structure, and if they enter a 72-hour treatment unit they organize their work into this time frame. Staff likewise use the time structure to determine how they will work, and what issues have to be dealt with and when. The time limit of the program thus provides the skeleton for the program elements and guides the staff and patients in their work together.

INTENSITY

The use of time limits in treating schizophrenia necessitates that a vast quantity of work be accomplished in a short period of time. A high staff-to-patient ratio is required to accomplish this. One way of creating an intensive treatment program is to use what Claudwell Thomas (Thomas & Weisman, 1970) called the "structured day." The clients' time is structured to keep them actively involved in various therapeutic interactions throughout the day and evening. This is accomplished by scheduling 3–5 hours of therapeutic groups or sessions a day plus several hours in the community working on survival issues such as finances and housing. Those times not scheduled used by the residents to become involved in the daily life of the household as members of that family or community. Eating, preparing meals, and household maintenance chores become major socializing experiences that validate the residents' experience of themselves as functional and useful to the family/community. Much of any remaining time is spent interacting with other community members, a therapeutic involvement countering isolation and facilitating the residents' development of mutual helping interactions. This intensive approach works, in part, because the patients are in a state of crisis and consequently open to learning less painful and more functional ways of reorganizing their thoughts and life. The program structure, values, and expectations become available to meet these needs.

The high activity level of the day is specifically effective in interrupting pathological ruminations. Structure and activity oriented toward participation in the life of the "home" displaces the patient's disorganized thinking or depressive rumination. Richard Almond (1974) notes that "the individual healing process begins by drawing the sufferer out of his isolated subjective and objective position and getting him to attend to a new environment; the healing community." He refers to social, physiological, and psychological saturation early in the healing process by which the individual is moved from inner self-absorption and passivity to interaction and activity.

CRISIS TEAMS

Crisis teams have been used in diverse clinical settings, including inpatient units, residential programs, emergency services, and outpatient clinics. They are small, multidiciplinary units organized so as to provide the varied services needed for crisis resolution within the time frame of a crisis. The team has both medical and nonmedical components. Often the only medical person is a psychiatrist who functions as a consultant and deals with issues such as medication, diagnosis, and assessment. The main body of the team consists of a mix of licensed and unlicensed mental health professionals, such as social workers, nurses, psychologists, paraprofessionals, and psychiatric technicians. The psychiatrist participates with other team members in developing treatment plans, program development, training, and supervision. The psychiatrist is responsible to ensure that adaquate medical services are provided.

Leadership on the team can be provided by any team member having the skills to run such a program. No specific degree is needed, and qualified individuals from any relevant work experience background can be highly effective. This may include people with experience such as work in public service programs, social workers, and counselors.

Central to the team concept is the proposition that the team as a whole can provide services more effectively than any one individual. One team member functions as case manager and has overall responsibility for implementation of the treatment plan. On a given case, one person may be assigned to do the individual counseling, another may run a group, another may consult about financial problems, and the psychiatrist may deal with arranging for treatment of a medical issue.

THE USE OF PARAPROFESSIONALS

One common and highly effective feature of crisis teams is the use of paraprofessionals. In some crisis programs 90% of the staff are paraprofessionals. A paraprofessional's role on a team is carefully defined by his or her abilities, past experience, and specialized training. Paraprofessionals are usually identified as counselors and, depending on their ability, function in areas such as: individual, group and family counseling, case management, treatment and discharge planning, activities, and coordination with community agencies and services.

A major advantage of using paraprofessionals in crisis work is that they can be hired from the same population as the patients and consequently share similar cultural, racial, and sexual identities. This facilitates forming rapid, empathic relationships by bypassing cultural and racial barriers. It can take many weeks or months for the best-trained professional to form a trusting relationship with someone from another culture or social class. Such barriers are prohibitive in crisis intervention because of its time-limited nature. Similarly, certain aspects of an individual's crisis situation may be unfamiliar or unknown to someone who does not share the same sexual orientation or racial background. These issues may be even more important when dealing with the patient's family because the culturally unique aspects of family interaction can be overlooked by the therapist.

NORMALIZING ENVIRONMENTS VERSUS INSTITUTIONS

Perhaps the most disruptive environments in which to place schizophrenics are psychiatric institutions. When patients are in a psychotic state they experience their world as frightening and chaotic. To counter this inner chaos they need an environment that they experience as safe and predictable. Placing them in an acute psychiatric hospital often not only fails to meet these needs but compounds the problems. In contrast to this, treating schizophrenia in a home environment has a rapid calming effect. In addition, residential settings create an entire set of normalizing expectations that directly prepares the individual for functioning in the community. In a home, patients quickly adapt to normative behavior patterns appropriate to family life rather than the type of behavioral latitude that is tolerated in a locked psychiatric ward. As Rosenhan's study (1973) of behavior in a mock prison setting has shown, the implicit expectations of the setting and the roles of those involved profoundly affect the attitudes, behavior, and nature of the ensuing interaction. A third normalizing feature of residential treatment is that a patient can receive treatment for severe mental illness without having to develop the identity inherent in the experience of having been in a mental institution.

The combination of crisis intervention for schizophrenia and residential treatment enhances the normalizing effect of each modality. Normalization of the treatment environment directly facilitates crisis resolution through its reintegrative, calming, identity-stabilizing effect. Both crisis intervention and residential treatment maintain the individual in a normative frame work and minimize the disruption of the current episode on the patient's daily life. The time-limited aspect of crisis intervention is itself normalizing in that it does not provide the time needed to crystallize a pathologic patient itentity. For those schizophrenics who are able to maintain jobs despite episodic decompensations, the brevity of the treatment is much less likely to lead to termination from work. Everyday living skills such as cooking or cleaning are retained or relearned in residential programs. By maintaining a normalizing treatment environment such as the patient's home, foster homes, and group residential homes, the disruptive effect of the illness process on identity and autonomous functioning is minimized or reversed.

CONTRACTS AND THE CONTROL OF DANGEROUS BEHAVIOR

The use of alternatives to hospitalization, such as homes and apartments, which contain potentially self-injurious opportunities and objects such as knives, creates a danger of harming self and others that appears formidable.

Despite the influence of environment on behavior and the calming effect of medication, some patients still have only a tenuous grasp on their violent or self-destructive impulses. It is usually helpful for such individuals to develop personalized contracts with the primary therapist. These contracts are based on the patients' willingness to negotiate a personal written contract with a staff member whom they trust. The general content of a "no violence" (or "no suicide") contract includes the following: (1) The patient agrees to talk to staff about violent feelings as soon as such feelings arise. (2) The patient agrees not to act on violent impulses while in the program. Such contracts are also used for screening out patients who require hospitalization. While negotiating the contract with the patient, the counselor assesses the patient's willingness and ability to comply with the contract.

The overall effect of these approaches is to provide a greater degree of voluntary control over destructive impulses than can be achieved in the hospital. The limitation to these approaches is that a small percentage of patients cannot be controlled adequately in residential settings. Such patients can usually be identified prior to admission, but for others, control of these impulses breaks down only after admission, and transfer to a hospital is necessary. Usually the residents are able to let staff know if they are having difficulty controlling themselves, or the staff picks up on this through non-verbal cues. Such patients can than be calmed down adequately or transferred to the hospital before losing control. In the La Posada residential crisis program there were no serious suicide attempts in over 2000 admissions, despite the fact that 30% of those admitted were suicidal. In the same program, minor staff injury occurred only three times in 10 years. Thorough staff training and ongoing supervision are essential in crisis residential programs in order to make work with these patients safe outside the protection of a hospital.

PARTICIPATORY PROBLEM IDENTIFICATION, PROBLEM SOLVING, AND TREATMENT PLANNING

Much of the treatment process in crisis intervention is organized around the patient's active participation in problem identification, problem solving, and treatment planning. Daily involvement with these issues provides the resident with active control over the treatment. Increasing the patient's participation in this process is a major therapeutic goal. Usually, a specific crisis team member serves as case coordinator/counselor and engages the patient in this process on a regular basis. Some group residential programs also have morning group meetings that address and revise plans daily. Treatment planning and/or implementation is a significant part of each patient's day. For example, instead of watching TV on a hospital ward, the patient is immersed in implementing a plan developed in the morning meeting, such as interviewing therapists in the community or trying to untie some financial knot at the welfare office.

By making problem solving and treatment planning the resident's responsibility, not only are solutions generated, but the individual learns to handle life problems effectively. Thus, a new way of coping is experienced and can to some degree be internalized. This approach requires a major shift in the way staff members see themselves. Staff must learn that their function is to empower the patient. Initially, staff members may experience this shift of responsibility to the patient as a threat to their own power or value.

INITIATION OF ALTERNATIVE COPING MECHANISMS

Problem identification is followed by identifying possible solutions and initiating these new ways of approaching problems. For example, solutions to family problems may lie in family therapy or financial problems may be addressed through the appropriate social agency. Initiating these new coping mechanisms while the individual is still in the program reduces the danger of the resident's not following through after discharge. By overlapping services, the trauma of separation at discharge is reduced, thus allowing for a smoother transition to the community and minimizing the discontinuity inherent in treating various phases of schizophrenia in different settings.

INVOLVEMENT OF FAMILY, AGENCIES, AND THE COMMUNITY

Schizophrenic patients often present with problems which initially appear to be theirs alone but which, upon further examination, are interconnected with one or more social systems. Consequently, effective crisis intervention usually entails considerable social system intervention (Polak, 1978).

For those patients living with their families, roommates, or in board-and-care homes, the major crisis often involves these social systems. For example, a family may be dealing with a death or a financial problem and, as a result, become increasingly dysfunctional as a unit. The schizophrenic member will react to the same stress experienced by the family as well as the secondary stress of the family's becoming dysfunctional. During this process the schizophrenic patient can begin to decompensate, creating a new stress for the family, who may then want that individual hospitalized so they are freer to deal with the original stress. Langsley et al. (1968) effectively treated schizophrenics living in families with family crisis intervention and produced results at least equivalent to hospitalization.

In the process of developing solutions to problems, the crisis program must work closely with involved agencies and therapists to guarantee continuity of treatment. Where these connections do not already exist the crisis team may need to refer the patient for such services. The use of other less formal community resources, such as clubs and ethnic social groups, helps create a social matrix for the individual. Community reentry is greatly simplified when the crisis residential program is in the neighborhood and can readily facilitate such connections.

TERMINATION

Because crisis intervention is short-term and separation issues are central to serious psychopathology, termination issues need to be addressed throughout treatment. Due to the intensity of the treatment and the vulnerability of patients in crisis, and despite the short duration of crisis treatment, strong bonds are formed to the crisis team and specific staff members.

Termination can be particularly difficult if patients are being returned to the life situation that initially overwhelmed their coping abilities. In order to minimize the effect of such transitions, it is important to initiate the postdischarge treatment while the individual is still in the crisis program. Aftercare can further lessen the severity of this transition. In the crisis inpatient program at the Connecticut Mental Health Center, a 30-day outpatient follow-up helped move the patient from the intensive inpatient program back into the community, spreading the termination over an additional month.

TRANSITION TO SERVICES SUBSEQUENT TO CRISIS RESOLUTION

Successful crisis intervention in its purest form implies a return to the previous level of functioning, a reestablishment of the equilibrium. While this is true in some cases of schizophrenia, in others a less intensive level of treatment beyond crisis intervention is necessary before the individual can return to a precrisis level of functioning. The crisis can be the first part in an episode that may take many weeks or months to stabilize. For example, 42% of the patients discharged from La Posada were referred for further, although less intensive, residential treatent (Weisman, 1985a,b). Other patientsneeded ongoing treatment in a day treatment program or an outpatient clinic. The availability of a coherent system of services of various types and levels of intensity provides for the additional treatment often necessary for resolving the acute schizophrenic episode after the crisis phase.

CRISIS INTERVENTION PROGRAMS FOR ACUTE SCHIZOPHRENIA

This section describes five crisis programs, each utilizing a different treatment modality, including: (1) crisis-oriented residential treatment, (2) family crisis therapy, (3) crisis foster homes, (4) crisis inpatient treatment, and (5) crisis day treatment. In addition, a sixth program containing a continuum of crisis services is also presented. These programs use many of the techniques described earlier, but each has selected those elements most appropriate to the modality used and the needs of the population served.

CRISIS RESIDENTIAL TREATMENT—LA POSADA

La Posada, a 10-bed crisis residential treatment program started in San Francisco in 1977, was developed primarily as a hospital alternative. The average length of stay was 9 days, with a maximum of 2 weeks. The program was based both on crisis intervention theory and on the social rehabilitation model developed in halfway houses over the preceding 20 years. First developed in England in the 1940s by Jansen (1980), the halfway house model uses the normalizing milieu of a home as a basis for retraining individuals discharged from the hospital for reentry into the community. Halfway houses enhance independent functioning and counteract regressive, dependent behavior. Because both crisis intervention and the halfway house model share the basic goal of returning the individual to the community, it was easy to combine the major principles of both modalities into a highly effective program.

From its inception, La Posada has been run by Progress Foundation, a nonprofit organization that contracts with San Francisco County Mental Health Services to develop and manage residential treatment programs. It has become an integral component of a countywide network of residential programs designed to provide services to individuals with varying levels of psychologic disturbance (Weisman, 1985a). La Posada has operated smoothly for the past 10 years and has become the prototype for 15 similar programs throughout California. Its ready replication differentiates it from programs that owe their success more to the leadership and skills of those who developed and ran it than to the soundness of the model. Its practicality is also related to its cost-effectiveness, which represents a 57% saving over the cost of a hospital day ($171 versus $400).

La Posada primarily serves severely disturbed chronic mental patients. The average patient has had four previous hospitalizations. Twenty percent of those admitted have a schizophrenic diagnosis, 16% have paranoia and other psychoses, and 35% have bipolar disorders or major depressions. La Posada diverts people from hospitalization in three ways:

1. Alternative to hospitalization: Referring clinicians judged that 30% of those admitted to La Posada would have been admitted directly to the hospital had a bed not been available.
2. Alternative to continued hospitalization: Another 28% are patients who have been discharged early from the hospital after a short stay for stabilization. The referring clinicians judged that these patients would have stayed longer in the hospital were La Posada not available.
3. Preventive intervention: An additional 28% are patients seen in the emergency room who are in the process of decompensation but are not yet disturbed enough to require hospitalization. Many of these would have continued to decompensate and would have been admitted to the hospital. Of those admitted to La Posada, 6% could not be maintained in the program and were hospitalized.

Suicidal patients are admitted if they are willing to contract with staff not to hurt themselves while in the program. Nonviolence contracts are also required if violence is an active problem.

La Posada is located in a home that is indistinguishable from others around it in a residential area of San Francisco. Its staff most often live in the neighborhood and reflect its ethnic and racial mix. The atmosphere in the house is warm, and there is an immediate sense that those who live there care about it. A part-time cook/counselor works with the residents in preparing meals. Home-style cooking in abundant quantities helps to rapidly form a therapeutic alliance. Upon entering the program, residents quickly learn that all the people in the house are responsible for their living space and spend some of their time daily in shared housecleaning and cooking responsibilities. By the time they leave, all the residents are encouraged to plan a meal for the house and to be in charge of preparing it, an accomplishment residents consider beyond their ability at the time of admission.

Residents at La Posada participate in an intensive treatment program with high functional expectations. These expectations are carefully geared to the individual's clinical state and functional potential; for example, expectations of someone who is acutely psychotic are minimal compared with those for a resident nearing discharge. The high expectations are communicated by the community as a whole and include programmatic expectations and expectations of the patient group. By virtue of the highly supportive patient group and the example of "old-timers" who have been in the program over a week, the new resident is drawn into becoming a functional member of the household. The high intensity involves the use of a structured day in which the individual has numerous scheduled activities and responsibilities. A high staff–patient ratio of 1 to 3 during the day and evening is required to accomplish this. The usual day involves a mixture of groups, individual counseling, family therapy, and other activities. Many activities require the individual to go out of the house alone or accompanied by another resident to attend to personal and survival issues, such as seeing the therapist, searching for a rooming situation, or visiting family. Such activities are the individual's way of learning to function autonomously in the community, and although it may appear that much of the resident's time is devoted to discharge planning and implementation rather than to therapy, these issues are intertwined with the resident's problems. For example, it can be more productive to help someone learn to deal with authority issues with the landlord than with the ward nurse. Likewise, in group therapy developing a plan for ongoing treatment subsequent to discharge is emphasized more than group process. While intrapsychic issues receive considerable attention, the program frequently does this through a focus on functioning in real-life situations and on how these relate to dynamic issues. Problems relating to roommates, landlords, and social agency employees are usually permeated by the residents' interpersonal conflicts.

Individual counseling is provided by the counselor assigned to be the resident's primary therapist. Part of the individual counseling is also focused on treatment planning, with the counselor and resident developing the plan together. Assessment of family and preliminary family counseling is also done by the primary therapist.

The resident's personal experience of La Posada is a significant factor in its success. Residents are strong supporters of La Posada because they experience it as a house rather than as an institution, and they feel personally involved in its vital functions. The personal attention available in a small program allows a focus on the individual's specific needs and facilitates a bonding between the resident and the program. Such meaningful and therapeutically useful connections are not readily formed in larger programs.

Residents discharged from La Posada usually have chronic problems, and recurrences of symptomology are anticipated. An annual readmission over several years occurs in some cases. Residents who previously rotated in and out of the hospital often no longer use the hospital but still need La Posada when they have a recurrent psychotic episode. Often there is gratifying progress in these patients over the years since most are kept actively involved in treatment programs between episodes. Labeling such readmissions as treatment failures does not take into account the long-term nature of the schizophrenic process. The fact that these patients are able to avoid rehospitalization has an important effect on their sense of identity, self-esteem, and autonomy.

FAMILY CRISIS THERAPY

In 1964 Langsley and Kaplan established the Family Treatment Unit at the Colorado Psychiatric Hospital (Langsley et al., 1968; Langsley & Yarvis, 1976). The program provided crisis family therapy in the office and home as an alternative to hospitalization. A controlled study was done comparing the outcome of treatment on 150 families randomly assigned to this program and 150 families assigned to hospital inpatient treatment. Inclusion in the study required an intact family that lived within an hour of the hospital. Seventy percent of those admitted to the hospital met this criterion. The results of the study showed numerous advantages to those assigned to crisis family therapy. None of the patients in the crisis group required hospitalization during the active treatment phase, and only 13% required hospitalization in the 6 months following treatment, compared with 29% of the group treated in the hospital.

The family crisis model views the patient's decompensation as a result of the family's failure to deal with a hazardous life event and an ensuing family crisis. The request to hospitalize the patient is one of the family's methods of dealing with the current crisis. Langsley states that "the request for hospitalization does not underestimate the importance of the patient's psychopathology or the influence of his heredity and physiology." The family crisis intervention consequently focuses on dealing with the family crisis as well as with the psychiatric problem.

The crisis therapy occurs both in the office and at home. Services are provided by "a clinical team consisting of a psychiatrist, a clinical psychologist, a psychiatric social worker, a psychiatric public health nurse, and two clerical personnel." The treatment lasts an average of 3 weeks and includes "five offices visits, a home visit and a few telephone calls." In addition to focusing on the family crisis, treatment includes efforts to help the family avoid scapegoating and labeling one individual as a mental patient. "Drugs are used for symptom relief in any member of the family. Tasks are assigned for resolving the crisis and returning each member to functioning. With this directive and supportive approach, symptomatic relief occurs very quickly (in hours or days)."

In 1976 Langsley reported on his efforts to set up a similar program in Sacramento County, California. He soon realized that the Denver pilot project had limited practicality in a new setting. In Denver he had been able to select and limit the size of the population studied. When he attempted to apply the family crisis approach in Sacramento County, his efforts were hampered by factors such as the large population needing services, the diversity of the problems, the lack of intact families, and staffing problems. Providing family therapy as described requires the patient to be living with his or her family, which is often not the case, particularly with more disturbed and chronic schizophrenics. Also, for chronic schizophrenics living at home, it is sometimes in the patient's best interest to provide treatment outside the home, particularly when ties between the patient and the family are pathologic and an integral part of the patient's problem.

CRISIS FOSTER HOMES—ALTERNATIVE HOME PROGRAM

A recent innovation in crisis intervention, the crisis foster home is based on one of the oldest innovative models of psychiatric treatment, the psychiatric community care system in Gheel, Belgium. The foster care model initially found its place in American psychiatry as a modality for providing long-term residential treatment, but more recently it has been modified to provide crisis residential treatment. Such programs are based on the normalizing milieu provided by a family system and a home environment. Families are hired and trained to provide housing, meals, and a family atmosphere to one or two acutely disturbed adults. A crisis team works closely with the resident and family to provide necessary consultation and direct services. Again, as with the La Posada model, the efficacy of a crisis team approach is combined with a specific residential treatment model to form a new modality. The use of an actual family to relate to the resident establishes a normative set of relationships as well as a normal environment. Patients frequently cannot be treated by a crisis team in their own homes because of conflicts, stress, or burnout in the family as a result of dealing, perhaps for many weeks or months, with an increasingly psychotic individual. Treatment in a family-based crisis home thus provides an optimal experience for some patients by preparing them for reentry into their own families or the community.

In 1972 the Southwest Denver Mental Health Center began the first family-based crisis residential program (Polak, 1978; Polak & Kirby, 1976; Polak et al., 1979). This was a component of "a comprehensive system of alternatives to psychiatric hospitalization." Based on the assumption that individuals are best treated in their natural environments, the program treats patients in their own homes whenever possible. If for clinical or practical reasons this is not an option, the patient is considered for other crisis programs. In the Denver program they have found that "over 80% of clients requiring temporary or permanent separation from their natural-life setting can be treated in the alternate home system, thus avoiding hospital admission."

These foster families usually consisted of older couples whose children had already left home. Polak describes the family sponsors as "warm, outgoing, healthy people, who are rich in life experience." Families are paid a base fee of $7.50 a day for room, board, and client care working with up to two acute psychiatric patients at a time. "Each family has a staff coordinator responsible for family supervision and support, and home sponsors meet regularly to learn from each other and from the staff." The patients are expected to participate in the functioning of the household, to the extent that their problems allow them, in much the same manner as a family member. The nonprofessional nature of the family facilitates a natural and personal quality in the relationship to the patient. To varying degrees the patients are integrated into the life of the family, joining them in activities and getting to know them on a personal level. The relationship to the family provides a major healing force in the treatment. By carefully selecting, training, and supporting sponsoring families, a healing environment is created that is dramatically different from a psychiatric ward. Various types of families are available within the program, thus giving further specificity to the treatment setting. This is particularly useful in treating patients from other cultures where the language, food, and social relationships of the matched foster family enhance the chances of the treatment program to therapeutically engage the client.

Crisis intervention is provided by a treatment team that includes a clinical case coordinator, a nurse, and a psychiatrist. The clinical staff member visits the home daily to conduct sessions with the client. The staff member functions as a case manager and has ongoing responsibility for crisis intervention, social-systems work, and treatment activities. The case management function continues after the individual leaves the home. At the time of placement the clinician can remain in the foster home with the client and sponsors for up to 24 hours in order to stabilize the patient. One or two volunteers can also be used in this manner. Certain patients are stabilized in the hospital for several days prior to placement in the home. Twenty-four-hour nursing coverage is provided by psychiatric nurses using a paging system. On-call psychiatric coverage is also available 24 hours a day. At the time of admission the psychiatrist does a psychiatric and physical examination. The Southwest Denver CMHC has developed a specific procedure for rapid tranquilization using high-loading doses of phenothiazines (Polak et al., 1979), which they feel "facilitates early crisis intervention and direct social-system intervention."

Polak describes crisis intervention and social system intervention as a central part of treatment. "Family problems pertinent to both the symptoms of the client and the referral for treatment are focused on intensively both during the client's stay and following discharge from the home."

The overall success of this model has led to its replication in other parts of the United States and in other countries. The cost at the Denver program is $98 a day. Stroul (1987) found that the average cost in six similar programs was $90 per day. As in the La Posada program, client satisfaction was found to be high. The use of a home-family environment not only is effective clinically but has important meaning to the person's sense of worth and identity as a functional member in a family.

AN INPATIENT 72-HOUR CRISIS TREATMENT UNIT

Although crisis intervention in the treatment of schizophrenia is predominantly used in programs developed as alternatives to hospitalization, there is general agreement that some patients require hospital treatment. The first inpatient program to be based on crisis intervention principles was the Emergency Treatment Unit at the Connecticut Mental Health Center (Thomas & Weisman, 1970; Weisman et al., 1969). This small, richly staffed unit provided intensive intervention for 72 hours followed by a 30-day outpatient treatment commitment. Such inpatient crisis programs can treat those who cannot be managed in community alternatives.

The Emergency Treatment Unit (ETU) was located in a small five-bed ward adjacent to the lobby in the Connecticut Mental Health Center. The program was staffed by Yale University's Department of Psychiatry. The ETU treated 450 patients a year, 80% of whom were discharged to the outpatient component of the ETU, usually in conjunction with other extended therapy. The remaining 20% were transferred to longer-term inpatient treatment programs. The staff was divided into two multidisciplinary crisis teams and included nurses, psychiatric technicians, a social worker, a part-time psychiatrist, and a psychologist. Each day was highly structured with multiple therapeutic interventions. The treatment, designed to be intensive without being intrusive, was based on the concept that the openness of the patient's identity during crisis motivated the individual to seek new ways of understanding and responding to problems. The program's intensity was thus experienced as helpful, because it filled a void created by the failure of pathologic coping mechanisms. Each day included individual counseling sessions, groups, planning meetings, and family therapy when indicated. By the end of the 72 hours a strong bond developed between the treatment team and the patient. This bond played an important role at termination when the patient had to choose between continuing with the team as an outpatient or being transferred to another inpatient hospital for longer-term treatment. Many patients seemed to pull themselves together in order to be ready for outpatient care so as to avoid termination with the crisis team. This contrasts with the usual hospital situation in which discharge means termination and often leads to a temporary regression.

The treatment program was carefully structured to eliminate or minimize the institutional and impersonal elements of hospital treatment. The concern was that the diffusion of the individual's identity during the crisis led the hospitalized patient to readily acquire a "patient identity" as a functional replacement for a dysfunctional identity. To avoid this, each element in the ETU program was designed to maximize autonomy and functional responsibility rather than to enhance compliant patient behavior. Autonomy was facilitated by having patients participate in treatment planning and all decisions made about their stay. Patients participated in staff discussions of their cases, except around potentially disruptive issues such as emerging homosexual panic. The patient essentially became a part of the treatment team rather than being a passive recipient of its services.

The 72-hour time limit was also developed as a way to help avoid the formation of a patient identity. Focusing treatment on resolving problems in the external world that have disrupted adaptational functioning kept the patient oriented to the world outside the hospital. In hospital treatment considerable time is often spent helping the patient become part of the ward milieu before shifting the emphasis to issues of discharge and functioning in the community. In the ETU both adapting to the milieu and being involved in crisis resolution and discharge planning are less differentiated processes. Learning to be a good patient on the ETU meant learning to leave the hospital and function in the community.

On the ETU the use of phenothiazines was no different than in other inpatient programs in the area. Rapid tranquilization was used to control disorganized thinking and dysfunctional behavior. Each patient also was given a complete physical examination and routine laboratory work was performed.

Families were involved in the assessment of each case, and where indicated family therapy was initiated. For those patients who were returning home or leaving home, the family work was crucial to the efficacy of the treatment. Ongoing family therapy was also made available during the outpatient phase of the treatment.

Crisis inpatient treatment combines the essential features of hospital treatment and of crisis intervention, thus compensating for many of the limitations of each treatment modality. Despite the success of the ETU over a 4-year period, the model was not replicated until recently, when several similar programs began to emerge. The American Psychiatric Association's Gold Medal award for 1987 was given to a similar program, the Emergency Psychiatric Treatment Unit at the Baystate Medical Center in Springfield Massachusetts (Kaskey, 1987).

CRISIS DAY TREATMENT—PARTIAL HOSPITALIZATION

Although day treatment is usually used as a long-term treatment modality, it can be structured to provide intensive crisis intervention. The author has had several years' experience in a crisis day treatment program developed in the early 1970s at the Mission Mental Health Center in San Francisco. The program was designed with a time-limited stay of 3 weeks and the possibility of a one-time renewal of this contract.

Staff was divided into two multidisciplinary teams, each including a nurse, a social worker, a mental health worker or psychiatric technician, and a part-time psychiatrist. Six to eight patients were assigned to each team. Team members had a case load of two patients for whom they were the primary therapist. This position included functions of a crisis therapist as well as case management responsibilities. In addition to team members, staff included an occupational therapist, a recreational therapist, and a clerk/typist.

Each treatment day began with a 45-minute morning group meeting of the team and its patients. This meeting updated all concerned on how the past 24 hours had gone, and it functioned as a crisis-oriented group therapy. Issues discussed included family issues, survival issues, individual conflicts, medication, and community survival problems. Later in the day the staff of each team had a wrap-up meeting in which each patient was reviewed. These two meetings were a framework for much of the treatment for both patients and staff. The primary therapist also provided individual counseling several times a week or on a daily basis if needed. Both the individual and team meetings served as a forum for developing, implementing, and revising a treatment plan on a daily basis.

Other elements of the program were typical of active day treatment programs: OT, assertion groups, men's and women's groups, music, outings. Time was made available for the individual to go into the community to handle the necessary survival tasks, such as housing, finances, and family-related business, outpatient therapy sessions, and other normalizing activities. Families were evaluated and family therapy was provided where indicated.

One of the limitations of the program in terms of acute treatment was that it did not function on the weekends, evenings, or nights. A close working relationship with the emergency service at the mental health center was developed in order to provide for drop-in visits at those times. The emergency room staff would be notified to expect a patient and were briefed on the clinical status and issues at hand. Another way of providing such coverage would have been to have an on-call staff available. Similarly, adding a supervised residential component to the program could fill in these gaps. The lack of 24-hour availability made the day treatment program unable to handle the more severe cases. Nonetheless, many patients can be diverted from hospitalization to a crisis-oriented day treatment program, and a large number of patients can be discharged to such a program from the hospital after a few days of stabilization. Crisis-orientated day treatment can also be highly effective in preventing hospitalization by working with patients who are beginning to decompensate.

THE "CONTINUUM OF CRISIS SERVICES" MODEL

One of the major issues for crisis programs is that each has its limitations. For example, a crisis residential program may provide too much stimulation for patients who might do quite well if placed in a crisis foster home. Likewise, a paranoid patient who has difficulty living with more than one person might function best in an apartment with one-to-one attendant care. In 1985 the Kent County Mental Health Center in Warwick, Rhode Island, developed a program that uses a series of crisis programs in order to provide the diversity of services necessary to meet these needs (Doherty-Holmlund, Rehm, & Salhany, 1986; Kent County Mental Health Center, 1986). The program, called Acute Care Alternatives to Hospitalization (ACA), provides a continuum of crisis services for adults at risk for hospitalization. It was based on the models of the Southwest Denver Community Mental Health Center and the Dane County Mental Center in Madison, Wisconsin. The primary goal was to keep clients out of the hospital and at home whenever possible or, as an alternative, in the least restrictive environment. This was to be accomplished by aggressively intervening with patients at risk for hospitalization rather than by emptying the hospital. Hospital admissions and hospital days have decreased each year since the program was begun.

The efficacy of the Kent County program is based both on the structure of each of the program elements and on the integration of these elements into one comprehensive program. Central to the program is the use of a mobile crisis intervention team that provides service in a series of crisis facilities. The sites for these programs include the patient's home, a crisis apartment, crisis beds in an adult crisis foster home in the community, an emergency room, and a crisis-oriented hospital program. The crisis team is the intake portal for the patient and is prepared to provide comprehensive crisis services for 60 days. Once the crisis team has evaluated an individual and placed him or her in a program element, they then continue to work with the person at that site. If the patient improves or worsens and requires transfer to a different type of crisis program, the team continues to provide continuity of care for the patient throughout the crisis episode.

The Kent County Crisis Intervention Team is multidiciplinary and includes psychiatrists, nurses, social workers, specialists in drug abuse, and a unique type of paraprofessional referred to as a "special." The function of the special is to be a caring, monitoring, and observing person who is able to spend entire work shifts with an individual in crisis. The specials can be assigned a patient in any of the crisis programs on an around-the-clock basis if the level of care needs intensification. A special can be sent into a patient's home to help the family manage the patient during a period of serious disruption or can be sent to one of the crisis residential facilities run by ACA. In this way, not everyone in a specific program need receive the same level of care, and the intensity of the monitoring can be changed without shifting the patient to another treatment program. Psychiatric services are available to the team, as are "crisis medication monitoring services" by on-call nurses.

Three types of crisis residential programs are available within the system: home treatment, adult foster care homes (community crisis beds), and a community apartment (intensive community treatment apartment). Each of these programs depends on the crisis team to provide services for individuals placed there, although the apartment program has some of its own staff who work in conjunction with the crisis team.

The community crisis bed program recruits homeowners to take clients into their homes and integrate them into their families. The homeowners receive the same training as the specials. The crisis team provides treatment and is available at all times to come to the home to consult with the family or see the patient if problems arise.

The third residential crisis setting is the intensive community treatment apartment. This unit was modeled after the Training in Community Living program in Madison (Stein & Test, 1978a,b). The apartment provides 24-hoursupervision by specials and regular visits by other team members. Psychiatrists make rounds daily. The apartment accommodates up to four patients. This program element is for patients too disturbed to be maintained at home or in a community crisis bed. It is the most intensive component of the program short of hospitalization.

Through the three different residential crisis programs, workers can treat patients according to their specific clinical needs rather than trying to meet all needs within the scope of one program. Patients requiring separation from their families can be treated in the foster care home, while those requiring 24-hour supervision can be worked with in the apartment. The least intensive programs may be particularly useful for patients reentering the community subsequent to hospitalization.

For patients who need hospitalization despite the availability of these alternatives, the hospital also offers a crisis-oriented approach. The same psychiatrist who runs the hospital crisis inpatient program also works on the crisis teams and provides hospital treatment with a philosophy consistent with the other program elements. Consequently, the average hospital stay is 5 days. The psychiatrist, like other team members, is able to follow each case throughout its course, even if the individual shifts from one program element to another.

CONCLUSION

Crisis intervention, initially developed 40 years ago to treat disaster victims, has developed into a powerful therapeutic tool for the treatment of acute schizophrenia, one that can be used in diverse clinical settings including home, residential, day treatment, and inpatient programs.

Perhaps the major question raised by the development of intensive crisis intervention as a treatment modality for acute schizophrenia is: To what extent can it replace the use of more traditional forms of hospital treatment? The controlled studies of Langsley et al., (1968, Stein and Test(1978a,b), and Polak and Kirby (1976) compared clients judged to be in need of hospitalization who were then randomly assigned to the hospital or crisis residential treatment. The results of these studies showed that very few of those admitted to the residential programs required transfer to a hospital. In addition, the Kent County program demonstrates that, if crisis-oriented inpatient treatment is an additional option, the percent requiring longer-term hospital treatment is further reduced. In combination, these crisis-oriented modalities appear to be effective in treating over 90% of acute psychiatric problems.

However, the implications of crisis residential treatment as an alternative to hospitalization do not include the elimination of psychiatric hospitalization. Rather, the question is: Which patients are best handled in the hospital and which are best served in crisis residential treatment? In making this determination it is important to consider the severity of the regression, the need for restraint, involuntary status, and the need for concurrent intensive medical monitoring. The decision as to which modality to use is best based on a policy of using the least restrictive environment appropriate for the case.

One of the major advantages of crisis programs is their cost-effectiveness. Stroul (1987) found that the average daily cost in an acute crisis home was $90, and the average cost of 20 group crisis residential programs was $135 a day. Comparing these figures with the average cost for acute psychiatric hospitalization ($400 a day) reveals a 77% saving for crisis homes and a 66% saving for group crisis residential programs. Although local governments are anxious to cut the cost of mental health services, there is a perplexing lag in the development of crisis residential services. This may be, in part, because acute residential treatment is not covered by health insurance. Consequently, it costs the patient less to be treated in more expensive hospitals where insurance covers 80% to 100% of costs. However, as more research and clinical trials in various cities occur, local governments are likely to give strong consideration to such programs. Recent legislation in California facilitates the establishment of crisis residential treatment programs. This has played a part in the development of 15 programs in the state based on the La Posada model. The 1986 NIMH Community Support Program Conference on crisis residential services marked the beginning of direct NIMH involvement in crisis residential treatment. NIMH plans to disseminate information about these programs on a national level. The fact that NIMH designates such programs as a major component of relevant mental health services is certain to bring this model to the attention of local communities seeking improved and more cost-effective approaches to treating schizophrenia.

Another barrier to the expanded use of intensive crisis intervention is the lack of attention paid within psychiatry to using teams as a therapeutic tool. The psychiatrist's role in a treatment team is essential, but, as yet, there is little opportunity in medical training or psychiatric practice for psychiatrists to become familiar with this role. It is often difficult for psychiatrists to learn to empower other team members rather than taking on the central role in decision-making themselves.

One of the major advantages of crisis residential treatment over hospitalization is the opportunity such programs offer to personalize treatment and avoid institutionalization. Although the depersonalizing effect of institutions is a familiar concept in psychiatry, the importance of personalizing treatment in dealing with schizophrenia has received relatively little attention in the literature or in the design of treatment programs. It is not sufficient to teach the program staff how to be humanistic if the program design and setting contradict these efforts. It is important to remember that institutions institutionalize staff as well as patients. Some of the factors that allow crisis programs to reduce such institutionalization include their small size (usually less then 10 clients), minimizing the use of the medical model, and maximizing the use of paraprofessionals. These factors, combined with the family and homelike aspects of these programs, engender a sense of intimacy and personal respect rarely available in institutional and hospital programs.

The rapid development of crisis intervention into an intensive treatment modality capable of effectively treating acute schizophrenia presents an exciting opportunity in the delivery of mental health services. The use of a continuum of crisis services provides a comprehensive model effective even in large metropolitan areas. Given the adaptability of crisis intervention to existing treatment modalities, it is likely that the development of new combined models will continue. This will add to a growing list of intensive crisis intervention programs for the treatment of schizophrenia and other acute psychiatric disorders.

REFERENCES

Almond, R. (1974). *The healing community.* New York: Aronson.

Baldwin, B. A. (1977). *Phases of emotional crisis.* Unpublished training materials.

Bengelsdorf, H., & Alden, D. C. (1987). A mobile crisis unit in the psychiatric emergency room. *Hospital and Community Psychiatry, 38,* 662–665.

Burgess, A. W., & Baldwin, B. A. (1981). *Crisis intervention theory and practice.* Englewood Cliffs, NJ: Prentice-Hall.

Caplan, G. K. (1964). *Principles of preventive psychiatry.* New York: Basic Books.

Doherty-Holmlund, K., Rehm, D., & Salhany, J. (1986). *Acute alternatives to hospitalization.* Paper presented at the Riviera Hotel, Las Vegas, Nevada.

Foxman, J. (1976). The mobile psychiatric emergency team. In H. Parad, H. L. P. Resnik, & L. Parad (Eds.), *Emergency and disaster management* (pp. 35–44). Bowie, MD: Charter Press.

Goffman, E. (1961). *Asylums.* New York: Anchor.

Gruenberg, E. M. (1969). From practice to theory: Community mental health services and the nature of psychoses. *Lancet, 1,* 721–724.

Jansen, E. (1980). The halfway house in the United Kingdom and America. In E. Jansen (Ed.), *The therapeutic community* (pp. 377–386). London: Croom Helm.

Kaskey, G. (1987). Brief psychiatric inpatient care for acutely disturbed patients. *Hospital and Community Psychiatry, 38,* 1203–1206.

Kent County Mental Health Center. (1986). *Description of adult and children's comprehensive emergency services program (ACESS).* Warwick, RI: Author.

Lamb, R. H. (Ed.). (1979). *Alternatives to acute hospitalization.* San Francisco: Jossey-Bass.

Langsley, D. G., Pittman, F. S., Machotka, P., & Flomenhaft, K. (1968). Family crisis therapy—Results and implications. *Family Process, 7,* 145–158.

Langsley, D. G., & Yarvis, R. M. (1976). Crisis intervention prevents hospitalization—Pilot program to service project. In H. Parad, H. L. P. Resnik, & L. Parad (Eds.), *Emergency and disaster management* (pp. 25–34). Bowie, MD: Charter Press.

Lieb, J., Lipsitch, I. I., & Slaby, A. E. (1973). *The crisis team.* San Francisco: Harper & Row.

Lindemann, E. (1944). Symptomatology and management of acute grief. *American Journal of Psychiatry, 101,* 141–148.

Pasamanick, B., Scarpitti, F., & Dinitz, S. (1967). *Schizophrenics in the community: An experimental study in the prevention of hospitalization.* New York: Appleton-Century-Crofts.

Polak, P. R. (1978). A comprehensive system of alternatives to psychiatric hospitalization. In L. I. Stein & M. A. Test (Eds.), *Alternatives to mental hospital treatment* (pp. 115–138). New York: Plenum Press.

Polak, P. R., & Kirby, M. W. (1976). A model to replace psychiatric hospitals. *Journal of Nervous and Mental Disease, 162,* 13–22.

Polak, P. R., Kirby, M. W., & Deitchman, W. S. (1979). Treating acutely psychotic patients in private homes. In H. R. Lamb (Ed.), *New directions fof mental health services: Alternatives to acute hospitalization* (Vol. 1, pp. 49–64). San Francisco: Jossey-Bass.

Rosenhan, D. L. (1973). On being sane in insane places. *Science, 179,* 250–258.

Stein, L. I., & Test, M. A. (1978a). An alternative to mental hospital treatment. In L. I. Stein & M. A. Test (Eds.), *Alternatives to mental hospital treatment* (pp. 43–56). New York: Plenum Press.

Stein, L. I., & Test, M. A. (Eds.). (1978b). *Alternatives to mental hospital treatment.* New York: Plenum Press.

Stroul, B. A. (1987). *Crisis residential services in a community support system.* Rockville, MD: NIMH Community Support Program.

Thomas, C. S., & Weisman, G. K. (1970). Emergency planning: The practical and theoretical backdrop to an emergency treatment unit. *International Journal of Social Psychiatry, 16,* 283–287.

Weisman, G. K. (1985a). Crisis houses and lodges: Residential treatment of acutely disturbed chronic patients. *Psychiatric Annals, 15,* 642–647.

Weisman, G. K. (1985b). Crisis-oriented residential treatment as an alternative to hospitalization. *Hospital and Community Psychiatry, 36,* 1302–1304.

Weisman, G. K., Feirstein, A., & Thomas, C. (1969). Three-day hospitalization—A model for intensive intervention. *Archives of General Psychiatry, 21,* 620–629.

Wilder, J. F. (1966). A two-year follow-up evaluation of acute psychiatric patients treated in a day hospital. *American Journal of Psychiatry, 122,* 1095–1101.

6

Community Residential Treatment
Alternatives to Hospitalization

LOREN R. MOSHER

INTRODUCTION AND BACKGROUND

In a properly designed and functioning community mental health system, community residential treatment facilities should serve the vast majority of disturbed and disturbing individuals in need of intensive interpersonal care who cannot be adequately treated by in-home crisis intervention. Use of these small, homelike facilities in conjunction with 24-hour mobile crisis intervention will dramatically reduce the need for psychiatric beds in hospitals (Hoult, 1986; Langsley, Pittman, & Swank, 1969; Mosher, 1982; Stein & Test, 1985). That is, a 100,000 population catchment area will need, at most, a 10-bed adult ward in a general hospital. This estimate presumes the existence of separate facilities for children and adolescents, the addictions, and geriatric cases. We also presume there will be no backup state hospital beds. This estimate also presumes that the system will have affordable transitional (halfway, quarterway houses) and nontransitional (e.g., group homes, Fairweather lodges, foster care, apartments) supported (supervised) and unsupported housing readily available for its clientele's use after the intensive care phase. Without adequate numbers of these facilities users will get "stuck" at home, in hospital, in alternatives to hospitalization, or in shelters. This

---

LOREN R. MOSHER • Associate Director, Addiction, Victim and Mental Health Services for Montgomery County, 401 Hungerford Drive #500, Rockville, Maryland 20850.

is both clinically unwise and unnecessarily expensive (Mosher & Burti, 1988).

In contrast to hospital-based interventions where various treatments are administered to patients on wards, residential alternative facilities are themselves the treatment. That is, the total social environment (place and persons) is the healing intervention. In more traditional language, these environments are conceived of as "therapeutic communities" or "treatment milieus."

Research (Braun et al., 1981; Kiesler, 1982a,b; Straw, 1982; Stroul, 1987) and clinical experience has shown that approximately 90% of functional psychotics currently treated in hospitals can be equally well or better treated, at less cost, in intensive residential community care. Only patients who are seriously assaultive, are uncontrollably overactive, have complicating medical problems, or need special monitoring or diagnostic procedures should be treated in places called hospitals.

Seriously disturbed and disturbing persons can be arbitrarily separated into two groups: those who have been recently identified and not received much residential care (less than 3 months or so), and those who have been more or less continuously in the mental health system for a long time, usually more than 2 years, and have had more than 3 months of residential care (usually a year or more).

It is for the first group that community-based residential care is especially important. First, because these alternative facilities are minimally institutionalizing and maximally normalizing, they provide a means of preventing "institutionalism," a well-known iatrogenic disease (Barton, 1959; Wing & Brown, 1970) that contributes so much to what becomes labeled "chronicity." Second, because of their being relatively inexpensive (averaging about $100 a day), they provide a setting in which an adequate trial of a psychosocial treatment, without the use of neuroleptics, can be conducted. Being inexpensive is important to a trial of treatment without antipsychotic drugs because the initial episode in residence will likely be longer than is generally allowed at present in hospitals for the treatment of acute psychoses. That is, given the current pressure to shorten lengths of stay for economic (not clinical) reasons, use of neuroleptics becomes almost obligatory. In alternative settings, a 3-month average initial length of stay (usually adequate to allow remission to occur) is not economically prohibitive. Thus, these environments allow an attempt to avoid two of today's most recalcitrant mental health problems: "chronicity" and tardive dyskinesia.

The design, implementation, and results of the use of residential alternative care without antipsychotic medication with newly diagnosed psychotic patients has been well researched in random assignment studies (Matthews, Roper, Mosher, & Menn, 1979; Mosher & Menn, 1978; Mosher,

Menn, & Matthews, 1975). Interestingly, there is no random assignment study currently available to definitively support the usefulness of these types of facilities for "veteran" (our term to replace the onerous "chronic") clients. However, there are a number of clinical studies (Kresky-Wolff, Matthews, Kalibat, & Mosher, 1984; Lamb & Lamb, 1984; Weisman, 1985a,b) that consistently demonstrate that these types of social environments can be successfully adapted for use with longer-term clients.

DEFINING THE SOCIAL ENVIRONMENTS

Gunderson (1978, modified by Mosher) has defined the seven essential functions of treatment milieus (Table 1). These functions are served to varying degrees in all of our living and working environments. However, an intentional social environment whose focus is recovery from psychosis provides them consciously, explicitly, and with ongoing attention to their maintainence and adequacy.

The variables are basically self-explanatory, with the possible exception of validation. By validation we mean that staff are instructed to let clients know that what they are experiencing is quite real, even though it cannot sometimes be consensually validated. For example, hallucinations can be discussed for what they are, what they mean, and how they make the person feel, but they should not be labeled as "not real" (because they are) and "part of their illness." Relating to hallucinations as "not real" only serves to reify the fragmentation the client is already likely to be experiencing.

The literature also provides differing descriptions of how milieus should operate in dealing with newly identified acutely disordered persons (Table 2) and with long-term "veterans" (Table 3) of the system. These descriptions provide more specific approaches that are to be carried out within the overall generic milieu functions listed in Table 1. Although different in some respects, the two types of effective milieus have a number of overlapping

Table 1. Milieu Functions[a]

---

1. Support
2. Protection
3. Containment
4. Structure
5. Socialization
6. Validation
7. Respite (asylum)

---

[a]Modified from Gunderson (1978).

Table 2. Effective Milieus,
Acute Psychosis[a]

1. Small (6–10 patients)
2. High staff-to-patient ratio
3. High interaction
4. Real involvement of line staff and
   patients in decisions
5. Emphasis on autonomy
6. Focus on practical problems (e.g.,
   living arrangements, money)
7. Positive expectations
8. Minimal hierarchy

[a]Mosher and Gunderson (1979).

characteristics. In addition, the two types of milieus differ to some extent with regard to what should be done when. That is, time needs to be allowed for the gross disorganization associated with acute psychosis to begin to recede before focusing on practical problems or decision-making processes. With system veterans, this initial reorganization period may be either unnecessary or short, and practical problems may be focused on almost immediately. For long-term clients, we have found that often the presenting "acute" symptoms are really only a way of accessing help. Once help is assured by their being admitted to residential care, these symptoms often recede quickly to the background. If both acute and veteran clients are admitted to the same facility, staff will have to develop the skill necessary to distinguish between their differing needs. Of course, a number of clients will fall in a gray area between the two. Unfortunately, there are no research data and only limited clinical experience to address the issue of whether or not these two populations do better when mixed together or maintained in separate, more homogenous groups. The issue will likely be decided on

Table 3. Effective Milieus, Hospitalization Veterans ("Chronic")[a]

1. Clearly defined, specific behaviors requiring change
2. Action- (not explanation-) oriented, structured program
3. Reasonable, positive, *progressive*, practical expectations with increasing
   client responsibility
4. Continuation of residential treatment program into *in vivo* community
   settings
5. Continuity of persons
6. Extensive use of groups to facilitate socialization and network building

[a]Paul (1969), Paul and Lentz (1977).

practical grounds—that is, are there enough newly identified clients deemed in need of hospitalization to keep 10 alternative beds (6 in a surrogate peer facility and 4 in homes of surrogate parents) full in a catchment area of 100,000?

A calculation for the United States is almost impossible because of our two-track (public/private) mental health system and the lack of mobile crisis intervention. However, in Italy, with its universal national health insurance coverage and in-home crisis intervention, roughly 10 to 15 hospital beds per 100,000 population are used (Mosher, 1982). Assuming that 10 of these beds could be replaced by community residential alternatives and that they will have somewhat longer lengths of stay, it would seem that one 6- to 8-bed alternative facility per catchment area serving a mixture of clients would be the most practical arrangement. The 4 additional surrogate parent beds should probably be used mainly for clients coming from parental homes. Whatever configuration is decided upon, newly identified clients should be given first priority for use of these facilities.

IMPLEMENTATION ISSUES

Given the substantial body of research that consistently favors alternative over hospital care, it can be legitimately asked why such care is not widely available. Some of the reasons for this were detailed by Mosher (1983):

> First and foremost, because all alternative care is by definition not given in a hospital it is classified by third-party payers as outpatient treatment. There are limitations on, and disincentives to, outpatient psychiatric care in nearly all health-insurance plans (including Medicare and Medicaid). For example, the federal employees' Blue Cross/Blue Shield high-option plan currently covers nearly all the costs of 60 days of psychiatric hospitalization but limits outpatient visits to 50 per year, with a 30 percent copayment. However, the 50-visit limit includes all physician–outpatient contacts. Thus, even in a "generous" plan, the actual number of psychiatric visits per year that are paid for by the insurance will be fewer than the maximum allowable. For its part, Medicare treats care in psychiatric wards of general hospitals like other types of inpatient care but has a $250 maximal annual reimbursement for psychiatric outpatient care. Payment is based on a formula requiring that $500 worth of care be delivered for the patient to receive the maximal reimbursement. The disincentives to outpatient care in these two large reimbursement schemes are representative examples of third-party-payment plans. Alternative care is usually intensive and may involve a residential (but nonhospital) component; outpatient coverage is rarely sufficient to cover professional fees and never covers residential care, because outpatient means nonresidential by definition. Hence, psychiatric treatment that is offered instead of hospitalization is a true Catch-22 with respect to health-insurance plans.

Secondly, since early in our history American physicians, patients, and the public at large have come to expect that serious mental disorders will be dealt with in hospitals. After a century and a half or more, culturally sanctioned expectations are a powerful force and are not easily modified. An attitude of "out of sight, out of mind" is pervasive. Hence, alternatives to psychiatric hospitalization tend to be unacceptable because they run contrary to conventional wisdom.

Thirdly, today's psychiatry prides itself on being scientific. The *Diagnostic and Statistical Manual* is the obsessional person's dream and the medical student's nightmare. Psychiatry's research on brain pathophysiology uses the latest biomedical technology. Its clinical research, especially into drug efficacy, uses highly sophisticated methods. Over the past several decades psychiatry has experienced a rapprochement with the rest of medicine, partly because of its scientific achievements. The growth of psychiatric wards in general hospitals has been part of this process. To ask psychiatry to move many of its therapeutic endeavors out of hospitals would be regarded as a disruption of its new relation with the rest of medicine. Hence, data about the effectiveness of alternatives are not greeted with great enthusiasm by the profession.

In addition to the three reasons described above, alternatives to hospitalization have failed to be developed because of a combined training and critical mass problem. That is, those that exist are mainly in the public/community mental health system. The present-day image of community mental health is not a very positive one. It is fashionable to criticize it for having been irresponsible with the deinstitutionalization process and for not having given priority to serving the most disturbed and disturbing persons. This system traditionally pays less well and has more bureaucratic barriers to good care as compared with the private system. It serves the disenfranchised: minorities, the poor, the homeless, and the truly weird. It is, in sum, not very attractive. Training in social work, psychology, and psychiatry tends to be focused on preparing students to be private practitioners. Community mental health and, with it, alternatives to hospitalization have a double whammy—its clientele tends to be unattractive and few potential staff have training relevant to working with them.

This training issue is compounded in the case of residential alternatives to a hospital; there are so few of them that it is impossible to provide training sites for more than a handful of students (the critical mass problem). With rare exception, line staff in residential alternative programs have had no previous experience in a similar setting. Hence, they are all basically trained on the job. On-the-job training can be excellent if experienced supervision is available. Here again, because there are so few of these facilities, there are not substantial numbers of experienced professionals available to organize, administer, and supervise these programs—another aspect of the critical mass problem.

This problem could be addressed if professional schools recognized the existence of the phenomenon of alternatives and began to include them in curricula. Over time a cadre of trained persons would be developed to provide the leadership and expertise necessary to implement these programs. We have described elsewhere a model for such community-based training (Burti & Mosher, 1986). Until this image and training issue is addressed it will be difficult to plan, develop, and implement the types of intensive residential community-based care described in this chapter.

CLINICAL MODELS

There are two basic models available for intensive community residential treatment: the Surrogate Parent model developed in Southwest Denver (Polak & Kirby, 1976; Polak, Kirby, & Dietchman, 1979) and the Soteria/Crossing Place Surrogate Peer model developed by Mosher and co-workers (Mosher & Menn, 1977, 1979, 1983; Wendt, Mosher, Matthews, & Menn, 1983). The Polak and Kirby model has not been formally researched in a random assignment study. The Soteria portion of the Soteria/Crossing Place model has been intensively and extensively studied in a random-assignment 2-year follow-up design. Crossing Place has published a clinical (i.e., nonrandom, no controls) short-term outcome study of its first 150 clients (Kresky-Wolff et al., 1984).

THE SURROGATE PARENT MODEL

The Southwest Denver model was developed in conjunction with the program's use of mobile in-home interventions as their major form of emergency service. They found, logically enough, that a certain percentage of in-home crisis interventions were not successful enough so that they felt safe to leave all the parties at home. The program's leadership (principally Paul Polak) was moderately hospital-phobic, so they devised their surrogate parent program to be used in those instances where someone needed to be temporarily taken out of the home.

The program's design capitalizes on the empty-nest syndrome. By means of ads in local papers and word of mouth the CMHC recruited families whose children had grown up and left home. In this mostly suburban part of Denver many couples had substantial homes with two or more empty bedrooms. Couples who responded to the ad were interviewed by CMHC staff and, if accepted, provided with a modest amount of information about, and training for dealing with, disturbed and disturbing persons. There were no hard-and-fast selection criteria, but they preferred to use couples with a previous record of some type of community service whose children were leading reasonably successful lives (i.e., not in jails or the mental health system). Each couple was asked to set aside one or two bedrooms for use by CMHC clients. The rooms were paid for whether or not they were occupied.

The program's success (as it is judged by the CMHC and the families) was due to a variety of factors. First, the CMHC's mobile community team promised a 15-minute response time to any crisis that evolved in the surrogate parent homes. Early in the program's life this availability was tested several times. As the parent couples became more comfortable with their roles, the need to call the backup team became quite rare.

Second, all acutely psychotic patients admitted to one of the homes were treated vigorously with neuroleptics, often via intramuscular "rapid neurolepticization." Hence, the program attempted to minimize the occurrence of disruptive behavior through chemical restraint. Whether this type of high-dose neuroleptic treatment was still necessary when the parents became more experienced was never really tested.

Third, the parent couples who stayed with the program were natural healers. They approached their temporary children with a great deal of support and reassurance and gentle firmness. As they got to know their charges, the parents began to involve themselves in helping them with problem solving. They gradually integrated the clients into the family's ongoing life. Although there were no length-of-stay rules, most clients stayed 2 to 3 weeks and would leave gradually. Even after they were no longer sleeping there, ex-clients would be invited to visit, to dinner, or to a family event.

Fourth, the parent couples were highly respected by the CMHC staff. They were seen as an integral part of the program. They were identified and highlighted as the persons responsible for the CMHC's ability to use only one bed (average) in the nearby state hospital, a statistic many people found astounding given a 75,000-person catchment area. Parent couples were sent to professional meetings to speak. They were visited by professionals, officials, and dignitaries of various types. All in all, they felt themselves to be important contributors to a groundbreaking, innovative program. The parents became advocates for better community-based care.

Fifth, it provided the couples with a new career to be pursued during their retirement years. In addition, the predictable income from the program allowed many of them to keep and maintain family homes that might otherwise have had to be sold.

In a sense the program provided preventive mental health care to the parent couples by refilling the empty nest. To us, the Polak-Kirby model is ideal for use in areas with low population density: i.e., semirural to rural areas. It is very economical even if the beds are not filled. Current replications provide stipends to the couples of $800 to $900 per month per bed.

With this model excellent care can be provided in the client's own, or a very nearby, community, thus minimizing disruption of ties with the natural support system. There are many rural areas where the nearest psychiatric inpatient care is 100 or more miles away; in this context hospitalization is extremely disruptive for patient, family, and network.

Although they are particularly well suited to rural settings, we also believe that good urban and suburban community programs should have two or more (i.e., four beds) of these settings available per 100,000 population. Clinically they would seem to be best suited to the treatment of unemancipated psychotic persons: i.e., in the 16- to 22-year-old age range with whom in-home family intervention has not been successful. The opportunity to live in an alternate family environment is one that affords many opportunities for these young people to experience, relate to, and learn from less highly emotionally charged parent figures. Properly done, these settings can also provide the client's parents with an opportunity to share their difficulties with another set of parents, get support and understanding, and perhaps learn new ways of coping with their offspring from surrogate parent examples.

Utilizing empty-nest parents allows the community program to actually address a problem with many seniors who are feeling put out to pasture too soon and unnecessarily. These parents constitute a much underutilized natural resource—the experience, knowledge, and wisdom that accrues to people as they get older. Successful child-rearing capabilities should be a highly prized commodity. Yet these qualities are rarely explicitly acknowledged and used for the benefit of others. This is an excellent illustration of a principle of good community psychiatry—using already available community resources for the program. These include school and recreational programs, libraries, gyms, and personal skills.

SURROGATE PEER MODEL

Background. The model developed by Mosher and co-workers has its roots in the era of moral treatment in psychiatry (Bockoven, 1963), in the psychoanalytic tradition of intensive interpersonal treatment (especially Sullivan, 1931; Fromm-Reichmann, 1948), therapists who have described growth from psychosis (Perry, 1962), research on community-based treatment for schizophrenia (Fairweather, Sanders, Cressler, & Maynard, 1969; Pasamanick, Scarpitti, & Dinitz, 1967), and to some extent in the so-called antipsychiatry movement (Laing, 1967). The Soteria project opened its first house in the fall of 1971. A replication house, Emanon, opened in another northern California town in 1974. The original house closed because of lack of funding in October of 1983. The replication had closed on January 1, 1980, for the same reason.

The basic notion behind the project was that the first treated psychotic episode was a critical intervention point. That is, the project's developers believed that the way that the first episode of psychosis is dealt with would likely have great impact on long-term outcome. The project selected young, unmarried, newly diagnosed DSM-II schizophrenics because, statistically, the literature clearly indicated that they are the most likely to become disabled (Klorman, Strauss, & Kokes, 1977; Phillips, 1966; Rosen, Klein, & Gittelman-Klein, 1971). Hence, the project took clients with whom a successful intervention might save society a great deal of money over the long run in terms of hospital days, medications, and welfare costs.

An additional reason the project took only newly identified patients was to avoid having to deal with the learned mental patient role that experienced patients have often acquired. Neuroleptics were not given for an initial 6-week period so that a fair trial of a pure psychosocial intervention could take place. In addition, no, or minimal, neuroleptic treatment is the only sure way to prevent tardive dyskinesia.

Although the program's individual elements were not new, bringing them under a single roof in a 1915-vintage six-bedroom house on a busy street in a suburban northern California town was. The program was designed to offer an altenative not only to the hospital but also to neuroleptic drugs and professional staffing of intensive residential care. The program's psychiatrist, for example, was a consultant who did initial client interviews and staff training but had no ongoing contact with the clients. As the program matured the psychiatrists came to be seen, and saw themselves, as mostly peripheral.

Given the three areas in which the Soteria project was designed to provide an alternative (i.e., hospitals, neuroleptics, and professionals), it is not surprising that over its 13-year life-span the project was regarded by the field with ambivalence at best and suspicion and hostility at worst. Its research grant applications set NIMH records for numbers of site visits, reviews, and opinions sought. It was, and to some extent still is, viewed as a threat to psychiatry's current biomedical *zeitgeist*. Nevertheless, as a demonstration, Soteria and its successor, Crossing Place, have provided the field with successful alternative clinical models. At the present time the only Soteria replication (i.e., with newly identified psychotics) under way is in Berne, Switzerland, under the direction of Professor Luc Ciompi. There are a number of Crossing Place-like facilities (i.e., ones that deal with the whole spectrum of clientele). An accurate count is difficult because of definitional and identification problems, but there are certainly 20 or more, almost all in the public sector.

Program Elements. The 11 most important elements of the surrogate peer model we have identified are listed in Table 4. They are, for the most part, self-explanatory. However, a comment on the size issue appears warranted. We believe, in light of our extensive experience, the Soteria data, and the literature on extended families, communes, experimental psychology task groups, group therapy, and the Tavistock model, that for a community to be able to maximize its healing potential no more than 8 to 10 persons should sleep under the same roof. Larger groups require more space than most ordinary houses provide, and the interaction patterns and organizational goverance needed are very different. Hence, economy of scale (i.e., 12- to 15-bed facilities in this situation) is *false* economy. Ideally, 6 clients, 2 staff, and 1 or 2 others (e.g., students, volunteers) should sleep in the facility at any one time. Eight clients can be accommodated, but this begins to tax the limits of the size of the social group and begins to stretch staff availability if half or more of the clients are in acute distress. Actually, we believe that a 50-50 mix of disturbed and disturbing persons with nondisturbed persons is about ideal for the functioning of the house as a therapeutic community. In this equation 6 clients, 2 or 3 of whom have been in residence long enough to have reorganized sufficiently to appear undisturbed, and 2 or 3 quasi-normal staff (including students) make for an optimal mix.

There are a number of residential alternatives in existence that have 15 or so client beds (Lamb & Lamb, 1984; Weisman, 1985b). We believe that the homelike atmosphere is so absolutely crucial to the therapeutic functioning of community-based alternatives that we would not include such programs as being examples of the Soteria/Crossing Place model. It is likely that when the NIMH or state departments of mental health get involved in the development of these facilities they will like the cost saving possible in these

Table 4. Soteria and Crossing Place:
Essential Characteristics

1. Small (6 clients), homelike
2. Nonprofessional staff
3. Peer/fraternal relationship orientation
4. Preservation of personal power valued
5. Open social system (easy access and departure)
6. Participants responsible for house maintenance
7. Minimal role differentiation
8. Minimal hierarchy
9. Use of community resources encouraged
10. Postdischarge contacts allowed/encouraged
11. No formal in-house "therapy"

larger units. However, it seems clear from Rappaport's research (Rappaport et al., 1986) that they sacrifice clinical effectiveness when they grow to the size of small hospital units, especially if they are located on hospital grounds. Their noninstitutional character is compromised, and with it, the treatment milieu is changed. To reiterate: To be family-like, the critical and unique characteristic, these facilities should have no more than six, or at most eight, client beds and must be real *community* homes.

We would also like to comment on what we mean by minimal role differentiation, since this is sometimes misunderstood and responded to by comments like "What these clients need are examples of clear roles and boundaries." What we mean is that, for the most part, each line staff member will be able to do anything needed by a particular client. For example, the same staff member may accompany a client to apply for an apartment, on the way home go with the client to the welfare office to see about SSI benefits, and meet with the client's family that evening. Only the program director and psychiatric consultants have different, and differentiated, roles.

A comment is also in order about the absence of formal in-house therapy. As noted elsewhere, we view the entire facility "package" as providing the therapeutic social environment. Hence, everything that goes on in and out of it can be viewed as potentially therapeutic. However, there are no time-limited in-office therapy sessions—individual, group, or family—*in the facility*. We believe that because of this policy client fragmentation and community suspicion about what's going on behind closed doors is prevented and a treatment value hierarchy cannot become established. That is, for the environment to be the treatment, the "real" treatment cannot be a one-to-one hour in the office with a therapist. Individual clients may be referred out, as indicated, to receive these types of therapy away from the setting itself.

Specific therapies can be made available in the house to persons living there so long as these therapies are brought in with the approval of a majority of the participants and are made available to everyone who wishes to become involved. Hence, art therapy, bibliotherapy, yoga, massage, acupuncture, and special diets have come and gone in the various settings depending on the group's wishes and their availability.

There are a number of group meetings held at the houses. Some, like the house meeting, occur on a regularly scheduled basis. Others, like family meetings, usually occur soon after the client is admitted and irregularly thereafter. Morning "what are you doing today" and evening "how was your day" meetings occur regularly but are not formalized. The Crossing Place brochure describes well the social environment that should characterize this type of intensive residential community care:

The basic therapeutic modality is one to one, intensive interpersonal support. Specially selected and trained staff members are with the client for as long as intensive care and supervision are required. The non-professional staff members all have experience in crisis-care.

The program's home-like environment is also an important therapeutic element: it minimizes the stress of going into residential care and re-entry into the community because it resembles the client's ordinary environment. Individuals focus on coping with their life-crisis in a real-life setting. In addition, the environment minimizes the potential for severe acting-out by being small, intimate, and rapidly responsive. This setting tends to elicit the best from clients by regarding them as responsible members of a temporary family.

The staff members work closely with the director and psychiatrists to help individual clients formulate goals and plans. The entire staff meets regularly to discuss problems encountered in the helping process. The program director and psychiatrists are available to give individual attention to clients with particularly difficult situations.

The length of stay varies from a few days to several months, depending on individual needs. Discharge is effected when the crisis has subsided and adequate plans have been worked out for important aspects of post-discharge living and treatment.

CLINICAL COMPARISON OF SOTERIA AND CROSSING PLACE MODELS

Soteria House was a carefully designed research project that limited its intake to young, newly diagnosed schizophrenic patients. Crossing Place takes adult clients of all ages, diagnoses, and lengths of illness. Soteria House existed mostly outside the public treatment system in its city. Its clients came from only one entry point and were carefully screened to be sure they met the research criteria before being randomly assigned to Soteria House or to the hospital-treated control group. Because of its restrictive admission criteria—about 3 or 4 of 100 functional psychotic patients admitted per month met research criteria—Soteria House was not seen as a real treatment resource within that system. Crossing Place is firmly embedded in the Washington, DC public mental health system. It was founded by Woodley House, a long-established private nonprofit agency whose programs include a 25-bed halfway house, a 50-bed supervised apartment program, and a thrift shop with a work adjustment program. Because of contractual arrangements with St. Elizabeth's Hospital and the District of Columbia Mental Health Department, Crossing Place accepts referrals from a variety of entry points. Its clients are system veterans whose care is paid for by one of these contracts. Although it officially excludes only persons who have medical problems or whose primary problem is substance abuse, it has little control over the actual referral criteria used by a variety of clinicians. Thus, in contrast to Soteria House, Crossing Place clientele are a less well-defined, more heterogeneous group. They *may* be less ill, violent, or suicidal (unfortunately it's not possible to know for sure) than those sent to St. Elizabeth's Hospital, the main residential treatment setting for public patients in Washington, DC. Crossing Place clients are older (32 versus 21), come more frequently from minority groups, and have extensive hospitalization experience (4.5 versus no admissions) as compared with Soteria subjects. Thus, although the characteristics of the Crossing Place client population are not as precisely known as those of the Soteria patients, the former group can be characterized as "veterans" ("chronic") and the latter as newly identified ("acute").

In their presentations to the world, Crossing Place is conventional and Soteria is unconventional. Despite this major difference, the actual in-house interpersonal interactions are similar in their informality, earthiness, honesty, and lack of professional jargon. These similarities arise partially from the fact that neither program ascribes the usual patient role to the clientele. Both programs use male/female staff pairs who work 24- or 48-hour shifts.

Soteria's research funding views length of stay as a dependent research variable. This allows it to vary according to the clinical needs of the newly diagnosed patients. The initial lengths of stay averaged just over 5 months. Crossing Place's contract contains length-of-stay standards (1 to 2 months). Hence, the initial focus of the Crossing Place staff must be: What do the clients need to accomplish so they can resume living in the community as quickly as possible? This focus on personal responsibility is a technique that Woodley House had used successfully for many years. At Soteria, such questions were not ordinarily raised until the acutely psychotic state had subsided—usually 4 to 6 weeks after entry. This span exceeds the average length of stay at Crossing Place (32 days). In part, the shorter average length of stay at Crossing Place is made possible by the almost routine use of neuroleptics to control the most flagrant symptoms of its clientele. At Soteria, neuroleptics were never used during the first 6 weeks of a patient's stay and were rarely given thereafter. Time constraints also dictate that Crossing Place will have a more formalized social structure than Soteria.

The two Crossing Place consulting psychiatrists evaluate each client on admission, and each spends an hour a week with the staff reviewing each client's progress, addressing particularly difficult issues, and helping develop a consensus on initial and revised treatment plans. Soteria had a variety of meetings but averaged one client-staff meeting per week. The role of consulting psychiatrists was more peripheral at Soteria than at Crossing Place. They were not ordinarily involved in treatment planning and no regular treatment meeting was held.

In summary, compared with Soteria, Crossing Place is more organized, structured, and oriented toward practical goals. Expectations of Crossing

Place staff members tend to be positive, but more limited than those of Soteria staff members. At Crossing Place, psychosis is frequently not directly addressed by staff members, while at Soteria, the client's experience of acute psychosis was an important subject of interpersonal communication. At Crossing Place, the use of neuroleptics limits psychotic episodes. The immediate social problems of Crossing Place clients (secondary to being system veterans and also because of having come from lower social class minority families) must be addressed quickly: no money, no place to live, no one with whom to talk. Basic survival is often the issue. Among the Soteria clients, because they came from less economically disadvantaged families, these problems were present but much less pressing. Basic survival was usually not an issue.

Crossing Place staff members spend a lot of time keeping other parts of the mental health community involved in the process of addressing client needs. The clients are known to many other players in the system. Just contacting everyone with a role in the life of any given client can be an all-day process. In contrast, Soteria clients, being new to the system, had no such cadre of involved mental health workers. While in residence, Crossing Place clients continue their involvement with other programs. At Soteria, only the project director and house director dealt with the rest of the mental health system. At Crossing Place, all staff members negotiate with the system. The house director supervises this process and administers the house itself. Because of the shorter lengths of stay, the focus on immediate practical problem solving, and the absence of most clients from the house during the daytime, Crossing Place tends to be less consistently intimate in feeling than Soteria. Individual relationships between staff members and clients can be very intimate at Crossing Place, especially with returning clients, but it is easier to get in and out of Crossing Place without having a significant relationship than is the case at Soteria.

One aspect of the Crossing Place program that deserves special mention is the graduates' evening. It is based in part on the Soteria experience, but it also grew out of the emphasis at Crossing Place and Woodley House on alumni involvement. An art therapist supervises the session, to which graduates and current residents are invited. Attendance varies considerably, but the formal time, place, and nature of the activity make returning much easier for persons who might otherwise not be sure they are "really" welcome. The evening provides social contact, a place to find friends, and a chance to meet new people. Art seems to be an ideal medium around which to focus a meeting of long-term clients. Almost anyone can draw, and the critical comments of others can be easily deflected by saying, "Well, I've never drawn before." Although a large, informal social network of clients

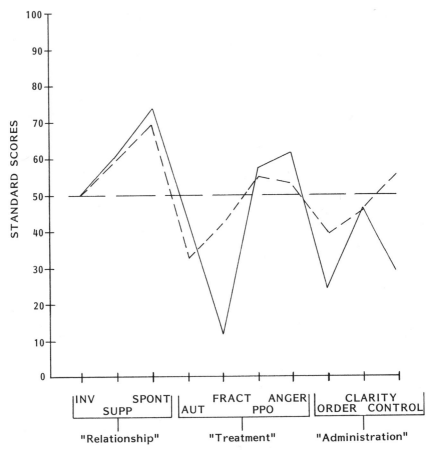

Figure 1. Program comparisons: Staff at Soteria and Crossing Place. Key: ———— Soteria, September 1976, *N* = 8; - - - - - Crossing place, March 1983, *N* = 9.

existed around Soteria, the house never had a formal arrangement with graduates. Again, this program difference would appear to be best explained by differences in clientele.

SYSTEMATIC RESEARCH MILIEU COMPARISON OF SOTERIA AND CROSSING PLACE

Moos' Community Oriented Program Environment Scale (COPES; Moos, 1974, 1975), a 100-item true/false measure of participants' perceptions of their social environment, was administered at regular intervals to staff and clients in both programs. This measure has both "real" (i.e., "How do you see it?") and ideal (i.e., "How would you like it to be?") forms.

Although staff and client real and ideal data were collected, only staff real data are reported here (see Figure 1). According to these data, Crossing Place staff members, as compared with Soteria staff members, are 3 standard deviations higher on the practical orientation variable and 2 standard deviations higher on the variables of order and organization and staff control. Both programs are 1 or more standard deviations lower than norms derived from other community-based programs on autonomy, practicality, and order and organization. They are 1 or more standard deviations higher on the three psychotherapy variables—involvement, support, and spontaneity—and on the treatment variables of perceived personal problem orientation and staff tolerance of anger. The overall shapes of the two profiles have almost point-by-point correspondence on six variables and similar profile shapes on the other four. The congruence between clinical descriptive and standardized assessment findings is both noteworthy and gratifying (Mosher, Kresky-Wolff, Matthews, & Menn, 1986).

It is noteworthy that the two programs conform well by both clinical description and systematic assessment to the literature-derived descriptions of effective therapeutic milieus for acute and "veteran" clients outlined earlier.

OUTCOME DATA

The clients in the Soteria control group were all treated with neuroleptics for an average of 28 days on a 30-bed ward in a community hospital that was used as a training site by a nearby university medical school. Forty-three percent were maintained on them for the entire study period.

Despite minimal neuroleptic use (57% never received neuroleptics and 4% were maintained on them during the 2-year study period), experimental group patients were less often readmitted, were more often able to leave home to live on their own or with peers, and had higher-level jobs as compared with control group patients.

These data support our contention that all newly identified psychotics deserve a trial of pure psychosocial intervention if a proper therapeutic environment can be provided.

PROGRAM STAFF

RECRUITMENT

Community residential treatment settings have usually used non-degreed paraprofessionals as staff. Some of these staff may, in fact, have college or graduate degrees, but these are usually not required. These facilities seek staff who are interested, invested, and enthusiastic about the type of work they anticipate doing, independent of credentials. The down side of this practice is that there is often no career ladder available to them. Hence, staff turnover is usually a consequence of returning to school to get graduate degrees, most frequently MSWs.

Our experience is that the more accurately the reality of the job is described, the less likely a misfit between job and person will occur. Thus, we like to make very explicitly clear exactly what will be expected of staff in ads and job descriptions provided them. This will not, of course, prevent a number of people from applying who will be operating from their own perception of what the program and its demands will be, unrelated to the reality as depicted by the job description. An accurate job description does provide a means of screening out potential staff who are not able to address the job for what it is, as compared with what they want it to be. Residential alternatives should not hire staff who, given an accurate program and job description, distort it substantially to suit their own needs. It is likely that such persons will behave similarly in the milieu and cause unnecessary problems.

The job description should contain sufficient substance to allow candidates to easily identify the major activities that will be part of their job. These include the following:

Client Assessment. Staff are required to evaluate each client's strengths and weaknesses, with an emphasis on expandable areas of strength. Psychopathology will be factored in, but in a manner that preserves the focus on health, positive assets, and normalization of functioning. This assessment will also include a future planning element since in these transitional programs the process of leaving begins at entry.

Relationships ("Being With"). Staff will be expected to form some modest relationship with most clients. It is expected that they will form close relationships with a minority of clients. The relationships are expected to be peer-oriented, fraternal, nonexploitative, attentive but not intrusive, warm, nurturant, supportive, and responsive. Staff are not expected to like everyone, nor are they expected to have a close relationship with the majority of clients. Neither are they expected to see themselves as psychotherapists, even with the clients with whom they form close relationships. Quiet, attentive, nondemanding support is highly valued.

Advocacy/Empowerment. Staff will work with clients on *their* goals. If this requires involvement outside the facility, they will be involved as required. Client goals are always primary, even if they require staff to go out of their way. They will take clients to the welfare, vocational, housing, socializing, and recreation systems and stay with them, if necessary. Their goal vis-à-vis the clients' goals is to facilitate the process of normalization and integration back into the mainstream of society. They are to view themselves as being the clients' employee and should treat them as "the boss" insofar as the clients' requests are at all reasonable. Even seemingly unreasonable (if not dangerous to anyone) requests should be pursued. Staff are not to see themselves as knowing what is "best" for the client. If a request is truly unreasonable, the world at large will make it clear soon enough that this is the case. The staff need not be involved in defining this "reality", nor should they necessarily attempt to protect (assuming no real risk of serious harm) clients from its impact. To do so would deprive the client of an *in vivo* learning experience.

Basically, staff should be able to put themselves, flexibly and nonjudgmentally, into the client's shoes. This ability will allow them to accept a variety of wishes, needs, and goals from the client without a predetermined, staff-derived hierarchical scale of importance or "rightness."

SELECTION

There are, of course, no absolute criteria for selecting staff. A great deal depends on the precise nature of the alternative setting, the overall context, and the salaries offered. Over time, however, a number of variables important in the selection of staff for residential alternatives have been identified (Hirschfeld, Matthews, Mosher, & Menn, 1977; Mosher, Reifman, & Menn, 1973). These are guides, not recipes. Each locale must modify them to suit its own situation and types of persons who respond when hiring takes place. What we espouse here presumes that the candidates have available an accurate description of the program and their duties. We have found that the single most important factor in selecting staff is their *self-selection* in applying for a position.

Some characteristics that we have identified as predisposing to being good program staff are the following:

Long Lives. A variable we've identified as important in persons working with psychotic clients is "having led long lives in relatively few years" (Mosher et al., 1973). What, in a selection process, does this mean?

Simply put, staff candidates who have experienced significant difficulty in their lives—whether self- or other-generated—that they have dealt with successfully are good job candidates. In our experience, nonminority, upper-middle-class, suburban-raised, intact, no-problem family offspring have not proved to be, in general, very good staff members. Princes and princesses do not generally thrive in these environments.

We found in our original group of Soteria staff a surprisingly large number we could characterize as the invulnerable children in "vulnerable," problem-laden families. That is, they were frequently the rather neutrally regarded (by the problem parent in particular) caretaker child in the family. For example, one staff member was his fatherless family's principal housekeeper while his mother was nonfunctional because of an 18-month-long episode of unlabeled and untreated psychosis. His older brother, who was much closer to the mother and involved with her, grew up with serious psychological difficulties, while our staff member developed into a highly competent person without serious problems.

It is this type of overcoming of serious adversity in their lives that we now look for in the backgrounds of potential staff members. Although it is obviously not always present, we are more confident in our selection when it is. We believe that the test-measured personality trait of high ego strength (Hirschfeld et al., 1977) that we found in the Soteria staff is also related to the process of successfully coping with these difficult life experiences. These experiences also seemed to have helped them develop the responsiveness, flexibility, and tolerance needed to work in these settings. Without such experiences we found that staff had substantial difficulties relating to unmedicated psychotic clients for prolonged periods. If they could be helped, by peer support and supervision, to stick with it, the Soteria experience seemed to become their time of adversity and learning to deal with it. At Crossing Place this type of on the job learning can go on over a longer period of time because the amount of externally manifest madness is less than was the case at Soteria, primarily owing to the use of neuroleptics.

Practical Problem-Solving Orientations. One idea behind our deciding not to require professional degrees to work in these settings was to attempt to avoid, as much as feasible, staff who had been taught theories of the etiology or treatment of psychosis. We believe it is easier to interact with mad persons from a phenomenologic stance (i.e., open, accepting, without preconceptions) if previous learning does not have to be unlearned.

Hence, when interviewing potential staff we asked about their ideas on the nature and treatment of madness. We found, not surprisingly, that most people have some theory of madness. In our experience, however, tentative, open-minded, nonexclusive theoretical preconceptions did not create difficulties, but doctrinaire adherence to a particular theory, no matter what its content, did create subsequent interactional difficulties.

In the job interview we also routinely assessed the nature of the person's motivation. To our surprise and pleasure, we found that most of our applicants were genuinely interested in trying to be of help to fellow human beings. Certainly, the salaries offered, at the level of psychiatric aide or technician, were not great motivators. Hence, we had to conclude that altruism is a personality trait that is still alive and well.

If we believe, in light of our interview and whatever other information we have, that the potential staff person is motivated by the rescue fantasy, we are likely to screen out that individual. Using the metaphor of St. George, the knight in shining armor setting out to rescue the damsel from the dragon, we take the position that it could be that the damsel does not want to be rescued—at least just yet. The kind of activist, doing to, controlling intrusiveness that the rescue fantasy tends to engender is not a kind of activity we want to have, or reinforce, in these settings.

When we ask the questions How do you see your role with the clients? What will your overall orientation toward them be? we like to hear some version of a practical problem-solving approach. Responses like "Those folks have real-life problems; maybe I can help them deal with them" or "Life seems to have dealt them a bad hand; maybe I can help them learn to play their cards better" are ones we used as positive selection criteria. Responses indicating a psychotherapy view of their role with clients (e.g., "I'd like to help them understand how they got that way") are ones we used in deselecting individuals.

In our experience, potential staff members who have been able to leave home and establish an existence for themselves, separate from their parents, without the process having been underwritten financially by their families, will likely have had to face enough real-life problems of their own to be useful to the clientele.

BURNOUT

Definition. Although a precise definition of this psychological state is difficult, it seems to be ubiquitous among mental health workers, especially those in direct face-to-face contact with mad persons for substantial segments of their workdays. It is a state that everyone seems to recognize and be seriously cognizant of, yet its precise description, cause, and treatment remain elusive. Its description involves various depressionlike symptoms: low energy, lack of interest, touchiness, unhappiness, and physical illnesses.

The symptoms of burnout generally parallel, in a less severe way, those of the clientele; low energy, lack of motivation, demoralization, and hopelessness are generally *sine qua non*s of being a patient in the public mental health system.

Causes. The conventional view is that burnout stems, for the most part, from working with this difficult population, from the sense of powerlessness, helplessness, and frustration experienced by staff in their day-to-day work. While this is clearly a factor, our experience has taught us that a more complete explanatory view is that it is an interactional product of setting, staff person, and client. Conventional wisdom attributes it almost exclusively to the client. In contrast, we ascribe great causal significance for burnout to the way in which the setting structures the staff's day-to-day working relationship with it and the clients it serves. The major issue is whether or not staff perceive themselves as being empowered to make, and feel responsible for, on-the-spot clinical decisions. The degree to which this empowered state is experientially validated (thus preventing burnout) is closely tied to the size of the setting and number of layers in the organization's hierarchy.

For intensive residential treatment settings the two ends of the hierarchy/size continuum are the large state hospital at one pole and small community alternatives at the other. Twenty to 30 bed wards in general hospitals fall midway on the continuum. In the large hospital hierarchy the lowest level of personnel ("aides," "technicians") have most direct contact with patients and least power. Decisions must be cleared with a series of more powerful persons: the nursing staff, the head nurse, the ward administrator, the multiunit administrator, and the hospital superintendent (occasionally). Hierarchies like these tend to engender paralysis in the lowest-level staff. They fear making important on-the-spot decisions, for they may misstep, and they fear taking responsibility, for they may subsequently be blamed for a mistake. This externally determined inability to make decisions about clinical situations is analogous to that experienced frequently by their clients, and it results in a similar psychological state: learned helplessness, dependency, demoralization, and lack of motivation to participate actively in the planning and treatment processes.

Treatment and Prevention. The "treatment" of burnout, given this analytic paradigm, is fairly straightforward but very problematic, because it would involve a major restructuring of most existing organizational units dealing with very disturbed and disturbing clients. What is required is small size, minimal hierarchy, and staff empowerment. It is very difficult for staff to feel empowered unless the other two conditions are met. To prevent burnout, staff at all levels must experience themselves as empowered, responsible decision makers while in the setting.

A touching example of what can happen when staff feel empowered and able to make decisions based on current circumstances is worth recounting:

A 30-year-old woman came to Crossing Place after having been picked up wandering in a daze around the bus station. She arrived still dazed, very tired, uncommunicative, and quasi-catatonic. She was able to tell us she was from a midwestern city and give a name and address. Her folks (mother and uncle) had no phone, so staff contacted the nearest police station and asked them to have family call Crossing Place. The relatives were overjoyed when they called because they thought our client was dead when her purse had been found in New York City some days before. The uncle came by bus the next day; our client came out of her daze when she saw her uncle. Staff offered them a ride to the bus station. In a simple, extraordinarily human gesture, a staff member asked the uncle if he'd ever been to D.C. before. He said no. The staff member then took uncle and client on a whirlwind tour of the monuments, White House, and Capitol Hill before dropping them at the bus station!

This is an example of a truly therapeutic interaction that occurs frequently in these settings. The staff member's kindness, humanity, and generosity were subsequently acknowledged and complimented by staff-peers, director, and consultants. A major psychological principle underlying helpful interventions is that remoralization and restoration or maintanence of self-esteem and self-confidence is derived from visible and acknowledged accomplishments or successes. Without feeling empowered, neither staff nor clients will be very willing to try things that might result in noticeable accomplishments. Hence, staff burnout is also prevented by their feeling empowered in a way that their actions can facilitate success experiences with a notably unsuccessful clientele. In turn, they must both acknowledge the client's accomplishments, however small, and be acknowledged by peers and supervisors for having facilitated the client's success.

For example, a client tells a staff person that he doesn't feel able to negotiate the process of getting into an apartment program (often based on previous failure experience in trying to do so). On the basis of their judgment of that person's clinical state and knowledge of the nature of the application process to the apartment program, staff decide that the client will probably be successful if accompanied. If the process is then successfully negotiated, everybody wins; both staff and client have accomplished something that is real and visible. The staff person delivers a lot of "positive strokes" to the client for his accomplishment (and the client is also, one hopes, stroked by client-peers and other staff), and the staff person's role in the success is acknowledged by the client, the supervisor, and staff-peers. Remoralization is the outcome for client, and maintainence of morale is the outcome for staff and setting.

Another strategy for preventing burnout involves activities that both provide "feeding" of the staff and build mutual respect and cohesiveness among them.

In the matter of in-house burnout prevention, we have found three different types of in-house "feeding" helpful. First, didactic training exercises focused around a specific topic, such as incest or spouse abuse. In our experience, it has been useful to have them led by outside "experts" brought in specifically for the occasion(s).

Second, regular staff-only meetings focused on problems that have arisen between staff members. These meetings can be led by the program director, but if similar issues keep resurfacing over time, it is usually more helpful to invite an outside facilitator to lead a series of such meetings.

Third, user-oriented group consensus development meetings focused on perplexing and difficult clinical problems as related to individual and group relationship issues with clients and between staff. This meeting should be problem-focused, relationship-building-oriented, and supportive of both individual positions and differences among staff, while operating with the overall expectation that a consensus will eventually emerge. In our experience, this user-oriented meeting is best led by the psychiatric consultant because it is focused on developing individualized approaches to each user's particular problems. In other settings these occasions would be called treatment planning meetings. Because of our emphasis on a collaborative planning and goal-setting process we have tried, at times, to have clients attend these meetings. We have tried having one client at a time present, but this was experienced by many clients as an inquisition or at least as overwhelming (there are usually 12 to 15 persons in the room because of students, split positions, and other factors). We have also tried having all clients in attendance; this is difficult logistically and proved rather inefficient. It also made it impossible to discuss certain background facts about clients (e.g., incest, abuse) in front of the other clients because of issues of confidentiality. Our current practice is to have individual clients attend these meetings when there is a consensus that it would be useful to hear their point of view firsthand.

The first two types of meetings (training and staff group with an outside facilitator) should be scheduled in response to problems as they arise within the setting. It is part of the program director's job to be sure these needs are addressed in a timely and appropriate fashion. What must always be remembered is that if the needs of clients are to be met, the staff must feel they have an accessible reservoir of energy from which to draw. Hence, meeting staff needs is no less important than meeting client needs. In fact, to avoid staff exploitation of clients, acting out against them, or being unresponsive to them requires constant attention to staff's own reasonable demands in the setting.

As for burnout prevention and treatment outside the setting, these activities are really just another way to ensure cohesion, trust, and mutual respect among staff. The basic paradigm is simple: parties held away from the clinical setting. In the early phases of programs they are best organized by the power figures—the program director or consultants. As a program becomes more settled and routinized, these events are best rotated among willing staff, whatever their programmatic role. We have found that two to three evening parties a year are important for maintence of morale.

Outside the setting, staff relationships represent another means by which staff treat or prevent burnout in themselves. These generally will evolve naturally. They should be regarded by the program's leadership as outside their direct purview. Our experience is that a number of pairings begun in these family-like settings have produced enduring relationships.

REFERENCES

Barton, R. (1959). *Institutional neurosis*. Bristol: Wright.

Bockoven, J. S. (1963). *Moral treatment in American psychiatry*. New York: Springer.

Braun, P. B., Kochansky, G., Shapiro, R., Greenberg, S., Gudeman, J. E., Johnson, S., & Shore, M. F. (1981). Overview: Deinstitutionalization of psychiatric patients: A critical review of outcome studies. *American Journal of Psychiatry, 138*, 736–749.

Burti, L., & Mosher, L. R. (1986). Training psychiatrists in the community: The Italian experience. *American Journal of Psychiatry, 143*, 1580–1584.

Fairweather, G. W., Sanders, D., Cressier, D., & Maynard, H. (1969). *Community life for the mentally ill: An alternative to institutional care*. Chicago: Aldine.

Fromm-Reichmann, F. (1948). Notes on the development of treatment of schizophrenics by psychoanalytic psychotherapy. *Psychiatry, 11*, 263–273.

Gunderson, J. G. (1978). Defining the therapeutic processes in psychiatric milieus. *Psychiatry, 41*, 327–335.

Hirschfeld R., Matthews, S., Mosher, L. R., & Menn, A. Z. (1977). Being with madness: Personality characteristics of three treatment staffs. *Hospital and Community Psychiatry, 28*, 267–273.

Hoult, J. (1986). The community care of the acutely mentally ill. *British Journal of Psychiatry, 149*, 137–144.

Kiesler, C. A. (1982a). Mental hospitals and alternative care: Noninstitutionalization as potential public policy for mental patients. *American Psychologist, 37*, 349–360.

Kiesler, C. A. (1982b). Public and professional myths about mental hospitalization: An empirical reassessment of policy-related beliefs. *American Psychologist, 37*, 1323–1339.

Klorman, R., Strauss, J., & Kokes, R. (1977). Premorbid adjustment in schizophrenia: Concepts, measures, and implications. Part III. The relationship of demographic and diagnostic factors to measures of premorbid adjustment in schizophrenia. *Schizophrenia Bulletin, 3*, 214–225.

Kresky-Wolff, M., Matthews, S., Kalibat, F., & Mosher, L. R. (1984). Crossing Place: A residential model for crisis intervention. *Hospital and Community Psychiatry, 35*, 72–74.

Laing, R. D. (1967). *The politics of experience*. New York: Ballantine.

Lamb, H. R., & Lamb, D. (1984). A nonhospital alternative to acute hospitalization. *Hospital and Community Psychiatry, 35*, 728–730.

Langsley, D. C., Pittman, F. S., III, & Swank, G. F. (1969). Family crisis in schizophrenics and other mental patients. *Journal of Nervous and Mental Disease, 149*, 270–276.

Matthews, S. M., Roper, M. T., Mosher, L. R., & Menn, A. Z. (1979). A non-neuroleptic treatment for schizophrenia: Analysis of the two-year post-discharge risk of relapse. *Schizophrenia Bulletin, 5,* 322–333.

Moos, R. H. (1974). *Evaluating treatment environments: A social ecological approach.* New York: Wiley.

Moos, R. (1975). *Evaluating correctional and community settings.* New York: Wiley.

Mosher, L. R. (1982). Italy's revolutionary mental health law: An assessment. *American Journal of Psychiatry, 139,* 199–203.

Mosher, L. R. (1983). Alternatives to psychiatric hospitalization: Why has research failed to be translated into practice? *New England Journal of Medicine, 309,* 1479–1480.

Mosher, L. R., & Burti, L. (1988). *Principles and practice of community mental health.* New York: W. W. Norton.

Mosher, L. R., & Gunderson, J. G. (1979). Group, family, milieu and community support system treatment for schizophrenia. In L. Bellack (Ed.), *Disorders of the schizophrenic syndrome* (pp. 399–451). New York: Grune & Stratton.

Mosher, L. R., Kresky-Wolff, M., Matthews, S., & Menn, A. (1986). Milieu therapy in the 1980's: A comparison of two residential alternatives to hospitalization. *Bulletin of the Menninger Clinic, 50,* 257–268.

Mosher, L., & Menn, A. (1977). Lowered barriers in the community: The Soteria model. In L. Stein & M. A. Test (Eds.), *Alternatives to mental hospital treatment* (pp. 75–113). New York: Plenum Press.

Mosher, L. R., & Menn, A. Z. (1978). Community residential treatment for schizophrenia: Two-year follow-up. *Hospital and Community Psychiatry, 29,* 715–723.

Mosher, L., & Menn, A. (1979). Soteria: An alternative to hospitalization for schizophrenia. In H. R. Lamb (Ed.), *New directions for mental health services—Alternatives to acute hospitalization* (Vol. 1, pp. 73–84). San Francisco: Jossey-Bass.

Mosher, L., & Menn, A. (1983). Scientific evidence and system change: The Soteria experience. In H. Stierlin, L. Wynne, & M. Wirsching (Eds.), *Psychosocial interventions in schizophrenia* (pp. 93–108). Heidelberg, West Germany: Springer-Verlag.

Mosher, L. R., Menn, A. Z., & Matthews, S. M. (1975). Evaluation of a home-based treatment for schizophrenia. *American Journal of Orthopsychiatry, 45,* 455–467.

Mosher, L. R., Reifman, A., & Menn, A. (1973). Characteristics of nonprofessionals serving as primary therapists for acute schizophrenics. *Hospital and Community Psychiatry, 24,* 391–396.

Pasamanick, B., Scarpitti, F., & Dinitz, S. (1967). *Schizophrenics in the community. An experimental study in the prevention of hospitalization.* New York: Appleton-Century-Crofts.

Paul, G. L. (1969). The chronic mental patient: Current status—Future directions. *Psychological Bulletin, 71,* 81–94.

Paul, G. L., & Lentz, R. J. (1977). *Psychosocial treatment of chronic mental patients: Milieu vs. social-learning programs.* Cambridge, MA: Harvard University Press.

Perry, J. W. (1962). Reconstitutive process in the psychopathology of the self. *Annals of the New York Academy of Sciences, 96,* 853–876.

Phillips, L. (1966). Social competence, the process-reactive distinction and the nature of mental disorder. *Proceedings of American Psychopathology Association, 54,* 471–481.

Polak, P., & Kirby, M. (1976). A model to replace psychiatric hospitals. *Journal of Nervous and Mental Disease, 162,* 13–22.

Polak, P., Kirby, M., & Dietchman, W. (1979). Treating acutely psychiatric patients in privatehomes. In H. R. Lamb (Ed.), *New directions for mental health services—Alternatives to acute hospitalization* (Vol. 1, pp. 49–64). San Francisco: Jossey-Bass.

Rappaport, M., Goldman, H., Thornton, P., Moltzen, S., Stegner, B., Hall, K., Gurevitz, H.,

& Attkisson, C. (1987). A method for comparing two systems of acute 24 hour psychiatric care. *Hospital and Community Psychiatry, 38,* 1091–1095.

Rosen, B., Klein, D., & Gittelman-Klein, R. (1971). The prediction of rehospitalization: The relationship between age of first psychiatric treatment contact, marital status and premorbid asocial adjustment. *Journal of Nervous and Mental Disease, 152,* 17–22.

Stein, L. I., & Test, M. A. (Eds.). (1985). *Training in the community living model—A decade of experience.* New Directions for Mental Health Services, No. 26. San Francisco: Jossey-Bass.

Straw, R. B. (1982). *Meta-analysis of deinstitutionalization.* Doctoral dissertation, Northwestern University, University Microfilms, Ann Arbor.

Stroul, B. A. (1987). *Crisis residential services in a community support system.* Report prepared for the National Institute of Mental Health Community Support Program.

Sullivan, H. S. (1931). The modified psychoanalytic treatment of schizophrenia. *American Journal of Psychiatry, 11,* 519–540.

Weisman, G. (1985a). Crisis houses and lodges: Residential treatment of acutely disturbed chronic patients. *Psychiatric Annals, 15,* 642–644, 647.

Weisman, G. (1985b). Crisis-oriented residential treatment as an alternative to hospitalization. *Hospital and Community Psychiatry, 36,* 1302–1305.

Wendt, R. J., Mosher, L. R., Matthews, S. M., & Menn, A. Z. (1983). Comparison of two treatment environments for schizophrenia. In J. G. Gunderson, O. A. Will, Jr., & L. R. Mosher (Eds.), *Principles and practice of milieu therapy* (pp. 17–33). New York: Jason Aronson.

Wing, J. K., & Brown, G. W. (1970). *Institutionalism and schizophrenia: A comparative study of three mental hospitals 1960–1968.* Cambridge: Cambridge University Press.

7

Partial Hospitalization

MARGARET W. LINN

Although the concept of partial hospitalization has existed for over a half century, its growth has not reached its described potential. The first day hospital was established in Russia in the early 1930s (Wortis, 1950). The emphasis was on rehabilitating individuals in regard to work. Day programs were established next in England and Canada around 1946 along a psychosocial therapeutic model. Vaughn (1985) documents how, at that time, day centers were a revolutionary concept, and that the idea flourished in the optimistic climate of opinion emerging in psychiatry during the 1950s. Day hospitals were seen as potential substitutes for large mental hospitals.

The psychosocial club model was also prominent in the first centers established in the United States shortly after World War II. One of the first day centers grew out of the observations of staff at the San Diego Veterans Administration Medical Center. They observed that a number of the psychiatric patients treated in the outpatient center gathered in the waiting rooms long before and after their scheduled appointments. The obvious social support that the patients gained led staff to set aside a special place with minimal staffing and a few therapeutic activities to help promote social support networks among the patients. At about the same time, the Boston Psychopathic Hospital opened a day hospital with an open-door philosophy on the inpatient services, nonuniform dress for nurses and doctors, and various aspects of milieu treatment (Greenblatt, York, & Brown, 1955).

MARGARET W. LINN • Social Science Research Department, Veterans Administration Medical Center, and Department of Psychiatry, University of Miami School of Medicine, Miami, Florida 33125.

VARIABILITY OF PROGRAMS

Differences in terms used to describe partial hospital programs have led to confusion about their functions and to problems in comparing studies that deal with outcomes of their patients. Although partial hospitalization is defined as any program that is less than 24 hours, it can be a day, weekend, or night program. The overwhelming majority of the programs, however, are day programs. The confusion arises from the various goals of the programs and their patient populations. Some centers focused on rehabilitation of acute patients in areas of work and role adjustment, and often had time-limited programs where the goal was to return the patient quickly to the community and to employment if possible. Other programs focused more on the chronic mental patients, who needed social support and a structured program in order to stay out of the hospital. For many of the chronic patients, return to employment or independent living in the community was less likely a major goal than with the acute patients. In addition, some centers were established primarily as aftercare programs, whereas others developed as alternatives to inpatient admission. Labels used to describe the programs were those such as day hospital, day treatment, or day care. For the most part, *day care* and *day treatment* described centers that treated longer-term chronic patients. *Day hospital* usually described brief intensive treatment rehabilitation centers. The ambiguity of labels and types of patients selected by the centers influenced comparison of the results of studies that were reported.

In addition, the different kinds of treatments and programs emphasized within each center increased variability among centers even further. Depending on the philosophy of the center, some used individual psychotherapy or group therapy more than others; some emphasized a variety of manual arts, occupational therapies, and social activities; others provided family therapy, social skills training, or other behavior modification programs. It is, therefore, little wonder that day programs soon reflected some of the same diversity in programming as that found in mental hospitals, and studying and comparing outcomes of day programs was akin to studying and comparing mental hospital effectiveness. This background is important in understanding the problems faced by day hospitals in being accepted in the field. It is also important because the ultimate success of day centers depends on demonstrating their intrinsic and comparative value and on establishing their widespread acceptance.

DEVELOPMENTAL HISTORY

The first major effort toward better definition of day programs and establishment of standards occurred as a result of a meeting of the Federation of Partial Hospitalization Study Groups, Inc., in 1976. The meeting led to publication of a report on the objectives of partial hospital care as an alternative to traditional full-time hospitalization. Models for third-party coverage and utilization review were also suggested. The outlook for the future of day hospitals, at that time, was optimistic. At present, however, that hope has been only partly transformed into a reality (Klar, 1982). There is still resistance to partial hospital utilization, as evidenced by lack of referrals from practitioners other than those who have had some direct experience with day hospitals. On the other hand, progress has been made, as evidenced by the fact that (1) formal standards have been set for partial hospitalization within the American Psychiatric Association, (2) there has been the continued growth of the American Association for Partial Hospitalization (AAPH), and (3) the *International Journal of Partial Hospitalization* was launched in 1981 and has been published biannually since that time. Furthermore, the Community Mental Health Centers (CMHC) Construction Act of 1963 mandated day hospitals as one of the required elements of the centers. There are more than 1,000 CMHC-affiliated and free-standing partial hospital programs, as well as 35 day hospitals and 47 day treatment centers in the VA system.

Taking an overview of the studies that have been done over the years, it is apparent that the majority of the efficacy studies started in the mid-1960s and peaked in the late 1970s. Few large-scale randomized studies have taken place in the 1980s. Despite the differences in day programs and their patients, these studies showed that partial hospital programs were generally as effective as inpatient units in treating psychiatric patients who were not at risk for suicide or violence. Furthermore, day programs were usually superior to outpatient treatment for chronic schizophrenic patients. Most of the studies focused on comparing patients randomly assigned or matched for partial hospitalization with those sent for inpatient treatment. Thus, the day hospital was studied as an alternative to inpatient hospital admission and care. Fewer of the studies evaluated the efficacy of day hospitals compared with other forms of outpatient care. If most of the studies occurred a few decades ago and showed favorable results for partial hospitalization programs, one may well ask what is new and whether, in fact, new studies are needed.

CURRENT ENVIRONMENTAL PRESSURES

Several things have happened to place day hospitals in a different environmental context. Studies that clearly demonstrated the effectiveness of partial hospitalization as an alternative to inpatient care may no longer be very relevant. There is little opportunity for inpatient care today. Two major forces have operated to shift the locus of care for the mentally ill from hospital to community. The deinstitutionalization movement, based on the philosophy that institutionalization was detrimental, led to psychiatry's move to community treatment and establishment of programs in the community rather than in large mental hospitals. Unfortunately, the community programs could not be developed quickly enough to handle the mass exodus of patients from state hospitals. Short-term admissions and the "revolving door" syndrome were soon prominent in a large segment of the deinstitutionalized population. A second major force, occurring somewhat later in conjunction with hospital care in general, has been the cost-containment programs that revolutionized general hospital care with prospective payment systems. Specification of criteria for diagnostic-related groups (DRGs) reduced length of hospital stay by placing hospitals at risk financially for keeping patients longer than the averages that were established for various diagnostic groups. Also, through more stringent utilization reviews, reductions in admissions and lengths of stay have also been achieved. Therefore, at the present time, there are fewer options for inpatient admission, and if patients are admitted, their length of stay for treatment is very brief. Brief treatment, in and of itself, is not bad. Caffey, Galbrecht, and Klett (1971) showed brief inpatient care (29 days) for schizophrenics to be as effective as care averaging three times as long. Furthermore, studies by Herz, Endicott, Spitzer, and Mesnikoff (1971) of brief treatment compared with standard hospitalization found no advantages for longer hospital stay. Planned brief hospital stay coupled with transition to a day hospital program is an attractive model for patients requiring stabilization in an inpatient setting. An even more attractive model is one that bypasses use of the hospital altogether. The fact remains, however, that a few decades ago it was possible to choose among alternatives of hospital or partial hospital, or longer or shorter hospital stay, as deemed necessary for a patient. Today, inpatient care often is not an alternative. Although it remains of clinical interest that partial hospitalization can be as effective as inpatient care and less expensive, the practical significance may be lost in the present health care scene.

Added to the complex economic climate, partial hospitals have had to expand and extend their function to encompass care for more divergent diagnostic groups. The growth of the elderly population and their medical care needs not only has changed the age ranges of the major psychiatric disorder groups but has increased, in particular, the treatment of dementia patients in day care centers. Furthermore, day hospitals are being established more than in the past for children, adolescents, and patients with various medical disorders.

In some ways, the partial hospital program has the potential of being the next target for cost containment in that it is next in order to hospitals in the high utilization of resources. With the economic pressures to reduce in-patient care, it is surprising that day hospitals have not come more recently to stand in the gap created by lack of hospital resources. One factor has been the difficulty in obtaining reimbursement from third-party payment sys-tems, and others have been lack of referrals by practitioners and restrictions by the centers themselves in whom they will accept for treatment. A large population of potential patients for partial hospital programs could be found among the homeless population of mentally ill. The homeless population, many of whom are schizophrenics discharged from mental hospitals, is at last receiving attention from the government as well as from mental health plan-ning groups. The question of the future would then seem to focus on how well partial hospitalization programs compare with other less restrictive and/or less costly outpatient methods of treatment.

FUNCTIONS AND PROGRAMS

According to the AAPH, partial hospitalization is an ambulatory treat-ment program that includes major diagnostic, medical, psychiatric, psycho-social, and prevocational treatment modalities designed for patients with serious mental disorders who require coordinated intensive, comprehen-sive, and multidisciplinary treatment *not* provided in an outpatient clinic setting (Casarino, Wilner, & Maxey, 1982). Excluded from the definition are self-help groups, social clubs, and social activity groups that may be thera-peutic but are not seen as forming a partial hospitalization function when operated exclusively as such. Day hospitals may give continuous or intermit-tent services. Their goals can be defined as providing: (1) an alternative to inpatient admission, (2) a transition from inpatient care to outpatient treat-ment, and (3) a maintenance supportive program for those at risk of mental illness or those who need a prolonged supportive environment in order to remain in the community. The AAPH believes that one of the primary functions of partial hospital programs is resolution or stabilization of short-term problems or crisis situations for decompensating clinical conditions that, if not arrested, would require 24-hour hospitalization (Casarino et al., 1982). Other functions include rehabilitation, maintenance, and diagnostic work, mainly with multiply impaired chronic patients.

In view of the diversity of programs and their patients, a question that needs to be addressed through research relates to indications and contraindi-cations for admission to partial hospitalization (Herz, 1982). Also, the ques-tion of patient mix needs to be addressed. Is it better to select either acute patients or chronic patients, or can patients best be served in some kind of case mix setting? For example, the more functional patients could be role models for chronic patients, and only one staff would be needed to care for all patients. On the other hand, does wide heterogeneity lead to the day program's being all things to all patients without clearly defined treatments? Furthermore, what are the effects of different diagnostic mixes? While some centers advocate labeling patients only in terms of their levels of care in regard to treatment needs, others would exclude patients with alcohol problems or those with dementia. The most pressing questions may not be those related to overall effectiveness of day programs with their diversity of approaches, but rather what treatment for what type of patient produces the best outcomes within the framework of partial hospitals. This book is concerned with treatments for schizophrenic patients. What do we know about treatment of schizophrenic patients in day hospitals?

DAY VERSUS INPATIENT STUDIES

Table 1 shows a number of major studies, listed chronologically, that compared partial hospitalization with inpatient care. There are several recent reviews on the studies of efficacy of day hospital programs (Mason, Louks, Burmer, & Scher, 1982; Moscowitz, 1980; Weiss & Dubin, 1982; Wilkinson, 1984). Almost all of the studies have included mixed diagnoses, including schizophrenia, but only a few singled out subgroups of schizophrenic patients for further analyses. Craft (1959), in a review of day hospitals, found diagnoses of schizophrenia among patients to range from 8 to 47%. Later, Glasscote, Kraft, Glassman, and Jepson (1969) reported schizo-

Table 1. Studies of Day Hospitals as Alternatives
to Inpatient Care

Authors	Sample
Kris (1961)	Mixed
Wilder et al. (1966)	Mixed
Michaux et al. (1970, 1972, 1973)	Mixed
Herz et al. (1971, 1975, 1977)	Mixed
Ettlinger et al. (1972)	Mixed
Washburn and Vannicelli (1976)	Mixed
Penk et al. (1978)	Mixed
Kecmanovic (1985)	Mixed
Dick et al. (1985)	Neurosis, personality disorders, adjustment reaction only

phrenia and depressive disorders as the most prominent diagnostic groupings of patients. It is apparent from early and more recent studies that schizophrenia is a diagnosis of many of the patients treated in day hospitals in this as well as other countries.

In regard to effectiveness of day hospitals as an alternative to inpatient care, Moscowitz (1980) has commented that critics of day hospitals have pointed to the fact that individuals often require hospitalization during the course of the day hospital treatment, indicating the failure of day hospitals to prevent hospitalization. However, he suggests that if we assume that most, if not all, of the patients treated by means of a day hospital program would require full-time hospitalization and would have been hospitalized on a 24-hour basis if the day hospital did not exist, then it could be argued that for any persons for whom day hospitalization avoided a full-time admission, the day hospital is a success rather than a failure.

All of the studies listed in Table 1 found partial hospitals to be as effective as, if not more effective than, inpatient care in regard to factors such as adjustment, relapse and readmissions, and cost for mixed patient groups. Those who further analyzed outcomes of schizophrenic patients were generally also favorable in regard to its superiority over full-time hospital care. One exception was the study of Michaux, Chelst, Foster, Pruim, and Dasinger (1973), which concluded that inpatient care provided more symptomatic relief for schizophrenic patients than did day hospital care. Unfortunately, the study did not employ a randomized design. To the contrary, Penk, Charles, and Van Hoose (1978) found greater improvement in vocational and social adjustment for schizophrenic than nonschizophrenic patients treated in day hospitals compared with matched and unmatched samples of inpatients. In the Wilder, Levin, and Zwerling (1966) study of patients followed up 2 years after admission, schizophrenic women treated in inpatient care had shorter intervals between admission and readmission than those treated in day hospitals, and schizophrenic men treated in day hospitals showed a trend toward earlier rehospitalization than men treated in full hospitalization. When number in the community at follow-up, number of readmissions, and median hospital stays were compared between day and inpatient groups, patients who profited most were schizophrenic women and those with neurotic or personality disorders. Although studies by Kris (1961), Herz et al. (1971; Herz, Endicott, & Spitzer, 1975, 1977), Ettlinger, Beigel, and Feder (1972), and Washburn and Vannicelli (1976) found day hospitals as effective as, if not more effective than, standard inpatient care, they did not analyze data separately by diagnosis. It can be assumed, however, that schizophrenic patients fared well, since most of the samples were composed of large proportions of schizophrenic patients. The recent British study by Dick, Cameron, Cohen, Barlow, and Ince (1985) showed that day hospital was as effective as inpatient treatment for nonschizophrenics. Many of the patients he studied had problems usually thought less amenable to treatment in day care, such as alcohol abuse and various forms of aggression. These are also problems prominent among many schizophrenic patients.

In a recent study in Yugoslavia, Kecmanovic (1985) compared matched groups of schizophrenics, patients with personality disorders, and neurotics treated as inpatients or in a day hospital. Data were collected for 18 months after discharge in regard to social adjustment, as reflected by work status, family role performance, and interpersonal relationships, as well as re-hospitalization. Fifty-eight of the 177 patients were schizophrenics. No significant differences were found with regard to outcome for the total group or for the schizophrenic subgroups, indicating that schizophrenics treated in day hospital settings did as well as those treated in inpatient care.

In general, favorable outcomes were achieved with lower financial costs in day care compared with inpatient care for schizophrenic patients. Thus, when acutely disturbed schizophrenics are suited to either inpatient or partial hospital care, these patients are likely to receive as good or superior treatment in a partial hospital, with less disruption to their role functioning, better social adjustment, and either lower readmission rates or shortened inpatient stays than those treated in the hospital.

PARTIAL HOSPITALIZATION AND OUTPATIENT CARE

Table 2 lists those studies that focused on day hospitals as alternatives to other kinds of outpatient care. Overall, day hospitals were usually superior to other forms of hospital aftercare. Again, most of the studies used mixed samples in regard to diagnosis. One study used a sample of schizophrenic

Table 2. Studies of Day Hospitals as Alternatives
to Outpatient Care

Authors	Sample
Meltzoff and Blumenthal (1966)	Mixed
Guy et al. (1969)	Mixed
Shafar (1970)	Mixed
Linn et al. (1979)	Schizophrenic
Fenton et al. (1979)	Mixed
Weldon et al. (1979)	Mixed
Tyrer and Remington (1979)	Mixed
Glick et al. (1986)	Schizophrenic and major affective

patients, and a few analyzed data separately for schizophrenic patients.

Meltzoff and Blumenthal (1966) showed that partial hospitalization was superior for marginally adjusted schizophrenic patients in areas of self-concept, family relationships, and mood compared with other forms of outpatient care. Furthermore, there were fewer readmissions for the day hospital group over an 18-month follow-up. Guy, Gross, Hogarty, and Dennis (1969) found that schizophrenic patients benefited more from day hospital than they did from outpatient treatment with medication. Chronic schizophrenic patients did poorly, as a whole, compared with other diagnoses, but those in the partial hospital had better outcomes than those treated as outpatients. Similar findings of less impressive results for nonschizophrenics were reported for a replication of the Guy et al. study done by Tyrer and Remington (1979) in Britain. Weldon, Clarkin, Hennessy, and Frances (1979) also found that a subgroup of schizophrenic patients fared better in day hospitals than in outpatient care when they were compared 3 months after hospital discharge in the areas of symptoms, mood, and community adjustment; the day hospital was partially effective in returning patients to work earlier.

Linn, Caffey, Klett, Hogarty, and Lamb (1979) conducted a randomized study of 162 schizophrenic patients in which they controlled for medication and specified the treatment approach used. Schizophrenic patients referred for day treatment at the time of discharge from 10 hospitals were randomly assigned to receive day treatment plus drugs or to receive drugs alone. They were tested before assignment and at 6, 12, 18, and 24 months on social functioning, symptoms, and attitudes. Community tenure and costs were also measured. The 10 day centers were described on process variables every 6 months for the 4 years of the study. Some centers were found to be effective in treating chronic schizophrenic patients and others were not. All centers improved the patients' social functioning. Six of the centers were found to significantly delay relapse, reduce symptoms, and change some negative patient attitudes. Costs for patients in these centers were not significantly different from costs for the group receiving drugs only. More professional staff hours, group therapy, and a high patient turnover treatment philosophy were associated with poor-result centers. More occupational therapy and a sustained nonthreatening environment were more characteristic of successful outcome centers. High-risk patients were those characterized by intropunitiveness, motor retardation, anxious depression, and disorganized hyperactivity. It appeared that good-outcome programs were able to offer an environment that provided an equilibrium between too much stimulation, which produces relapse, and too little stimulation, which fosters apathy.

A recent study by Glick et al. (1986) randomly assigned nonchronic schizophrenics ($N = 37$) and major affective disorder patients ($N = 42$) to day hospital or weekly outpatient therapy. About half of each group received individual psychotherapy, and 10 to 30% of the groups had group therapy. Compliance with medications was similar between groups. No differences were found between groups in dropout rates, overall pathology, role performance, or social adjustment. Furthermore, day hospital costs were much more than outpatient treatment costs. The nonchronic schizophrenic patients did not benefit more from day hospital than from other, less costly forms of outpatient care. However, only 70% of the original sample of schizophrenic patients were assessed at 6 and 12 months (14 in day and 10 in outpatient). Since power calculations for sample size were not provided, it is difficult to judge whether the sample was large enough to detect significant differences between day and outpatient groups for the schizophrenic patients.

Overall, chronic schizophrenics appear to fare better in day hospitals than in other outpatient care, and good outcomes can be obtained in day centers that operate on a cost-effective basis in regard to staffing and programs. It is, however, more costly than other forms of outpatient care. There is some question about whether day hospitals produce better outcomes than other outpatient treatment for nonchronic schizophrenics. There appears to be a need for a controlled study of a larger number of nonchronic schizophrenic patients to replicate the results of Glick et al. (1986) before firmly concluding that day hospitals are not cost-effective for this group. In essence, day hospitals as an alternative to other outpatient care must demonstrate superior outcomes to be effective because they will always cost more than other outpatient care.

OTHER STUDIES OF DAY HOSPITAL EFFECTIVENESS

Table 3 presents examples of other efficacy studies of day hospitals. Most are follow-up studies of day patients where assessments were done at time of discharge from the program and/or at specific intervals during or

Table 3. Other Studies of Efficacy
of Day Hospitals

Authors	Sample
Fottrell (1973)	Mixed
Rubins (1976)	Acute schizophrenics
McDonnell (1977)	Mixed
Davis et al. (1978)	Mixed
Edwards et al. (1979)	Mixed
Turner et al. (1982)	Mixed

after treatment. Assessments may be related to psychosocial adjustment or to readmission to the hospital. They do not involve comparisons of the patients in the day hospital with patients treated in other programs. The studies reported effectiveness rates for day hospitals in the range of 50 to 88%. One of the studies (Rubins, 1976) dealt only with acute schizophrenic patients. Evaluation was by means of staff ratings and psychological assessments. Results showed that 88% of the patients had moderate to high improvement in symptoms and 72% improved in feelings about self. Also, 67% showed improved cognitive functioning. Moreover, it has been reported that about 80% of the patients discharged from a day hospital program did not require psychiatric hospitalization during 2 years following treatment (Fottrell, 1973). Likewise, McDonnell (1977) found that over half of 225 patients followed in day care improved in symptom relief, social and leisure activities, and disruptive behaviors. In a study by Edwards, Yavis, and Mueller (1979), patient and therapist ratings of the patient's well-being changed positively after day hospital treatment.

In one other study (Davis, Lorei, & Caffey, 1978), 1,400 patients in 34 VA day hospital (acute treatment) centers were followed up 3 months after admission in relationship to treatment goals. Significant improvement occurred in perceptual-cognitive functioning, antisocial behavior, hygiene, assaultiveness, drinking, and anxiety. There was no change in economic dependence. However, schizophrenics improved less than nonschizophrenics. Therefore, the day programs generally were considered less effective in promoting well-being for schizophrenics 3 months after entry. It is possible that 3 months was too short a period of time to observe dramatic changes in the schizophrenic patients.

Turner, McGovern, Donneson, Sandrock, and Burstein (1982) evaluated admissions to 13 partial hospitals over an 8-month follow-up with unobtrusive assessments involving clinical outcomes. Analyses showed that the centers were most effective with chronic and acute schizophrenic conditions, paranoid schizophrenia, and affective disorders. They were least effective with adjustment disorders.

The limitations of the methodology of follow-up studies, particularly when evaluations of outcome are done by the therapists in the program, have been pointed out by others (Guy & Gross, 1967). The consistency of reported rates of improvement, however, lend support to findings that day hospitals are effective.

STUDIES OF PREDICTORS OF OUTCOME IN DAY HOSPITALS

Table 4 shows some of the studies that have attempted to identify responders to day hospital care. In regard to the importance of diagnosis,

Table 4. Studies of Predictors of Outcome
in Day Hospitals

Authors	Sample
Beigel and Feder (1970)	Mixed
Erickson (1972)	Schizophrenic vs. nonschizophrenic
Niskanen (1974)	Mixed
Heineman et al. (1975)	Mixed
Fink and Heckerman (1979)	Mixed
Falloon and Talbott (1982)	Mixed
Thompson (1985)	Mixed
Vidalis and Baker (1986)	Mixed

Beigel and Feder (1970) found diagnosis to have little prognostic significance. They compared those who completed an intensive 90-day hospital program with those who withdrew. Although history of prior hospitalization was not associated with outcome, grouping of patients as acute versus chronic at time of admission was an important predictor. Patients with acute onset of symptoms or acute illness were more likely to complete the program than those who were considered chronic (with no crisis situation or recent onset of symptoms). Thus, diagnosis itself was not as important as current symptomatology.

Erickson (1972) compared schizophrenic and nonschizophrenic patients in regard to length of day treatment and improvement 90 days after admission. Schizophrenic patients improved in depression, anxiety, interpersonal relationships, alcohol abuse, and employment. Nonschizophrenics improved in the same areas, except for interpersonal relationships, and also improved in cognitive function. Longer stay was predictive of greater improvement in both groups.

Niskanen (1974) found positive patient and family attitudes to predict improvement. Heineman, Yadin, and Perlmutter (1975), in a study in Finland, found that diagnosis and demographic factors were not associated with functional outcome of day hospital patients, but that being married and not living in a boarding home were related to improved social function. Fink and Heckerman (1979) found treatment failures (dropouts within 2 weeks) to be more frequent among women, those with psychotic diagnoses, and those referred by private psychiatrists.

More recently, Thompson (1985) studied the characteristics of 519 patients in a large midwestern partial hospital program. Twelve characteristics were associated with treatment outcome. The strongest predictors were previous state hospitalization, age at admission, age at onset, and parental incidence of mental illness. Schizophrenic patients (71% of the sample) were found to have the best outcomes in the program; however, the author points out that staff had higher expectations for benefits for these patients than they did for other diagnostic groups. In a British study of day hospital effectiveness (Vidalis & Baker, 1986), 100 admissions to the partial hospital program were followed and outcomes evaluated in regard to attendance, transfer to inpatient care, and return to employment. No significant predictors of outcome were found among variables such as age, sex, diagnosis, or living arrangements.

In general, diagnosis does not appear to be a major predictor of outcome. The patient's motivation for change of behavior, independent of diagnosis, may be the important factor (Falloon & Talbott, 1982). Niskanen (1974) concluded that clinical condition and diagnosis were of comparatively little significance in determining therapeutic results of day hospitalization, but that motivation for treatment was essential because of the nature of the outpatient setting. Day hospitals have successfully treated patients with severe psychopathology. Admission criteria based on attitudinal and motivational factors, rather than diagnosis, seem to be warranted.

TREATMENT OF SCHIZOPHRENICS IN PARTIAL HOSPITAL PROGRAMS

Test and Stein (1978) describe several characteristics of chronic psychiatric patients that could be applied to schizophrenia: a high vulnerability to stress, deficiencies in coping skills, extreme dependency, difficulty in working in competitive jobs, and difficulty managing interpersonal relationships. Mosher and Keith (1980) pointed out that extended social networks and natural support systems protect schizophrenic patients from stress. It is possible to view the day hospital as a social support system. Within the supportive framework of day hospitals, a number of treatment modalities described elsewhere in this book offer potential for treatment of schizophrenic patients.

Neuroleptic drugs for schizophrenic disorders made deinstitutionalization possible. Yet most schizophrenic patients show extensive social deficits, despite control of symptoms pharmacologically. Liberman, Mueser, and Wallace (1986) have emphasized the need for improving social functioning through social skills training, where patients are taught interpersonal skills to facilitate community survival and help meet their emotional needs. Social skills training, including modeling, behavior rehearsal, homework, feedback, and contingent reinforcement, is a methodology easily incorporated into partial hospital settings. In fact, social skills training for schizophrenic patients is a major element of treatment in most partial hospital programs today (Bellack & Hersen, 1979; Hersen & Luber, 1977). Targeted behaviors can range from basic instrumental activities of daily living, such as shopping or preparing meals, to higher levels of functional activities, like financial planning or interpersonal relationships. The goal of treatment is to help patients correct deficits in functioning so that they can cope better with everyday stress in the community. Training is usually carried out in a highly structured group setting and uses role-playing and feedback. Often, video-taping is used to facilitate learning. Skills are taught very slowly in small components repeated frequently, and positive attempts are reinforced. There is considerable evidence that social skills training is effective for schizophrenic patients (Wallace et al., 1980); however, there is less evidence that generalization of the newly acquired behaviors occurs.

Closely related to social skills training are problem-solving training as described by Kanfer and Goldstein (1975) and life management training (Hersen & Luber, 1977). The goals of both of these approaches are to help patients learn skills required to function effectively in the community. The problem-solving training focuses on cognitive function and helps the individual define a problem, formulate alternative solutions, make a decision, and verify the decision.

Day hospitals have sometimes used token economy systems to provide effective management, particularly in areas such as attendance and participation in programs. Token economy can provide instant feedback concerning progress that could help patients develop self-assessment skills.

Expressed emotion in families of schizophrenics has also been implicated in their relapse (Wallace et al., 1980). Various forms of practical, educationally oriented family intervention, as well as social skills training—both alone and in combination—have been shown to forestall relapse significantly (Hogarty et al., 1986; Leff & Vaughn, 1985). Hogarty et al. (1986) studied a patient-centered behavioral treatment and a psychoeducational family treatment. The family approach was designed as an education and management strategy intended to improve the emotional climate of the home while maintaining reasonable expectations for patient performance. Through the provision of formal education about the disorder and strategies for managing it more effectively, family members become allies in the treatment process as their anxiety and distress are decreased. More traditional attempts to promote disclosure, "insight," or direct modification of family systems, including the resolution of intergenerational and marital issues, were, for the most part, avoided. The goal was to reduce both the positive and negative symptoms of schizophrenia that might be associated with the extremes of stimulation contained in either the therapeutic process or family life. The principles of social skills training employed were those described above. Following hospital admission, 103 patients residing in high expressed emotion households who met research diagnostic criteria for schizophrenia or schizoaffective disorder were randomly assigned to a 2-year aftercare study of (1) family treatment and medication, (2) social skills training and medication, (3) their combination, or (4) a drug-treated condition. First-year relapse rates among those exposed to treatment demonstrate a main effect for family treatment (19%), a main effect for social skills training (20%), and an additive effect for the combined conditions (0%) relative to controls (41%). Effects are explained, in part, by the absence of relapse in any household that changed from high to low expressed emotion. Only the combination of treatment sustains a remission in households that remain high in expressed emotion. Continuing study, however, suggests a delay of relapse rather than prevention.

Liberman et al. (1986) also believe that family therapy, while reducing propensity for relapse, will not yield improved social vocational adjustment in patients without concomitant skills training. They also point out that the primary action of neuroleptics is on positive symptoms, and that social skills training has a direct effect on social competencies; therefore, the two treatment strategies for schizophrenia tend to complement each other.

The milieu itself provides a source of treatment, particularly for schizophrenic patients. The degree of stimulation can be titrated to meet the patient's needs. For schizophrenic patients in particular, certain environments actually may be toxic. Linn et al. (1979) showed that patients with symptoms of motor retardation, emotional withdrawal, and anxiety were a high-risk group for day treatment. Findings support differential effects of environments on patients who differ in their vulnerability. Ideally, one ought to be able to define characteristics of the psychological environment of the chronic schizophrenic that would protect against disorganization. It is suggested that process schizophrenics, who have nuclear, core, or poor premorbid histories, suffer from an inability to distinguish and filter out vast amounts of irrelevant stimuli. Too much stimulation results in a high level of arousal, which patients attempt to reduce by restricting their cognitive field to a size they can manage. Venables and Wing (1962) found hyperarousal to be related to withdrawal in chronic schizophrenics. Brown, Birley, and Wing (1972) suggested that when the patient is unable to withdraw, latent thought disorders manifest themselves in delusions or odd behavior. They also cautioned that too enthusiastic attempts at reactivating long-term patients have been shown to lead to sudden relapse of symptoms.

Along these same lines, May, Tuma, and Dixon (1976) pointed out that milieu therapy can have toxic, antitherapeutic effects, particularly when techniques and methods developed for neurotics and those with character disorders are indiscriminately applied to psychotic patients. In their review and critique of studies that combined drugs and sociotherapies in aftercare, they concluded that helping schizophrenics with limited social and vocational goals appeared to be of value, but they found no support for combining drug therapy with insight and deeper psychological understanding. It is possible that the less intensively personal and more object-focused activity therapies produce better outcomes than intensive interpersonal stimulation. Finding the environmental equilibrium between too much stimulation, which produces relapse, and too little stimulation, which fosters apathy, is a critical issue. Acute patients may need intensive programs utilizing group and individual therapies, and chronic patients may need a less intensive treatment focus and less stimulation in the environment.

Methods for matching patients to treatments in day hospitals are a major need. Hersen (1979) suggests that "Does partial hospitalization work?" is the wrong question to ask about day hospitals. The more appropriate question is "What treatment, by whom, is more effective for this individual?"

MATCHING PATIENTS AND TREATMENTS

Partial hospitals often have been accused of providing all types of treatment to all types of patients, with no attempts to match treatments to patient characteristics. Matching first requires some system of classifying needs of the patient and levels and types of treatments. Various matches could then be studied in regard to treatment efficacy. There have been a few attempts either to classify patients by some typology system or to classify environments in regard to what they offer.

McCreath (1986) suggested a patient typology for partial hospitals based on four variables: (1) ability to conform, (2) capacity for task management, (3) level of motivation, and (4) level of supervision. He believed that the patient population (case mix) has a major impact on the "personality" of milieu programs. Patients in a day center were rated high or low on the four variables and, when ratings were combined, six types emerged that described performance of patients in the milieu. The six types were then ranked according to how disruptive or supportive each was in the environment. Although no attempt was made to match patients and environments, the typology, based on patient behaviors, is one example of a classification system.

Capurso (1986) described a method, based on the cognitive-developmental literature, for changing the environment in order to stimulate motivation for participation in day hospital programs. Rather than simply trying to change the individual, goals can be directed toward changing environments as well. Since it is the interaction between person and environment that promotes development of cognitive structures, environmental manipulation provides optimal levels for psychological growth. The necessary and sufficient conditions for therapeutic change were described in areas of challenge, involvement, support, structure, and feedback. A program functions best when it is directed by a set of principles and a conceptual framework. The partial hospital has the potential for being a powerful treatment modality when variables such as these can be manipulated to meet the individual needs of a given patient.

Wing and Furlong (1986) discuss treating the severely disabled in the community and propose a patient classification system based on ratings of low, moderate, and high dependency needs in three areas: occupation, residence, and recreation. The term *dependency* indicates a level of need for care. There are many causes of high dependency, but usually it is associated with multiple impairments, social disadvantages, and adverse personal reactions. Because each person's pattern is unique (and often changes), each needs an individually oriented program of care. A stairway analogy is used to classify dependency. For example, residency need is rated on seven steps from low dependency (maintaining one's own home) to high need (placement in a secure unit). Staff who act as gatekeepers to services have to try to assess such factors and allocate priority to each. They also classify treatment environments according to open versus custodial settings, in regard to power and staff attitudes, boundaries, stigma, outside influences, and milieu. They point out that custodial care cannot be equated with inpatient care, nor open care with nonhospital alternatives, and that "restrictiveness" carries a connotation of arbitrary authority and may be unjustified. The proper question, they conclude, is whether help is being given that will reduce the causes of social disability to the minimum possible level and keep it there.

To help mental health professionals make informed decisions when matching specific treatments to specific patient characteristics, Klar, Frances, and Clarkin (1982) defined three kinds of partial hospitals—intensive care, chronic care, and rehabilitative care—and proposed selection criteria for referral to each model. The *intensive care* partial hospital is defined as the alternative to inpatient care and provides many of the same services as found on inpatient units. The intensive model provides diagnosis and assessment, stabilization of acute symptoms, and identification of precipitating environmental factors in the patient's illness. The goal will focus on short-term care, with transition to more definitive treatments after discharge from partial hospitalization. The *chronic care* model is characterized by lower expectations, high symptom tolerance, and a concrete and practical approach. There is no expected length of stay, and the door is always open for patients to return. The *rehabilitation* model lies between the other two types of programs and serves patients with severe impairments in social and vocational functioning who need more intensive treatment than can be found in the usual outpatient treatments. The goals, however, are for change, and there is low tolerance for disruptive symptoms. Treatment would again be time-limited but somewhat longer than for acute care. Patient classifications are provided in terms of relative indications, enabling factors, and relative contraindications for each of the models. For example, indications for intensive care are patients who otherwise would have to be admitted for acute psychotic care or supervised diagnostic tests and medications. Enabling factors are motivation to attend, sufficient organization or social network to ensure compliance, history of rapid treatment response to medication, and good outcome if treated previously in partial hospitalization. Contraindications include significant organic mental syndrome, suicidal/homicidal behavior, severe medical illness, requirement of 24-hour diagnostic tests, and other management problems. The question again arises as to whether a single center can accommodate all of these models or whether different models need to operate separately. This has not been resolved. As the authors point out, these classifications represent hypotheses to be tested. These kinds of tests are greatly needed.

INNOVATIONS AND FUTURE DIRECTIONS

One of the most interesting recent innovations in day hospitals was described by Gudeman, Shore, and Dickey (1983). A similar approach has been described by Ferber, Oswald, Rubin, Ungemack, and Schane (1985). In these programs, the day hospital becomes the entry point for all psychiatric services. For example, the day hospital in the Massachusetts Mental Health Center (Gudeman et al., 1983) was reorganized so that all psychiatric patients who were believed to require inpatient hospitalization are instead admitted directly to a day hospital program. The day hospital serves as the locus of care for the seriously ill who require hospitalization. Those who do not have a stable outside environment to which they can return at night sleep in a dormitory/inn on the center's premises. Patients who require 24-hour hospitalization because they are a danger to themselves or others are cared for in a psychiatric intensive care unit and returned to the day hospital as soon as they have improved.

The reorganization began by replacing the inpatient services with three components of psychiatric care, all located in the same or connected buildings. There were two day hospitals, each staffed with a psychiatrist, a chief resident and five first-year residents, nurses, mental health assistants, social workers, occupational and recreational therapists, and a psychologist. The day programs operated 8:00 a.m. to 4:00 p.m. 5 days a week. The second component was an intensive 28-bed inpatient unit under the direction of a psychiatric nurse/clinician. The third component was a domiciliary facility directed by a social work administrator and operated from 4:00 p.m. to 8:00 a.m. on weekdays and around the clock on weekends. The day hospital was the entry point for all patients and provided evaluation and offered treatments usually available for inpatients. Patients were assigned to first-year residents, and if 24-hour intensive care was necessary, the treatment responsibility remained with the day hospital psychiatric resident and social worker. This ensured continuity of care and discouraged dependency on intensive treatment. The dormitory/inn housed patients who required temporary residence as a transition to new living arrangements elsewhere or for those severely ill. It also provided brief respite care for families. On weekends, there were planned activities. Preliminary data on the program showed that inpatient care could be reduced and day hospital utilization increased without increasing average length of stay in the hospital or decreasing daily census. Cost of personnel was reduced. The inn provided cost-effective services for those who required shelter. Finally, different levels of care were provided in a cost-effective manner.

Although a number of studies, such as the one in Boston, have documented the clinical effectiveness and cost advantages of partial hospitals over other settings, future growth will be shaped to some degree by reimbursement by third-party insurers. Fink (1982) pointed out a number of clinical, administrative, and fiscal issues involving current partial hospital programming and the health care system in general that have led to limitations in reimbursements. Partial hospitals have described their programs as being too all-inclusive. Since the goals of third parties are to cover medical services that can be clearly defined and monitored, any lack of precision in defining services creates barriers to coverage. Another barrier is described as lack of standards that have left insurance companies without sufficient data to predict cost of care or number of individuals who will require payment of benefits. Fink urged a narrowing of the definition of partial hospital treatment and establishing standards that might imply levels of care, varying from intensive to transitional care, and with other levels separated out as those designed for rehabilitation or maintenance. He suggested further that standards include treatment plans, assessment and treatment services, staffing patterns, and clinical policies and procedures that address issues such as noncompliance, quality assurance, and utilization review. Prerequisites to pursuing third-party coverage are thus seen as being enhanced by redefinition of the scope of partial hospital services and development of detailed standards of treatment.

Another determinant of the future of partial hospitals lies with psychiatric practitioners. It has been found that most of the referrals from psychiatrists come from those who have had some experience with partial hospitals. Using the day hospital as a setting for residency training and affiliating partial hospitals with university medical center teaching programs could serve to change its image in the same way that the teaching nursing home model has been proposed for community nursing homes. Placing residents and medical students within the partial hospital could also draw on the possibility of involving community psychiatrists in the day hospital program as clinical teaching staff, and thereby could expose them to advantages that a day hospital has to offer.

Finally, the future of partial hospitals will also depend on research studies that are carefully designed to tease out effectiveness of the program as it relates to selecting the right patient for the right kind of treatment. Klar (1982) suggested that in an era that increasingly demands cost-effective, minimally restrictive treatments, partial hospitals make good common sense. He continues that partial hospitals provide a glimpse of what an effective, flexible outpatient program can offer many different patients, and concludes that recognition of their potential must be accompanied by a convincing body of scientific data. Otherwise, it will be hard to persuade third-party payers to reimburse programs and equally difficult to persuade reluctant colleagues to refer their patients to partial hospitals—regardless of the dictates of our common sense.

REFERENCES

Beigel, A., & Feder, S. (1970). Patterns of utilization in partial hospitalization. *American Journal of Psychiatry, 126*, 1267–1274.

Bellack, A. S., & Hersen, M. (Eds.). (1979). *Research and practice in social skills training.* New York: Plenum Press.

Brown, G. W., Birley, J. L. T., & Wing, J. K. (1972). Influence of family life on the course of schizophrenic disorders: A replication. *British Journal of Psychiatry, 121*, 242–258.

Caffey, E., Galbrecht, C., & Klett, C. (1971). Brief hospitalization and aftercare in the treatment of schizophrenia. *Archives of General Psychiatry, 24*, 81–86.

Capurso, R. J. (1986). Using a potent developmental environment as a means of improving attendance at a day-treatment center. *International Journal of Partial Hospitalization, 3*, 159–167.

Casarino, J. P., Wilner, M., & Maxey, J. T. (1982). American Association for Partial Hospitalization (AAPH) standards and guidelines for partial hospitalization. *International Journal of Partial Hositalization, 1*, 5–21.

Craft, M. (1959). Psychiatric day hospitals. *American Journal of Psychiatry, 116*, 251–254.

Davis, J., Lorei, T., & Caffey, E. (1978). An evaluation of the Veterans Administration day hospital program. *Hospital and Community Psychiatry, 29*, 297–302.

Dick, P., Cameron, L., Cohen, D., Barlow, M., & Ince, A. (1985). Day and full time psychiatric treatment: A controlled comparison. *British Journal of Psychiatry, 147*, 246–250.

Edwards, D., Yavis, R., & Mueller, D. (1979). Evidence for efficacy of partial hospitalization: Data from two studies. *Hospital and Community Psychiatry, 30,* 97–101.

Erickson, R. (1972). Length of stay and adjustment and role skill changes of day hospital patients. *VA Newsletter of Research Psychology, 14,* 31–33.

Ettlinger, R., Beigel, A., & Feder, S. (1972). The partial hospital as a transition from inpatient treatment: A controlled follow-up study. *Mt. Sinai Journal of Medicine, 39,* 251–257.

Falloon, I. R. H., & Talbott, R. E. (1982). Achieving the goals of day treatment. *Journal of Nervous and Mental Disease, 170,* 279–285.

Fenton, F., Tessier, L., & Struening, E. (1979). A comparative trial of home and hospital care. *Archives of General Psychiatry, 36,* 1073–1079.

Ferber, J. S., Oswald, M., Rubin, M., Ungemack, J., & Schane, M. (1985). The day hospital as entry point to a network of long-term services: A program evaluation. *Hospital and Community Psychiatry, 36,* 1297–1301.

Fink, E. B. (1982). Encouraging third-party coverage of partial hospitals. *Hospital and Community Psychiatry, 33,* 38–41.

Fink, E., & Heckerman, C. (1979). Predicting partial hospital treatment failures. In R. Luber, J. Maxey, & P. Lefkovits (Eds.), *Proceedings of the Annual Conference on Partial Hospitalization: 1978.* Boston: Federation of Partial Hospitalization Study Groups.

Fottrell, E. (1973). A ten year's review of the functioning of a psychiatric day hospital. *British Journal of Psychiatry, 123,* 715–717.

Glasscote, R., Kraft, A., Glassman, S., & Jepson, W. (1969). *Partial hospitalization for the mentally ill: A study of programs and problems.* Washington, DC: Joint Information Service.

Glick, I. D., Fleming, L., DeChillo, N., Meyerkopf, N., Jackson, C., Muscara, D., & Good-Ellis, M. (1986). A controlled study of transitional day care for nonchronically ill patients. *American Journal of Psychiatry, 143,* 1551–1556.

Greenblatt, M., York, R. H., & Brown, E. L. (1955). *From custodial to therapeutic care in mental hospitals.* New York: Russell Sage Foundation.

Gudeman, J. E., Shore, M. F., & Dickey, B. (1983). Day hospitalization and an inn instead of inpatient care for psychiatric patients. *New England Journal of Medicine, 308,* 749–753.

Guy, W., & Gross, G. (1967). Problems in the evaluation of day hospitals. *Community Mental Health Journal, 3,* 111–118.

Guy, W., Gross, M., Hogarty, G. E., & Dennis, H. (1969). A controlled evaluation of day hospital effectiveness. *Archives of General Psychiatry, 20,* 329–338.

Heineman, S., Yadin, L., & Perlmutter, F. (1975). A follow-up study of clients discharged from a day hospital aftercare program. *Hospital and Community Psychiatry, 26,* 752–753.

Hersen, M. (1979). Research considerations. In R. Luber (Ed.), *Partial hospitalization: A current perspective.* New York: Plenum Press.

Hersen, M., & Luber, R. (1977). Use of group psychotherapy in a partial hositalization service: The remediation of basic skill deficits. *International Journal of Group Psychotherapy, 27,* 361–376.

Herz, M. (1982). Research overview in day treatment. *International Journal of Partial Hospitalization, 1,* 33–44.

Herz, M., Endicott, J., & Spitzer, R. (1975). Brief hospitalization of patients with their families: Initial results. *American Journal of Psychiatry, 132,* 413–418.

Herz, M., Endicott, J., & Spitzer, R. (1977). Brief hospitalization: A two year follow-up. *American Journal of Psychiatry, 134,* 502–507.

Herz, M., Endicott, J., Spitzer, R., & Mesnikoff, F. (1971). Day vs. inpatient hospitalization: A controlled study. *American Journal of Psychiatry, 127,* 1371–1382.

Hogarty, G. E., Anderson, C. M., Reiss, D. J., Kornblith, S. J., Greenwald, D. P., Javna, C. D., & Madonia, M. J. (1986). Family psychoeducation, social skills training, and maintenance chemotherapy in the aftercare treatment of schizophrenia, I: One-year effects of a controlled study on relapse and expressed emotion. *Archives of General Psychiatry, 43,* 633–642.

Kanfer, F., & Goldstein, A. (1975). *Helping people change: A textbook of methods.* New York: Pergamon Press.

Kecmanovic, D. (1985). Post release adjustment of day and inpatients. *International Journal of Social Psychiatry, 31,* 74–79.

Klar, H. (1982). Partial hospitals: Refining the data. *Hospital and Community Psychiatry, 33,* 5.

Klar, H., Frances, A., & Clarkin, J. (1982). Selection criteria for partial hospitalization. *Hospital and Community Psychiatry, 33,* 929–933.

Kris, E. (1961). Prevention of rehospitalization through relapse control in a day hospital. In M. Greenblatt, D. Levinson, & G. Klerman (Eds.), *Mental patients in transition.* Springfield, IL: Charles C Thomas.

Leff, J. P., & Vaughn, C. E. (1985). *Expressed emotion in families.* New York: Guilford Press.

Liberman, R. P., Mueser, K. T., & Wallace, C. J. (1986). Social skills training for schizophrenic individuals at risk for relapse. *American Journal of Psychiatry, 143,* 523–526.

Linn, M. W., Caffey, E. M., Klett, J., Hogarty, G. E., & Lamb, H. R. (1979). Day treatment and psychotropic drugs in the aftercare of schizophrenic patients. *Archives of General Psychiatry, 36,* 1055–1066.

Mason, J. C., Louks, J. L., Burmer, G. C., & Scher, M. (1982). The efficacy of partial hospitalization: A review of recent literature. *International Journal of Partial Hospitalization, 1,* 251–269.

May, P. R. A., Tuma, A. H., & Dixon, W. J. (1976). Schizophrenia—A follow-up study of results of treatment: I. Design and other problems. *Archives of General Psychiatry, 33,* 474–478.

McCreath, J. (1986). A client-population typology for day programs. *International Journal of Partial Hospitalization, 3,* 137–146.

McDonnell, D. (1977). An evaluation of day centre care. *International Journal of Social Psychiatry, 23,* 110–119.

Meltzoff, J., & Blumenthal, R. (1966). *The day treatment center: Principles, application, and evaluation.* Springfield, IL: Charles C Thomas.

Michaux, M. H., Chelst, M. R., Foster, S. A., & Pruim, R. J. (1972). Day and full time psychiatric treatment: A controlled comparison. *Current Therapy Research, 14,* 279–292.

Michaux, M. H., Chelst, M. R., Foster, S. A., Pruim, R. J., & Dasinger, E. M. (1973). Post-release adjustment of day and full-time psychiatric patients. *Archives of General Psychiatry, 29,* 647–651.

Michaux, M., Chelst, M., Foster, S., & Schoolman, L. (1970). A controlled comparison of psychiatric day center treatment with full time hospitalization: An interim report. *Current Therapy Research, 12,* 627–638.

Moscowitz, I. S. (1980). The effectiveness of day hospital treatment: A review. *Journal of Community Psychology, 8,* 155–164.

Mosher, L. R., & Keith, S. J. (1980). Psychosocial treatment: Individual, group, family, and community support approaches. *Schizophrenia Bulletin, 6,* 10–41.

Niskanen, P. (1974). Treatment results achieved in psychiatric day hospital care: A follow-up of 100 patients. *Acta Psychiatrica Scandinavica, 50,* 401–409.

Penk, W. E., Charles, H. L., & Van Hoose, T. A. (1978). Comparative effectiveness of day hospital and inpatient treatment. *Journal of Consulting and Clinical Psychology, 46,* 94–101.

Rubins, J. (1976). Five-year results of psychoanalytic therapy and day care for acute schizophrenic patients. *American Journal of Psychoanalysis, 36*, 3–26.

Shafar, S. (1970). Follow-up of day patients. *British Journal of Psychiatry, 117*, 123–124.

Test, M. A., & Stein, L. L. (1978). Community treatment of the chronic patient: Research overview. *Schizophrenia Bulletin, 4*, 350–364.

Thompson, C. M. (1985). Characteristics associated with outcome in a community mental health partial hospitalization program. *Community Mental Health Journal, 21*, 179–188.

Turner, R. M., McGovern, M., Donneson, G., Sandrock, D., & Burstein, D. (1982). A naturalistic assessment of partial-hospital treatment. *International Journal of Partial Hospitalization, 1*, 311–326.

Tyrer, P. J., & Remington, M. (1979). Controlled comparison of day hospital and outpatient treatment for neurotic disorders. *Lancet, 1*, 1014–1016.

Vaughn, P. J. (1985). Developments in psychiatric day care. *British Journal of Psychiatry, 147*, 1–4.

Venables, P. H., & Wing, J. F. (1962). Level of arousal and the subclassification of schizophrenia. *Archives of General Psychiatry, 7*, 114–119.

Vidalis, A. A., & Baker, G. H. B. (1986). Factors influencing effectiveness of day hospital treatment. *International Journal of Social Psychiatry, 32*, 3–8.

Wallace, C. J., Nelson, C. J., Liberman, R. P., Aitchison, R., Lukoff, D., Elder, J., & Ferris, C. (1980). A review and critique of social skills training with schizophrenic patients. *Schizophrenia Bulletin, 6*, 43–63.

Washburn, S., & Vannicelli, M. (1976). A controlled comparison of day treatment and inpatient hospitalization. *Journal of Consulting and Clinical Psychology, 44*, 665–675.

Weiss, K. J., & Dubin, W. R. (1982). Partial hospitalization: State of the art. *Hospital and Community Psychiatry, 33*, 923–928.

Weldon, E., Clarkin, J. E., Hennessy, J. J., & Frances, A. (1979). Day hospital versus outpatient treatment: A controlled study. *Psychiatric Quarterly, 51*, 144–150.

Wilder, J., Levin, G., & Zwerling, I. (1966). A two-year follow-up evaluation of acute psychotic patients treated in a day hospital. *American Journal of Psychiatry, 122*, 1095–1101.

Wilkinson, G. (1984). Day care for patients with psychiatric disorders. *British Medical Journal, 288*, 1710–1711.

Wing, J. K., & Furlong, R. (1986). A haven for the severely disabled within the context of a comprehensive psychiatric community service. *British Journal of Psychiatry, 149*, 449–457.

Wortis, J. (1950). *Soviet psychiatry.* Baltimore: Williams & Wilkins.

8

Family Education

John F. Clarkin

INTRODUCTION

Providing information about the diagnosis and nature of schizophrenia to patients and their families seems such a reasonable (and ethical) procedure in the present climate that it is hard to imagine doing otherwise. However, this cross-sectional view would miss the paradigm shift that has occurred in the last several decades. It is only in the last 15 years that schizophrenia has come to be viewed as a disorder with prominent biological factors. Previously, the condition was seen as caused by the ills of society, or later by the interaction patterns of the family (Hatfield, 1987). Only as knowledge accrued concerning the biological factors in the illness was there a body of information to impart and a movement to do so.

In the 1960s and early 1970s, labeling (making psychiatric diagnoses) was seen as detrimental to the patients as they interacted with the family and their social world. Szasz was a loud, articulate, and often listened-to critic of the concept of mental illness. For him, mental illness was a myth because it was based upon an analogy between biological illnesses and problems in living that had no biological basis. It was his contention that the mistaken concept of mental illness resulted not only in confused thinking but in misuse of psychiatry (Szasz, 1960). More specific to schizophrenia and the family, many family theorists saw schizophrenia not as an illness condition but as a set of behaviors that results from interpersonal (family) struggles and triangles (Haley, 1969). If one assumes that the family is the cause of a condi-

---

JOHN F. CLARKIN • Department of Psychology, New York Hospital-Cornell Medical Center, 21 Bloomingdale Road, White Plains, N.Y. 10605.

tion or *is* the condition (Selvini, Boscolo, Cecchin, & Prata, 1978), then one will not label the patient but rather label the family as the locus of pathology, deviant, and/or the object to be changed. The family therapy movement has been against labeling or diagnosing of patients, for that was seen as scapegoating the patient, or as engaging in linear causality and missing the role that the sick behavior of the patient plays in stabilizing the whole family system (Wynne, Gurman, Ravich, & Boszormenyi-Nagy, 1982).

While not labeling the patient, family therapists have labeled the family as pathological, an orientation that is the subject of much bitter feeling among parents of schizophrenics. Ironically, the whole intent of the current movement to provide and explain the diagnosis of schizophrenia is to free the family from labeling on their own part—that is, attributing the behavior of the individual with schizophrenia to willful moral failure rather than to an illness condition. Accurate labeling, such as making a diagnosis of schizophrenia for patient and family, might assist in more productive coping rather than scapegoating.

But times have changed. Knowledge about the biology and stress-responsive nature of schizophrenia has progressed, and it is now possible to disseminate a body of information, not complete but growing, including probable mechanisms and biological parameters of schizophrenia. A quantum leap was made in the diagnostic system itself from DSM-II to DSM-III (and now DSM-III-R) with its observable, often behavioral criteria that are more reliable in assessment. Out of this changing social, political, scientific context came the rationale for different centers to develop what is called psychoeducation for patients with schizophrenia and their families.

Even in today's climate, however, there is not universal acceptance of the idea of delivering a dreaded diagnosis to a patient and family. In a recent survey (Green & Gantt, 1987), while 90% of the psychiatrists surveyed always or usually told the family and patient about an affective disorder diagnosis, only 76% told the family of the diagnosis of schizophrenia, and only 58% always or usually told the patient. Respondents' resistance to disclosing the diagnosis of schizophrenia included the lack of biological markers for the disorder, the fear that labeling stigmatizes, fear that patients and families lack competency to understand the meaning of the term, and fear of demoralizing patient and family. One should not naively ignore these fears, and possibly future research will give some answers to this debate.

Psychoeducation, narrowly defined, is the giving of information to the family and patient about a disorder and its etiology, symptoms, course, and treatment. Broadly defined (Anderson, Reiss, & Hogarty, 1986), psychoeducation is a whole approach to the long-term management of the disorder with educational workshops, guidelines for management, and other services. Since other chapters in this volume deal with aspects of the broader definition of psychoeducation, in this chapter we will review both the format and the educational content of psychoeducational programs in the narrow sense. The intent will be to provide the practicing clinician with the basic information and resources to begin such a procedure. In addition, we will review some of the empirical findings that relate to the impact of family education and suggest clinical guidelines.

There are a number of clinical research centers that have articulated and in some cases researched a psychoeducational approach (Anderson et al., 1986; Cozolino & Nuechterlein, 1986; Falloon, Boyd, & McGill, 1984; Leff & Vaughn, 1985; Snyder & Liberman, 1981). Since Anderson et al., Falloon et al., and Leff and Vaughn have not only researched their approach but also published the psychoeducational material in some detail, in this chapter we will concentrate on them. It should be noted, however, that in addition to those programs that have been put in writing, there are numerous clinical settings, especially hospitals with units that treat schizophrenic patients, that are utilizing pschoeducational methods in family group meetings and all-day workshops. It is our impression that settings using these approaches have found them very helpful and have received positive feedback from the participants.

Leff and Vaughn (1985) have a social treatment package for the schizophrenic and family that involves three components: education, a relatives' group, and individual family sessions. Anderson and colleagues (1986) have devised a treatment package that is composed of an initial survival skills workshop including psychoeducation, followed by regularly scheduled family sessions during the reentry phase for a year or more, and finally a social and vocational rehabilitation phase. Falloon and colleagues (1984) have likewise devised a multifaceted treatment program that includes psychoeducation, communication training, and problem-solving training. The similarities and differences should be noted. The programs vary in duration. The Leff program is the briefest one, covering some 20 weeks, while the Falloon and Anderson programs expand over several years' duration. All three programs introduce psychoeducation (in the narrow sense) at the beginning of the treatment package as a way to help the family conceptualize what is happening and to help shape the alliance between the mental health professionals and the family. As we will note in more detail later in the chapter, all three of these programs have been investigated and the results are quite promising. However, it is not always clear to what extent and in what precise manner the psychoeducational component is beneficial.

RATIONALE

It is quite interesting to follow the overlapping but somewhat different rationales for the provision of psychoeducation that the various clinical research groups have traversed. The rationale expressed by these groups provides an indication of the social context, both within the professional mental health world and in the world of the family members in today's society, that led to the current developments.

A rationale that came from the research community was based on the work of British investigators that began in the early 1960s (Brown, Monck, Carstairs, & Wing, 1962). Since the early studies showing that relapse of a schizophrenic family member is more likely in a family atmosphere characterized by criticism and overinvolvement (high expressed emotion or EE), Leff and Vaughn (1985) in England set out to lower EE by a psychosocial intervention package including psychoeducation. It was hypothesized that armed and supported with information about the etiology, symptoms, course, and management/treatment of schizophrenia, the family members might alter their behavior, especially those behaviors (high EE) that had been shown to be associated with higher relapse.

The rationale given by Anderson and colleagues in the United States is somewhat different, although related to that provided by researchers in England. In the mid- to late 1970s they began to suspect that the traditional approaches to "treating" families with a schizophrenic member were not only not helpful but actually injurious and antitherapeutic. Unstructured treatment approaches that stimulated expression of intense affect were noted to be correlated with increase in patient symptomatology. In the meantime, Hogarty et al. (1979) were involved with chemotherapy of schizophrenic patients and noted the relapse of many patients despite appropriate medication (e.g., 35% of patients on injectable fluphenazine decanoate). Evidence began to accumulate that the schizophrenic patient had a vulnerability to complex, vague, emotionally charged situations that seemed to trigger an emotional or cognitive dysregulation. Thus, the stage was set to articulate an intervention program composed of both medication and family support that was targeted to helping the patient and the family manage the specific deficits that the disorder involved.

Another rationale for psychoeducation came from the families themselves. In a questionnaire and interview study of members of the Schizophrenia Association of Greater Washington, Hatfield (1979) found that the families with a schizophrenic member were quite clear about what they perceived as their most salient need. Knowledge about the disease and practical techniques for coping with it were the first priorities.

More recently, Spaniol, Jung, Zipple, and Fitzgerald (1987) surveyed a national sample from the membership of the National Alliance for the Mentally Ill (NAMI). The subjects were predominantly white females, over 50 years of age, and highly educated. The patients were predominantly under 30 years of age, male, well-educated, unemployed, hospitalized more than five times with a diagnosis of schizophrenia. There was a large dissatisfaction with mental health services, especially treatment coordination, practical advice, information about the illness, emotional support, and referral assistance. In a parallel fashion, the families rated as their most important areas of need practical advice, information about the illness, and treatment coordination.

ASSUMPTIONS

Psychoeducational approaches have arisen with a group of common assumptions. McFarlane (1983, p. 10) points out that the new family psychoeducational approaches assume an important interaction between a specific deficit in the individual with schizophrenia and family variables. These therapists enlist the family as adjunct therapists with the goal of rehabilitation of the patient, rather than some more ambitious and vague goal of reversal of a hypothesized family schizophrenic process.

Likewise, Anderson (1983) has detailed the assumptions behind her psychoeducational program. These assumptions are worth noting because they form the foundation of both the content and the process of the education. The individual with schizophrenia is hypothesized to have a core deficit that increases his or her vulnerability to both internal and external stimuli. The patient is vulnerable to overstimulating home, work, and treatment environments. The major approaches to this vulnerability are the taking of medication and the careful management of the family environment so as to minimize overstimulation in this crucial environmental setting.

CONTENT OF FAMILY EDUCATION

While there is some variation in the educational content presented to the families in the different programs, there is a basic body of information that is communicated, including a discussion of the nature of schizophrenia (diagnosis, symptoms, etiology, and course of the illness), the treatment of schizophrenia (medication and family management), and the interaction of the family and schizophrenia (needs of patient and needs of family; Table 1).

DIAGNOSIS, SYMPTOMS, ETIOLOGY, AND COURSE

Most of the educational programs begin with a discussion of the diagnosis of schizophrenia. In their survival skills workshop Anderson et al., (1986) place schizophrenia in historical context with a discussion of early

Table 1. Content of Family Education

Anderson, Reiss, and Hogarty (1986)	Falloon, Boyd, and McGill (1984)	Leff and Vaughn (1985)
Schizophrenia: What is it?	Nature of schizophrenia	Diagnosis
History and epidemiology	Correcting misconceptions about schizo-	Symptomatology
The personal experience	phrenia	Etiology and course
The public experience	What, then, is schizophrenia?	Treatment
Psychobiology	Symptoms of schizophrenia	
Treatment of schizophrenia	Thought interference	
The use of antipsychotic medication	Delusions: False beliefs	
(how it works, why it is needed,	Hallucinations: False perceptions	
impact on outcome, side effects)	Unusual behavior	
Psychosocial treatments	Course of the illness	
Effects on course	Causes of schizophrenia	
Other treatments and management	Biological components	
The family and schizophrenia	Psychosocial components	
Needs of patient	Issues related to medication	
Needs of family	Rationale for maintenance on neuroleptics	
Common problems that patients and	Finding the optimal dose	
families face	Warning signals of relapse	
What the family can do to help	Side effects	
Revise expectations	Alcohol and drug abuse	
Create barriers to overstimulation		
Set limits		
Selectively ignore certain		
behaviors		
Keep communication simple		
Support medication regime		
Normalize family routine		
Recognize signals for help		
Use professionals		

descriptions down to current DSM-III criteria. The historical material is presented to give the audience a sense of the arbitrariness and limitations over time in understanding and classifying the symptoms of schizophrenia. It is then pointed out that the term *schizophrenia* is not a condemnation and a reason to despair, but rather a term that aids in communication. There is no ultimate test that gives a definitive diagnosis of schizophrenia, and, in fact, Anderson points out that some 10% of the patients in their program have a change in diagnosis over time.

Most programs also contrast what schizophrenia is with what it is not. The common myths (e.g., split personality, violence) are described and dispelled.

In the Anderson program, family members are next given information on the incidence and prevalence of schizophrenia in order to further the growing notion, which is often new to many family members, that they are not alone in their pain and frustration of dealing with this constellation of symptoms.

Most programs then describe in detail the common symptoms of schizophrenia, including thought disorder, delusions, hallucinations, withdrawal, and reduced feeling and affect. To get beyond a simply abstract understanding of the symptoms, both the Falloon and Anderson programs try to personalize the material. In the Falloon program, this is done by having the patient (who is present for the psychoeducation) and the family talk about which of these symptoms, and in what idiosyncratic ways, have been experienced by the patient. In the Anderson survival skills workshop, the patient is not present. Instead, the presenter uses autobiographical reports of the experience of schizophrenia, including the disturbing process of distraction, stimulus overload, intensified sensitivity to stimuli, and misperceptions of the environment.

In the Anderson survival skills workshop, this discussion of the personal and public symptoms of schizophrenia is followed by a presentation of the current understanding of the psychobiology of schizophrenia. This technical knowledge explained in terms appropriate for a lay audience with the use of visual aids (e.g., slides and photographs) is more extensive than in the other programs. An attention-arousal model of schizophrenic pathophysiology is described. The role of disturbance in neurotransmission is explained in some detail, and, simply put, it is suggested that too much dopamine and/or too many receptors may be causally related to the disturbances in attention and information processing. This gives a cognitive base for understanding some of the mechanisms underlying the day-to-day symptoms that are so obvious to the family members, and it provides a clear and concrete rationale for the subsequent use of medication that affects neurotransmission.

MEDICATIONS

Most programs have a detailed discussion of medications that are commonly used in the treatment of schizophrenia. The Falloon program emphasizes regular medication, the effectiveness of the neuroleptics, the effectiveness of low doses to protect from relapse, and the side effects of these medications. A very important discussion is the education of the family concerning the early warning signs of an impending psychotic episode and the need to alert the physician for possible change in medication.

Building upon their presentation of the pathophysiology of the illness, the Anderson program explains that all antipsychotic drugs block the action of certain neurotransmitters that play a role in normalizing the arousal level of the patient, and enable the patient to more appropriately attend to relevant environmental cues. Thus, family members have a rationale for medication usage that will assist them in encouraging patient compliance. The side effects of the medications are then explained to the family not only to give them this needed information but to enlist the family as a source of information about more subtle side effects that might be missed by the clinician.

Both the Falloon and Anderson programs talk about other substances that may be consumed by the patient with possible deleterious effects. After obtaining patient and family information regarding the use and abuse of alcohol and street drugs, Falloon and colleagues give information about the potential harmful effects of these chemicals with schizophrenics.

ETIOLOGY AND COURSE

One of the major goals of psychoeducation is to decrease the guilt of the family in presuming they have in some way caused the illness, and in developing a positive management alliance between the mental health personnel and the family. To this end, the discussion of the etiology, while confusing and not totally understood by anyone, is most germane and potent. The Anderson program emphasizes the genetic causes of the condition. The stress-diathesis model is presented. In the Falloon program it is stressed that both heredity and environment combine to influence the onset of schizophrenia. It is stressed that families do not cause schizophrenia but that the illness is a stress-responsive condition, and the family can play an important role in managing the stress on the patient and thus potentially improving the course of the illness.

THE FAMILY AND SCHIZOPHRENIA

The Anderson program gives the most extensive educational presentation concerning typical interaction between the family and the patient, and guidelines for how to cope with the situation. The common emotional responses of the family are discussed, including anxiety, guilt, stigma, embarrassment, frustration, anger, sadness, and loss. This is followed by a discussion of the common behavioral tactics that families try (often to no avail), such as coaxing and persuasion, attempting to make sense out of nonsensical communications, ignoring the patient's behaviors, providing constant supervision of the patient to the detriment of their own time, and ignoring the needs of other family members. This is followed by some guidelines that might help the family provide an atmosphere of delicate balance between too much and too little stimulation, a low-keyed but structured environment. Topics of discussion relevant to this goal include temporarily revising expectations, creating barriers to overstimulation, setting limits, selectively ignoring, keeping communication simple, supporting the patient's medication regimen, and recognizing signals for help.

EDUCATIONAL FORMAT

The format of the psychoeducation—that is, to whom is the education provided, in what location, for sessions of what frequency and duration, over what period of time—varies at the different centers (see Table 2). The Anderson group has a daylong survival skills workshop. Falloon and colleagues used two family sessions in the home for the psychoeducation component, the first session on the nature of schizophenia and the second ses-

Table 2. Format of Family Education

	Anderson, Reiss, and Hogarty (1986)	Fallon, Boyd, and McGill (1984)	Leff and Vaughn (1985)
Patient present	No	Yes	No
Group format	Yes	No	No
Held in home	No	Yes	Yes
Number of sessions	Daylong workshop	2	2
Timing of psycho-education	First	First	First
Education followed by:	Family sessions Social and vocational rehabilitation	Communication training Problem-solving skills	Relatives group Family therapy

sion on the issues related to medication. The number of sessions devoted to specific psychoeducation is usually two. The educational material can be presented either to a single family or to groups of three to four families. Some programs encourage the patient to be present and others do not. Patients are excluded from the Anderson survival skills workshop because it comes at the beginning of treatment when the patient is often not stabilized enough to attend and absorb a 7-hour meeting, and because family members at this early phase are perceived as more comfortable in discussing their anxieties and questions without patients present. In contrast, the Falloon program has the patient present for the psychoeducational presentation in order to use the patient as an important personal source of information about the symptoms and experience of the condition.

An important decision related to who should attend is the location of the psychoeducational presentation. Anderson et al. use a family group format at the hospital or institutional location. They argue that the group format is less threatening for the more shy and reticent family members, and it also helps families come out of their isolation in dealing with this illness. Right from the beginning the group setting allows families to compare experiences and develop a sense that they are not alone. They further point out that treatment is best done by a team of professionals, and this team is located in an institution. By holding the psychoeducational workshop at the institution, the home of the professional team, the family begins to develop a relationship with the team and its home base. In contrast, Falloon and colleagues chose to work with the individual family with the patient present in the family's home setting. They argue that families and patients are more relaxed in their own homes and that attendance by a wider group of family members is more likely if sessions are held in the home.

The style of presentation is usually a didactic one, and material can be presented via blackboard or slides, with handout material, or by similar methods. Programs vary as to the timing of psychoeducation from during the hospitalization of the patient, to following patient discharge, to when the patient has become stabilized on medication. Clearly, an important factor in the timing of the psychoeducational intervention is the availability of the patient and the family to the mental health system, and this often occurs during or immediately after a psychotic break that occasioned a hospitalization. However, one should probably also consider the impact of education in reference to the family's phase of coping with schizophrenia. Tessler, Killian, and Gubman (1987) have described nine phases in the family acceptance of the reality of the serious mental disorder. One could easily imagine differential family response to psychoeducation given the different phases of that cycle.

EMPIRICAL STUDIES OF PSYCHOEDUCATION

Psychoeducation is typically delivered as one part of a larger and multi-faceted treatment approach to the schizophrenic patient and family. Thus, while there is a growing number of studies that demonstrate the positive impact of various types of family intervention on the course of schizophrenia, there are few studies that delineate the precise impact of the psychoeducation itself.

There have been several investigations (Berkowitz, Eberlein-Fries, Kuipers, & Leff, 1984; McGill, Falloon, Boyd, & Wood-Siverio, 1983) on the rather straightforward question of whether and how much families increase their knowledge of schizophrenia following a psychoeducational program. McGill et al. (1983) provided two educational sessions in the home as part of a family treatment program to 39 patients and their families. Session 1 was focused on the nature of schizophrenia and Session 2 on medication. The amount of knowledge possessed by family members was assessed with a two-part questionnaire (open-ended questions and multiple-choice questions) at three specific times: baseline, 3 months, and 9 months. Parents who received the educational session possessed significantly more knowledge at 3 and 9 months, and there was no tendency for scores to decline over time.

Berkowitz et al. (1984) provided psychoeducation to relatives (classified as high and low EE) of hospitalized schizophrenic patients. The educational program consisted of two short talks in the home covering diagnosis, symptomatology, etiology, and treatment and course. Knowledge was assessed using a "knowledge interview," which was given at baseline, following the psychoeducation, and at follow-up 9 months after the patient's discharge. Berkowitz et al. (1984) found no differences at baseline between the high and low EE relatives. Following the education there was an increase in knowledge concerning diagnosis, symptomatology, and management of the illness. In addition, attitude changes emerged as related to EE in the relatives. While low EE relatives saw the patient as his or her usual self between illness episodes, the high EE relatives perceived the patient as always being sick and never having periods of relative normality.

The authors noted that the relatives retained only a small amount of what they had been taught. The absence of knowledge about the etiology of schizophrenia was quite pronounced, and all groups tended to retain their own personal views of the cause of the illness even after the psychoeducation. The major contribution of this research is that it begins to relate information and attitudes both prior to and after the learning experience with characteristics of the family members.

Barrowclough et al. (1987) have recently furthered our understanding of the nature and mechanisms of psychoeducation by distinguishing functional from nonfunctional knowledge. These investigators assessed not only the knowledge of the family about schizophrenia but also the *functional* knowledge—that is, knowledge that would have an impact upon the family's behavior toward the family member. There was a significant increase in knowledge following the educational program. Most interestingly, those family members who were rated low on criticism on the Camberwell Family Interview had significantly higher test scores (i.e., more knowledge) at both preeducation and posteducation testing. In contrast, relatives rated low on hostility or emotional overinvolvement did not show significant differences from those rated high on these variables.

This investigation is unique in two important aspects. First of all, it attempts to measure functional knowledge—that is, knowledge that is potentially instrumental in changing family members' behaviors toward the patient and not just abstract information. Second, there is an attempt to relate some characteristics of the family member to both preeducational knowledge and the amount of knowledge that is absorbed in the training program.

It has been our clinical experience that the impact of psychoeducation is different in regard to positive symptoms than it is in reference to the negative symptoms of schizophrenia. We have found families quite accepting of the idea that the positive symptoms are related to an illness and need understanding from the family and treatment. However, the acceptance of negative symptoms as part of an illness and not the "responsibility" of the patient and the annoyance level of these symptoms is a different matter. Hooley, Richters, Weintraub, and Neale (1987) hypothesize that patients' florid symptoms and marked behavioral excesses would more likely be perceived by their spouses as illness-caused and consequently associated with less marital discord than would negative symptoms. Consistent with this hypothesis, spouses of patients diagnosed as schizophrenic or affectively disordered with negative symptoms and impulse control deficits reported significantly lower levels of marital satisfaction than spouses of patients with positive symptoms.

FUTURE RESEARCH

It seems clear from the review of the research on the psychoeducational approach that these data are at a very primitive level of development. It is possible to assess the amount of information possessed before and after intervention by the individual members of the family. This leaves a number of questions unanswered. How does the information affect the patient's self-image, aspirations, hope for the future? While the individual family member may learn, how is this knowledge utilized by the family as a working unit? How does the knowledge influence the behavior of the individual and/or the family unit? How is the process of acquisition affected by characteristics of the individuals in the family (characteristics such as EE status, intelligence, SES) and characteristics of the family as a unit? Fears of the negative effects of labeling still exist. Is there any way that providing the diagnosis is harmful?

There are two lines of related research that so far have been ignored or forgotten by those investigating the impact of psychoeducation. Drawing on problem-solving literature in psychology and previous investigations of family problem-solving styles in families with a schizophrenic member, Reiss (1981) has investigated the problem-solving styles of families of normals, delinquents, and schizophrenics. While initially interested in the question of family cognitive style and the etiology of schizophrenia, Reiss (in the spirit of the times that has changed the approaches to family intervention that gave rise to family psychoeducation) shifted focus to concentrate on a general notion of the typologies of family information-seeking and digestion. However, his results (admittedly on very small N's) are interesting since they point up some factors that may be relevant to the clinical application of psychoeducation.

Reiss found that families with a schizophrenic member were characterized in a card-sorting task as relatively poor in group problem solving, consensus-sensitive during group problem solving, and ultimately functioning better as individuals than as a family group.

The Reiss investigation is important to the clinician implementing psychoeducation for several reasons. Enthusiasm for intervention programs with schizophrenics tends to decrease over time. There is currently great enthusiasm for the educational approach; it is innovative, fits the spirit of the age of consumer rights, and holds promise. However, as the novelty wears off and as it is found to be difficult with some families (not hard to imagine), enthusiasm may wane. We should anticipate this by investigations of how the information is absorbed differentially by individuals and family units. This will temper early enthusiasm and forestall premature disappointment. Furthermore, it may assist the clinician in doing psychoeducation differentially, depending upon the information-processing characteristics of the family involved.

Another tradition of research that has not been tapped by those in schizophrenia and psychoeducation is that of the medical sociologists. According to Mechanic (1978), it is consistently found in the illness-behavior research literature that individuals are more likely to take action for symptoms that in some fashion disrupt usual functioning. The individual's concept of help is affected as much by total functioning as by the nature of the symptoms that are experienced. Particularly relevant to psychiatric disorders, as well as to other physical disorders, is the way people attribute the locus of causality. Under what conditions, Mechanic asks, do people come to view their feelings or behavior as a consequence of a moral failure or of an illness for which they are not responsible? Attributions of causality by the afflicted persons, the families, and the health care delivery system have an important impact not only on the way the patients see themselves and their efforts at coping but also on the way they are perceived by the community in which they reside.

While there is currently much enthusiasm for the psychoeducational approach with some rationale, as mentioned earlier in this chapter, there is no overall model that helps to put the intervention in an explanatory framework. Recently, Hooley (1987) has articulated an attributional model for the explanation of high EE behavior that is quite relevant to the use of psychoeducation as an intervention strategy. Faced with schizophrenia (or other major psychiatric disorders), the family members must attribute the cause of the condition to an internal (blaming the patient) or an external (e.g., illness) cause. Data suggest that low EE families do not doubt the legitimacy of the patient's illness status, while high EE families tend to make internal attributions about the causes of the deviant behaviors. High EE behavior may, in fact, be efforts to get the patient to change behaviors attributed to the voluntary control of the patient. It is particularly negative symptoms, which typically involve an absence of normal functions and are thus more likely to be perceived as under voluntary control, that in this illness-attribution model would be associated with relatively high levels of family distress and EE.

Another interesting feature of this attributional model of EE is the prediction of which families will and will not benefit (possibly even be adversely affected) from psychoeducation. Toxic levels of EE may be reduced by psychoeducation that attributes the patient's behavior, especially negative symptom behavior, to an illness rather than to an internal, voluntary cause. However, in cases where the patient–family interaction was premorbidly poor, education about the illness without other interventions would be unlikely to be very successful. Furthermore, in cases where the family is overinvolved with the patient, education about the illness where relatives already hold strong beliefs about the illness model might simply foster more overinvolvement.

INDICATIONS

Given the state of the art in psychoeducation, what are the indications and contraindications for the clinical use of this approach with families having a schizophrenic member? First of all, with a patient clearly diagnosed as schizophrenic, there are data suggesting that families do increase their knowledge through a psychoeducational program, and that family intervention programs including psychoeducation lead to fewer relapses and hospitalizations in the patients.

Data to date do not yield any contraindications for the use of psychoeducation with the family of a schizophrenic member. As noted before, there were fears that labeling would further scapegoat the patient and solidify toxic family interaction involving the patient. There is no evidence to date of such deleterious effects, and the fears that labeling of patients would lead to further scapegoating seems unfounded. In the studies to date, the patients were carefully diagnosed, their symptoms were chronic and obvious to family members before the giving of a diagnosis, and the family members seemed relieved and assisted by the recognition of the disorder. Investigators have assumed that information would improve the attitudes of the family toward the patient, reduce family guilt and hostility, and stimulate realistic expectations of the patient. A critic and disbeliever might note that most of the investigators of psychoeducation to date seem inclined to perceive it as beneficial, and they may have not measured or observed subtle deleterious effects.

There may, of course, be families that resist the education or are unable to respond to the information, and the explication of those subgroups needs further study. Those subgroups may well need a different educational format than what has been established so far.

We are suggesting that psychoeducation is indicated for every case when the diagnosis of schizophrenia is relatively clear. It seems ethically appropriate for mental health professionals to provide as much information as possible to patients and families who are dealing with this serious and often chronic condition.

CLINICAL GUIDELINES

In light of the brief history of psychoeducation and the few research programs that have been done to date, it is possible to summarize a few clinical guidelines for those who intend to use this approach in their own clinical setting:

1. The content of the education is quite uniform across research groups, and available in publications for professionals to use (see Anderson et al., 1986; Falloon et al., 1984; Leff & Vaughn, 1985). In addition, there are lists of books written for the layperson that can be made available to those families seeking further information (e.g., Appendix A in Anderson et al., 1986).

2. The question arises as to when in the course of the disorder and the phase of a single-episode psychoeducation is most effectively introduced. It appears that earlier in the course of the disorder is better than later, before the family has had years to form their own theories of etiology. But the clinician has little control over when the family is available in the course of the disorder for psychoeducation.

More under the control of the clinician is the point during the present episode to begin psychoeducation. Berkowitz et al. (1984) argue that the anxiety and disruption of the hospitalization itself may distract from the intake of information. However, more data are needed on this question. Practicality (e.g., getting to the families available during a hospitalization episode) may win out over theoretical timing.

3. As Tarrier and Barrowclough (1986) have emphasized in their interactional model, there is a clinical need to take into account the patients' and relatives' own idiosyncratic views of the etiology of the disorder. Before giving information, it is important to find out the prevailing view or counterinformation of the particular family. Families who have dealt with the illness for a long time without the assistance of psychoeducation will probably have the most crystallized views.

4. While a number of authors mentioned previously in this chapter have utilized questionnaires or semistructured interviews both before and after a psychoeducational intervention to assess the impact of the interview, it may be *clinically* useful for other centers to assess the knowledge base at baseline as part of the educational package itself. Such baseline assessment may help focus the family members and highlight both for themselves and for the clinicians their areas of misinformation or lack of information. In this regard, it is interesting to review the knowledge interviews and questionnaires as published by the clinical researchers. Berkowitz et al. (1984) described a knowledge interview that includes 21 open-ended questions around topics including diagnosis, symptomatology, etiology, course of the condition and prognosis, medication, and wish of relative for more information.

Cozolino and Nuechterlein (1986) developed the UCLA "family interview," which was done following the educational interviews and therefore may be less applicable to baseline assessment. The questions vary in format, including asking patients to rate the amount of information they had prior to the sessions and open-ended questions. The interview questions cover previous knowledge, general impression of the UCLA psychoeducational program, diagnosis, etiology, effects of stress, symptomatology, family's role in rehabilitation, family etiology, medication, prognosis/recovery period, practical tips, and relating to doctors, clinical staff, other professionals, and other participants. These questions range in content from asking what information they had prior to the sessions, what information stands out from the psychoeducation, feelings about such things as disturbance about prognosis, and recollection of useful tips for management. And finally, Barrowclough et al. (1987) provided their knowledge about a schizophrenia interview (KASI) that was administered to each relative individually prior to and after psychoeducation. As with the Berkowitz and McGill instruments, diagnosis, symptomatology, etiology, medication, course, and prognosis and management were covered. However, in addition, a section on patient management with open-ended questions was utilized and rated to provide a quantification of the functional use of knowledge in patient management. Ratings range from 1 for negative value (relative reports information that may lead to potential detrimental acts in the patient's management) to 4 for positive value (wide knowledge that may lead to potential valuable actions in the patient's management).

5. The knowledge content that is provided should not be too general, theoretical, and factual, but should be specific and functional. Generalized knowledge is not found to be as useful as that which is applied to the specific family. The family often does not want general theories but rather prefers concrete guidelines. Furthermore, as Tarrier and his investigators have pursued, functional knowledge is probably more important than just knowledge *per se.*

6. Both the amount of information and the absorption rate of the material will vary across families. This, plus the interactional model mentioned in number 1, suggest that the psychoeducation must be tailored to the needs, perceptions, history, and experience of the particular family.

7. Psychoeducation in the narrow sense is not adequate in and of itself but should be integrated into a total management approach for the family and their ill member. The three major psychoeducational programs presented in this review do not stand alone but are embedded in larger programs, including communication training, problem solving, reentry, and later vocational foci. Families need to use the information, then come back and discuss some more. Most programs combine psychoeducation with skill development (e.g., Falloon) and specific family management guidelines (e.g., Anderson). Just as one cannot learn to play tennis by talking about it, one also needs to practice the management skills.

However, if local resources (e.g., a general hospital with facilites for brief hospitalization) are limited, psychoeducation for family and patient may be useful even delivered by itself. It may provide an introduction for the family so that they can seek further assistance when needed.

8. Clinically, questions do arise as to what form of psychoeducation to use when the diagnosis of the patient is uncertain (e.g., schizophreniform vs. schizophrenia, and affective disorder vs. schizophrenia vs. schizoaffective disorder). One alternative is to address and explain the uncertainty about the diagnosis in the psychoeducational material itself (Anderson et al., 1986).

9. There is no current reason to assume that the psychoeducational

approach need be limited to schizophrenics and their families. Other biolog-ically based disorders, such as bipolar disorder and recurrent depressions (e.g., Jacob, Frank, Kupfer, Cornes, & Carpenter, 1987), are likely candi-dates. The extent to which other disorders can be so addressed remains to be seen.

10. Since schizophrenia is a chronic disorder with the prospect of ups and downs, an important clinical element in the treatment is the develop-ment and nourishing of a therapeutic alliance between patient/family and clinician. Families today do not want a therapist who will assess and diagnose them as part of a systems problem. Families want a collaborative relationship in which they are supported in their efforts to cope. The psychoeducational approach provides the clinician with a method for initially approaching a family and shaping a collaborative enterprise. The search for a culprit is minimized and countered by information that decreases guilt and gives the family a handle on coping with the chronic condition of the patient.

REFERENCES

Anderson, C. M. (1983). Psychoeducational program for families of patients with schizophrenia. In W. R. McFarlane (Ed.), *Family therapy in schizophrenia* (pp. 99–116). New York: Guilford Press.

Anderson, C. M., Reiss, D. J., & Hogarty, G. E. (1986). *Schizophrenia and the family: A practitioner's guide to psychoeducation and management.* New York: Guilford Press.

Barrowclough, C., Tarrier, N., Watts, S., Vaughn, C., Bamrah, J. S., & Freeman, H. L. (1987). Assessing the functional value of relatives' knowledge about schizophrenia: A preliminary report. *British Journal of Psychiatry, 151,* 1–8.

Berkowitz, R., Eberlein-Fries, R., Kuipers, L., & Leff, J. (1984). Educating relatives about schizophrenia. *Schizophrenia Bulletin, 10,* 418–429.

Brown, G. W., Monck, E. M., Carstairs, G. M., & Wing, J. K. (1962). The influence of family life on the course of schizophrenic illness. *British Journal of Prevention and Social Medi-cine, 16,* 55.

Cozolino, L. J., & Nuechterlein, K. (1986). Pilot study of the impact of a family education program on relatives of recent-onset schizophrenic patients. In M. J. Goldstein, I. Hand, & K. Hahlweg (Eds.), *Treatment of schizophrenia: Family assessment and intervention* (pp. 129–144). New York: Springer-Verlag.

Falloon, I. R. H., Boyd, J. L., & McGill, C. W. (1984). *Family care of schizophrenia: A problem-solving approach to the treatment of mental illness.* New York: Guilford Press.

Green, R., & Gantt, A. (1987). Telling patients and families the psychiatric diagnosis: A survey of psychiatrists. *Hospital and Community Psychiatry, 38,* 666–668.

Haley, J. (1969). Toward a theory of pathological systems. In G. H. Zuk & I. Boszormenyi-Nagy (Eds.), *Family therapy and disturbed families* (pp. 11–27). Palo Alto: Science and Behavior Books.

Hatfield, A. B. (1979). The family as partner in the treatment of mental illness. *Hospital and Community Psychiatry, 30,* 338–340.

Hatfield, A. B. (1987). Families as caregivers: A historical perspective. In A. B. Hatfield &

H. P. Lefley (Eds.), *Families of the mentally ill: Coping and adaptation* (pp. 3–29). New York: Guilford Press.

Hogarty, G. E., Schooler, N. R., Ulrich, R. F., Mussare, F., Herron, E., & Ferro, P. (1979). Relapse analyses of a two year controlled study of fluphenazine decanoate and fluphenazine hydrochloride. *Archives of General Psychiatry, 36,* 1283–1294.

Hooley, J. M. (1987). The nature and origins of expressed emotion. In K. Hahlweg & M. J. Goldstein (Eds.), *Understanding major mental disorder: The contribution of family interaction research* (pp. 176–194). New York: Family Process Press.

Hooley, J. M., Richters, J. E., Weintraub, S., & Neale, J. M. (1987). Psychopathology and marital distress: The positive side of positive symptoms. *Journal of Abnormal Psychology, 96,* 27–33.

Jacob, M., Frank, E., Kupfer, D., Cornes, C., & Carpenter, L. (1987). A psychoeducational workshop for depressed patients, family, and friends: Description and evaluation. *Hospital and Community Psychiatry, 38,* 968–972.

Leff, J., & Vaughn, C. (1985). *Expressed emotion in families.* New York: Guilford Press.

McFarlane, W. R. (1983). Introduction. In W. R. McFarlane (Ed.), *Family therapy in schizophrenia.* New York: Guilford Press.

McGill, C. W., Falloon, I. R. H., Boyd, J. L., & Wood-Siverio, C. (1983). Family educational intervention in the treatment of schizophrenia. *Hospital and Community Psychiatry, 34,* 934–938.

Mechanic, D. (1978). *Medical sociology* (2nd ed.). New York: Free Press.

Reiss, D. (1981). *The family's construction of reality.* Cambridge, MA: Harvard University Press.

Selvini, M., Boscolo, L., Cecchin, E., & Prata, G. (1978). *Paradox and counterparadox.* New York: Jason Aronson.

Snyder, K., & Liberman, R. (1981). Family assessment and intervention with schizophrenics at risk for relapse. In M. J. Goldstein (Ed.), *New developments in interventions with families of schizophrenics* (pp. 49–60). San Francisco: Jossey-Bass.

Spaniol, L., Jung, H., Zipple, A. M., & Fitzgerald, S. (1987). Families as a resource in the rehabilitation of the severely psychiatrically disabled. In A. B. Hatfield & H. P. Lefley (Eds.), *Families of the mentally ill: Coping and adaptation* (pp. 167–190). New York: Guilford Press.

Szasz, T. S. (1960). The myth of mental illness. *American Psychologist 15,* 113–118.

Tarrier, N., & Barrowclough, C. (1986). Providing information to relatives about schizophrenia: Some comments. *British Journal of Psychiatry 149,* 458–463.

Tessler, R., Killian, L., & Gubman, G. (1987). Stages in family response to mental illness: An ideal type. *Psychosocial Rehabilitation Journal, 10*(4), 3–16.

Wynne, L. C., Gurman, A., Ravich, R., & Boszormenyi-Nagy, I. (1982). The family and marital therapies. In J. M. Lewis & G. Usdin (Eds.), *Treatment planning in psychiatry* (pp. 227–285). Washington, DC: American Psychiatric Association.

9

Behavioral Family Therapy

KIM T. MUESER

HISTORICAL INTRODUCTION

The family has long been thought to play a critical role in the etiology and course of schizophrenia. Early formulations based on psychoanalytic theory postulated that schizophrenia emerged as a defense against hostile or rejecting parental attitudes. Sullivan (1927) was one of the first pioneers to emphasize the interpersonal nature of schizophrenia and to explore the role of the family. He attempted to treat the illness by recreating the family in an inpatient setting, in order to provide patients with emotional experiences that would presumably correct early pathological family interactions. Fromm-Reichmann (1948) conducted extensive individual treatment with schizophrenic patients, and introduced the term *schizophrengenic mother* to describe a pattern of overbearing, emotionally insecure behavior observed in the mothers of some patients. While many of these speculations were not supported by later research, they served to draw attention to the families of schizophrenic patients and initiated the first systematic research into family factors and schizophrenia.

Research and treatment programs that evolved from the work of Sullivan, Fromm-Reichmann, and others continued to focus on the role of the family in the development of the illness. Bateson, Jackson, Haley, and Weakland (1956) theorized that children who are habitually exposed to "double-bind" messages (i.e., a communication from an important person in which one part of the communication contradicts another part, such as a

---

KIM T. MUESER • Department of Psychiatry, Medical College of Pennsylvania at EPPI, 3200 Henry Avenue, Philadelphia, Pennsylvania 19129.

mother saying, "I love you," while she scowls and pushes the child away) learn to avoid punishment by responding incomprehensibly, leading to the inability to distinguish meaning and, hence, schizophrenia.

Lidz, Fleck, and Cornelison (1965) extensively studied 17 families containing a schizophrenic member, and concluded that *all* the families were seriously disturbed, although a single pattern of pathological behavior was not identified. Lidz et al. believed that the families provided too little nurturance and structure to enable the formation of a stable personality, resulting in schizophrenia. Furthermore, such families were observed to have a high rate of marital discord, and to transmit "irrationality" to their offspring by denying obvious realities in order to subjugate the child's needs to that of the parent(s). Bowen (1961) also emphasized poor marital adjustment; he reasoned that schizophrenia develops as a consequence of immature parents' forcing their children to remain immature through adolescence and adulthood, bolstering the parents' self-esteem and preserving their marriage.

Wynne, Ryckoff, Day, and Hirsch (1958) identified the "pseudo-mutuality" of families with a schizophrenic person as a shared attempt to conceal serious conflict, inhibiting the child from establishing his or her own individual identity. They observed that the boundaries constraining the behavior of members of such families were like a "rubber fence," expanding when necessary but then constricting to pull members closer to the family, limiting external influences perceived as threatening the integrity of the family unit. Later, Wynne and Singer (1963) focused on the communication of thought disorder from parents to their children, using the term *communication deviance* to describe the "amorphous" or "fragmented" quality of family interactions with a schizophrenic.

Theories of the family's role in the development of schizophrenia stimulated systematic hypothesis testing and explorative trials of family therapy. As briefly summarized below, research failed to support the role of the family as a *cause* of schizophrenia, and instead pointed to a larger role for biological factors:

1. The proposition that families cause schizophrenia had difficulty explaining why schizophrenia tends to develop in one offspring, leaving other siblings relatively unscathed. Studies of communication style between parents and a schizophrenic offspring compared with a healthy sibling have not revealed expected differences (e.g., Waxler & Mischler, 1971). The incidence of childhood trauma has not been found to differ between schizophrenics and their siblings, although retrospective research suggests that the preschizophrenic may be more sensitive to such events (Prout & White, 1956). Other retrospective research has indicated that some preschizo-

phrenics manifest a variety of problems early in life. This includes pre- and postnatal complications, learning problems in school, and poorer social competence, suggesting that constitutional factors may predispose some children to schizophrenia (Lewine, Watt, Prentky, & Fryer, 1980; Pollack, Woerner, Goodman, & Greenberg, 1966).

2. The assumption that communication deviance in families with a schizophrenic member is responsible for the illness is unwarranted. Disordered communication or family strife could easily reflect the disruptive impact of the illness itself on the family, rather than the converse (e.g., Waxler, 1974). In addition, problems in communication have been found in families with a nonschizophrenic, mentally ill member (e.g., Farina & Holzberg, 1968), showing that disturbances in family communication are not specific to schizophrenia.

3. The accumulation of data from studies of twins and adopted-away offspring supporting a genetic contribution to schizophrenia (e.g., Farmer, McGuffin, & Gottesman, 1987; Tienari et al., 1985) made familial etiological theories untenable. Some researchers continue to look for communication patterns that may increase risk to develop schizophrenia in presumably vulnerable persons (e.g., Goldstein, 1985; Singer, Wynne, & Toohey, 1978), but faulty family communication is no longer viewed as *causing* the illness.

4. Family interventions based on theories of familial etiology failed to demonstrate any significant benefits (e.g., Massie & Beels, 1972). Terkelsen (1983) has argued that these therapies can be destructive by alienating family members from participating in their relative's treatment.

As evidence against the role of the family in the development of schizophrenia accumulated, there were changes in clinical and research priorities. The deinstitutionalization movement in the late 1950s and early 1960s, spurred on by the discovery of antipsychotic medications, resulted in increasing numbers of schizophrenic patients' returning to live at home or in community rehabilitation residences. Since the majority of these patients remained symptomatic and periodically required rehospitalizations, the search began for environmental influences on the *course*, rather than the *cause*, of the illness. The most significant research paradigm suggesting that the family may affect the course of schizophrenia concerns family "expressed emotion."

EXPRESSED EMOTION

The potential influence of such environmental factors as negative family affect on the course of schizophrenia was discovered serendipitously by

Brown and his colleagues (Brown, Carstairs, & Topping, 1958). Brown et al. found that male schizophrenics returning from a psychiatric hospital to live with siblings, distant relatives, or in hostels had better outcomes than patients returning to parental homes or their wives. A second study replicated the favorable effect of patients' living with siblings as compared with parents or wives (Brown, Monck, Carstairs, & Wing, 1962). Furthermore, the worse prognosis of schizophrenics living with their parents or spouses was not due to any differences in the severity or chronicity of their illness. Brown et al. hypothesized that patients living with close relatives might be exposed to higher levels of negative affect or intrusiveness, predisposing them to symptom relapses.

To evaluate this possibility, Brown and Rutter (1966; Rutter & Brown, 1966) constructed the Camberwell Family Interview to assess the affective climate of families with a psychiatric patient. The Camberwell Family Interview is a semistructured interview conducted with an individual relative of a patient who has recently been admitted to a hospital for treatment. This 1- to 2-hour interview is tape-recorded and later rated for expressed emotion (EE) by a trained rater. EE refers to the expression of critical, hostile, and/or emotionally overinvolved (e.g., dramatic, self-sacrificing) feelings about the patient. Ratings are made primarily on the basis of voice tone (e.g., pitch, emphasis, loudness), with content being of secondary importance. EE is not unique to families with a schizophrenic patient, and it can influence the course of other disorders as well, such as depression (Hooley, Orley, & Teasdale, 1986; Vaughn & Leff, 1976). Over seven carefully controlled, prospective, cross-culturally replicated studies have demonstrated that high levels of EE in one or more family members increases a schizophrenic's risk for relapse following hospitalization (e.g., Brown, Birley, & Wing, 1972; Karno et al., 1987). Schizophrenic patients returning to live in high EE households (defined as the presence of at least one high EE relative) are more than twice as likely to relapse than are patients returning to low EE homes. As with Brown's earlier studies, premorbid characteristics and severity of illness do not account for the differences in outcome (Miklowitz, Goldstein, & Falloon, 1983).

EE is rated on the basis of an interview with a key relative *in the absense* of the patient. High EE relatives are assumed to convey their negative feelings or emotional overinvolvement directly to the patient, who may lack the necessary skills to deflect these stressful communications. Some evidence supports the construct validity of measures of family EE. High EE relatives have been found to express more criticism and to be more intrusive in family problem-solving discussions with their schizophrenic offspring than low EE relatives (Miklowitz, Goldstein, Falloon, & Doane, 1984; Strachan,

Goldstein, & Miklowitz, 1986; Strachan, Leff, Goldstein, Doane, & Burtt, 1986).

The findings that EE is predictive of relapse in schizophrenics stimulated the first efforts to modify family EE through behavioral (Falloon et al., 1985) and psychoeducational approaches (Anderson, Hogarty, & Reiss, 1980; Leff, Kuipers, Berkowitz, Eberlein-Vries, & Sturgeon, 1982). However, the apparent role of EE in precipitating relapse must be viewed in the broader context of the family's response to the patient's illness. Similar to patients who may withdraw as a strategy to cope with stressful interactions with family members, relatives may resort to frequent criticism or extreme attempts to control as a means by which to cope with and improve the patient's symptomatic behavior. The burden of schizophrenia on the relatives must be addressed to underscore the need for family therapy that improves both patient *and* family functioning.

FAMILY BURDEN

Families have assumed a greater role in caring for chronic mental patients since deinstitutionalization. Goldman (1982) has estimated that 65% of patients return to live with their family after a psychiatric hospitalization. As a result, schizophrenic patients with varying degrees of residual symptoms often disrupt family life with their enigmatic behavior, requiring special accommodation at the cost of engendering resentment and despair in their relatives.

The effects of schizophrenia on the family have been described in surveys (Creer and Wing, 1974; Hatfield, 1978) and first-person accounts (Dearth, Labenski, Mott, & Pellegrini, 1986). Family members must develop strategies for coping with such diverse problems as medication management, aggressive or inappropriate behavior, poor self-care, and pronounced social withdrawal in their schizophrenic relatives (Spaniol, 1987). The negative symptoms of schizophrenia, such as apathy, withdrawal, and anhedonia, are particularly distressful to family members and are more likely to provoke criticism than are positive symptoms, such as delusions and hallucinations (Leff & Vaughn, 1985). The dissatisfaction of family members with patients' negative symptoms reflects the visible presence of these symptoms at home, which tend to be stable over time and to remit only slowly (Kay & Opler, 1987; Pogue-Guile & Harrow, 1985). Even when positive symptoms are present, they are not always apparent to family members, unlike the more prominant negative symptoms. The importance of deficit symptoms of schizophrenia to relatives is illustrated in a survey of 52 family members

(McElroy, 1987). These members reported that the most problematic patient behaviors were: (1) inability to achieve his or her potential, (2) lack of motivation, (3) inability to prepare for a vocation, (4) inability to work, (5) inability to adhere to or develop a predictable schedule (McElroy, 1987, p. 235).

Living with a symptomatic patient can disrupt the social networks of relatives, increase their vulnerability to physical illnesses because of stress, and create a range of negative emotions, including embarrassment, guilt, anxiety, depression, and anger. Successful family therapy must both reduce the burden of the illness on the family and allievate stress on the patient. Through work with the family as an extended part of the patient's own treatment team the rehabilitative potential of the family can be harnessed (Evans, Bullard, & Solomon, 1961; Kuipers & Bebbington, 1985) and more effective strategies for managing common problems and achieving goals can be taught.

BEHAVIORAL FAMILY THERAPY

THEORETICAL RATIONALE

The stress-vulnerability-coping skills model of schizophrenia (Zubin & Spring, 1977) serves as a guide for educational and behavioral interventions with families. This model postulates that individuals predisposed to schizophrenia have a *psychobiological vulnerability* to manifest symptoms when exposed to sufficient amounts of stress. This vulnerability is assumed to be determined primarily by genetic and early maturational factors, and it is reflected by such indices as poor information-processing ability and heightened autonomic reactivity (e.g., Nuechterlein & Dawson, 1984).

Environmental stress impinges on an individual to increase his or her vulnerability to the symptoms of schizophrenia, which can cause symptom exacerbations requiring temporary hospitalization. Some patients have a high level of vulnerability and are continuously symptomatic. Even with chronically ill patients stress can worsen the symptoms, necessitating increased medication. Stressors are environmental events or contingencies that require persons to adapt in order to minimize negative consequences. Common stressors that can increase vulnerability to schizophrenic symptoms include family EE, life events, and demanding or intensive psychosocial treatment (e.g., Drake & Sederer, 1986). Just as overstimulating environments can be stressful, an unstructured or socially impoverished setting can also worsen symptoms.

Coping skills or social skills mediate the negative effects of stress on vulnerability to schizophrenia. Social skills are behaviors that enable people to achieve goals and reduce stress effectively. Stress can be minimized either by pinpointing and eliminating the source of the stress itself (e.g., effective problem solving) or by coping more effectively with its noxious effects (e.g., stress management techniques). Thus, the outcome of schizophrenia is determined by the balance of biological vulnerability and environmental stress, with patient social skill mediating the noxious effects of stress.

The implications of the stress-vulnerability-coping skills model for treatment are that antipsychotic medications lower patient vulnerability and are usually essential to the treatment of schizophrenia. Social skills training can improve patients' ability to manage stress and achieve goals, lowering their vulnerability to symptoms. Behavioral family therapy strives to lower negative affect when it is present in the family and to improve the coping skills of all family members, including the patient. Through enhancement of the ability of the family to deal effectively with stress and achieve personal goals, the patient's prognosis should improve owing to reduced exposure to stress. Just as family members become more skillful, patients too may improve their social skills in family sessions, increasing their own ability to buffer stress and minimize symptoms.

OVERVIEW OF BEHAVIORAL FAMILY THERAPY

The model of behavioral family therapy presented here was developed over the past 15 years by Ian Falloon, Robert Paul Liberman, and their colleagues, primarily for schizophrenic patients returning to live with their families following a recent hospitalization (Falloon & Liberman, 1983; Falloon, Boyd, & McGill, 1984). The therapy is conducted in a teaching format in which the therapist acts as an instructor, providing information and teaching skills based on the principles of social learning, (Bandura, 1969): modeling, rehearsal, social reinforcement, and generalization. Treatment procedures are determined by two broad goals: The first is to improve the collective ability of family members to manage the patient's illness. This includes the awareness of early warning signs of symptom relapse, facilitating medication compliance, utilizing available resources in the community (e.g., psychiatrists, social services, hospitals, day programs), and participating in other aspects of patient rehabilitation. The second is to improve the ability of *all* family members to achieve their own personal goals, independent of the patient's illness.

These general goals are accomplished by three specific aims of therapy: (1) to provide information to the family about the illness of schizophrenia; (2) to teach communication skills that improve clarity and reduce negative affect among family members; and (3) to teach a structured approach for cooperative problem solving that facilitates stress management and goal attainment. The treatment can be divided into five sequential stages, although material from previous stages is repeated as needed: assessment, education about schizophrenia, communication skills training, problem-solving training, and special problems (e.g., anxiety, unassertiveness). Before a more detailed exposition of the stages of treatment, consideration is given to the selection of patients and families, logistics, and setting the stage for therapy.

Psychiatric patients with schizophrenic-spectrum disorders (schizophrenia, schizoaffective, schizophreniform, schizotypal personality) who are in contact with a relative or significant other can potentially benefit from family therapy. While the first rigorous treatment study of behavioral family therapy included only patients living with their parents (Falloon et al., 1985), anecdotal evidence suggests that it may also be therapeutic with different family constellations (e.g., the patient and his or her spouse or children) or for chronically hospitalized patients in contact with their families (Liberman, Mueser, & Glynn, 1987). In addition, the treatment procedures have also been applied to families meeting in multiple family groups (Liberman, Falloon, & Aitchison, 1984). Regardless of whether the patient lives with family members or elsewhere, the parties should have at least several hours of contact per week in order to practice the skills with each other outside of the therapy session and work cooperatively solving problems together.

Family therapy sessions can be conducted at any location convenient to the family and the therapist (e.g., home, clinic, hospital, boarding home). Therapy is usually provided over a limited period of time (6 months to 2 years) on a declining contact basis (e.g., weekly for 3 months, biweekly for 6 months, and monthly for 3 months). Session length is normally 45 to 60 minutes, but briefer sessions may be necessary with some symptomatic patients who have difficulty sustaining their attention for extended periods. A convenient time to initiate family therapy is following an acute symptom exacerbation requiring hospitalization, when both patient and family members are highly motivated to avoid or minimize future rehospitalizations. Patients' symptoms should preferably have subsided or be stabilized before starting therapy, although with severely ill patients this is not always possible.

Patients and family members can be engaged in treatment by presenting to them the goals of therapy: reduction of symptoms and rehospitalizations, and improved communication and problem-solving skills within the family. A few families may have had past negative experiences with therapy and may be wary of trying another approach. With such families it is important to highlight the differences between the therapies, and to stress the positive focus of learning to deal with day-to-day stresses in behavioral family therapy. Liberman (1981) has provided useful suggestions for stemming resistance to this therapy.

When beginning to work with a family, the therapist should establish clear positive expectations for treatment. The goals, components of treatment, and expectations for all participants can be arranged as a handout (Table 1) and discussed with the entire family. The length of treatment should be established, as well as the frequency of sessions, the location, and the need for a quiet working environment. The setting of expectations and working out the logistics of meeting can usually be accomplished in a half-hour session with the family after all members have tentatively agreed to participate in treatment. At the end of this meeting the therapist arranges to meet with each person individually, in order to begin assessment of the family.

Table 1. Orientation to Behavioral Family Therapy

Role of the therapist
    Coordinate, guide, and assist family members in learning new information
       and coping skills.
Goals and its treatments
    Reduce tension in family relationships.
    Improve family's internal communication.
    Increase family's understanding and acceptance of the illness.
    Assist the family in developing problem-solving strategies that are
       more satisfactory.
Format
    Provide assessment of each individual family member.
    Provide assessment of strengths and weaknesses of the family as a unit.
    Provide education about the nature of the illness and its treatment.
       Communication skills training
       Problem-solving training
       Development of new strategies for specific problems
Expectations of family members
    Regular attendance
    Active role-playing
    A quiet working environment (if conducted at home)
    Completion of all homework assignments
    Cooperation with each other and the therapist
Family can expect the therapist to provide
    Regular attendance
    Thoughtful systematic intervention
    Strict confidentiality (except with treatment team)
    A comfortable working environment (if conducted in clinic)
    Homework materials
    Crisis counseling (if applicable)

Assessment

Before therapy sessions begin, a careful analysis is made of the family's strengths and weaknesses in coping. This assessment serves as a guide to the therapist in targeting specific skills for change, and it is repeated throughout the treatment to monitor progress of the family. The assessment is organized to gather information about four general areas of family functioning: (1) the quality of family members' communication and problem-solving skills, (2) knowledge about schizophrenia, (3) the role that specific problem behaviors play in the functioning of the family, and (4) goals of individual family members. In addition, the therapist learns information about the family, such as a family genogram, the educational level of members, work history, and past medical and psychiatric treatment.

A variety of different methods are used to collect the relevant information, including individual family member interviews, questionnaires, naturalistic observation of the family during sessions, and structured family interaction tasks. These individual interviews usually take 1 to 2 hours to complete, and more than one meeting may be necessary in order not to fatigue some family members. During the interviews the therapist determines family members' knowledge of the patient's specific diagnosis, the perceived benefits and disadvantages of medication, compliance with past treatments, and the burden of the illness on each person. Members are asked to identify problems and are helped to formulate short-term personal goals (i.e., *not* patient-related) to work toward over the following 3 months. Previous steps already taken toward these goals are noted, as are past and anticipated obstacles, and family support or conflict regarding the goal. Each member's progress is routinely assessed in family sessions, and goals are revised and updated regularly at 3-month intervals. In addition to personal goals, the therapist learns each member's perspective on what family problems need attention.

For example, the 18-year-old brother ("John") of a patient set a goal of saving $200 over the next 3 months. John had already made some steps toward this goal, including having a job, opening a bank account, and saving $25. John had previously had trouble with his car, and he anticipated that this might prevent him from saving the money. He thought his family was supportive of this goal, since his mother had often told him he should save some of his money. He stated one family problem was that his mother and stepfather often had heated arguments, especially over financial matters, and this led to a tense atmosphere in the family.

In order to evaluate how the family solves problems together, the therapist observes their interaction in a structured task before treatment. This task is easy to administer and provides the therapist with a useful measure of family communication and problem-solving skill. A tape recorder is used to conduct the assessment. The therapist explains to the family that it is important for him or her to *directly observe* how they deal with problems together. A moderate-size problem or goal is identified, and family members are requested to express their opinions and attempt to solve the problem for a 10-minute period, during which time the therapist leaves the room. When 10 minutes have elapsed, the therapist returns to the room and inquires into the family's progress in solving the problem. Positive steps toward problem solving are praised, and the therapist elicits from the family how representative their interactions were of their usual approach to solving problems. Examples of how the family has attempted to solve problems in the past are discussed, and successful coping strategies are noted. After the session, the therapist listens to the family interaction and observes the quality of communication among the family members. Repeated problem-solving assessments (e.g., every 3 months) guide the therapist in teaching specific skills to the family.

Two final sources of information about communication and problem-solving skills are: (1) naturalistic observation of family interaction during sessions, and (2) the performance of family members on homework assignments to practice specific skills. By carefully observing the family during treatment sessions, the therapist can track the presence or acquisition of skills targeted for modification. Homework assignments are given at every session and involve family members' attempting to utilize taught skills outside of therapy, in their natural environment. Successful follow-through on homework suggests that the skill has generalized beyond the therapy session, although repeated practice is usually necessary to change deeply entrenched communication patterns.

EDUCATION

The educational material about schizophrenia can be covered in two to four family sessions. The goal of these sessions is to give families a primer in schizophrenia, in order to increase their ability to recognize, understand, and cope with the complexities of the illness. The teaching format of the educational sessions is primarily didactic, with the therapist providing handouts and using posters or other visual aids to present the material. The flow of information to the family begins with an introduction and description of basic concepts of schizophrenia. Following this, biological aspects and the role of antipsychotic medication in treatment are addressed, and then the family's role in managing the illness and facilitating psychosocial rehabilitation is presented.

In the first educational session the therapist begins by asking all the family members to describe how schizophrenia has affected their own personal lives. This serves to highlight the disruptive effects of schizophrenia on every family member, especially the patient, and to build their motivation to work together to improve their collective ability to manage the illness. Common myths are refuted early in the session, such as the patient's having a "split personality," the potential for violence, and families' "causing" schizophrenia. Information is presented on diagnostic procedures, and the specific symptoms are systematically discussed. The therapist solicits the patient's active participation in the session by connotating his or her role as the "expert" in the illness. As different symptoms of the illness are described, the patient is invited to share his or her personal experience with the symptom, and the therapist inquires into family members' awareness of this experience. Other, more basic information about schizophrenia is also given, including the prevalence, onset, and course of the illness, its presence in different cultural, ethnic, and socioeconomic groups, and the early warning signs of an impending relapse.

After an introduction to schizophrenia has been provided, the role of biological factors is considered. The dopamine hypothesis of schizophrenia is explained to family members, as well as the beneficial effect of antipsychotic medication on reducing acute symptoms and preventing symptom exacerbations. Side effects of the antipsychotics are described, and the patient's personal experiences with medication are elicited. The role of anticholinergic medications is discussed, as are strategies for coping with problematic side effects.

To illustrate the process of involving family members in an educational session, an excerpt from a transcript of a family session is presented here. The selection involves the impact of schizophrenia on family members' lives. The patient was a 38-year-old hospitalized chronic schizophrenic man who had spent most of the past 15 years in psychiatric hospitals. He was stabilized on medication but remained floridly psychotic. The family members present were the patient ("Ed"), his father ("Joe"), and one of his two brothers ("Tom"). The excerpt is taken from the first educational session with the family, after the initial greetings between the therapist and family members:

THERAPIST: Schizophrenia is a disorder that handicaps everyday functioning. People with schizophrenia have a hard time doing everyday tasks, such as writing a check, washing clothes, or holding a job, because they experience intrusive thoughts and have other upsetting experiences.

ED: Its very painful because you can't even have a good time. You can't let yourself have a good time because you have to separate things in your mind and it drains you of all your energy. For example, even though the shore is near here and I love the shore, I don't enjoy it anymore. You can ask my brother. We were a shore family. We all love the shore, but I can't even get enough energy to get to the shore.

THERAPIST: Well, Ed, that is a very good point that you raised. You have just described a very common symptom for people who have schizophrenia, and there is a term for it. It is called "anhedonia." Let me write it on the blackboard. It means that the person has difficulty experiencing pleasure. Activities that they used to find enjoyable, like going to the shore, are just not as enjoyable as they used to be.

ED: Or going to the movies and getting strange messages. I went to see the film *2010*. I went in there, and there was a lot of computer data on the screen—the actors were talking about the computer at the time. I got scary messages from that computer—names, numbers, and things like that. I had to get up and leave the movie.

JOE: You *thought* you got messages.

ED: Yea, I thought I got messages. Well, I don't know if I actually got messages, but I paid six dollars to see that movie, and I had to get up after ten minutes and leave.

THERAPIST: I am sure that was very frustrating.

ED: And I can't watch TV. I can't concentrate. I can't listen to the radio without changing the stations and picking out songs that I like to reduce the fear I get from messages coming across the airways.

THERAPIST: Ed, you are describing the influence that schizophrenia has had on your life, and I would also like to hear from your father and brother about what influence this illness has had on their lives. How about you, Joe?

JOE: Well, this is something that as Ed's father I've had to cope with. I have always had a very pressured job, and its totally consuming, unfortunately. So it's difficult for me to give Ed the time that I should give, and then when I am off of my job I, you know . . .

ED: He gets very tired. . . .

JOE: I do need the rest and relaxation to get away, because I've got problems and troubles day after day after day. So in that way, it has been difficult for me, and very sad for me to see Ed in this situation. Ed was always such an outstanding young man and conversationalist. He was intelligent and bright, cheerful and happy. And to see this illness come along and really destroy a life that had tremendous potential is sad. It's something we all have to live with. At the same time, I have to live with my situation, too.

THERAPIST: How about you, Tom?

TOM: How has it affected my life? It makes me feel guilty sometimes, because Ed will call me on weekends and want to do something. But in a lot of ways I really don't have a lot of control over my own life. In other words, there are so many activities going on during weekends, like children and things to do around the house. There's always something to do. So, when a weekend comes along it's almost depressing, because I have no time to think of relaxing. I have to go to work occasionally on Saturday mornings. So, when Ed calls, I can feel the sadness, but there are so many things going on that I just can't be available.

COMMUNICATION SKILLS TRAINING

Good communication among family members is essential to defusing a negative affective climate and promoting cooperative problem solving within the family. Four core communication skills are taught to families: attentive listening, expressing positive feelings, making positive requests, and expressing negative feelings. The early sessions in communication skills training focus on creating a warm milieu by teaching empathic listening, expressing positive feelings, and prompting mutually rewarding behavior between family members. Only when a positive supportive environment has been achieved in the family does the therapist address the communication of unpleasant feelings, and problem-solving training.

Training in communication skills emphasizes brief, direct, and specific verbal communication that is congruent with paralinguistic (e.g., voice, tone) and nonverbal (e.g., facial expression) features. Family members are encouraged to "take responsibility for their feelings" by using "I" statements, such as "I would appreciate it if you would clear the dishes off the table." Communication skills are taught to family members using the principles of social skills training. Each skill is broken down into small, manageable component behaviors (Table 2) in order to provide family members with specific instructions and feedback for their performance. The format for teaching these skills can be divided into seven steps, briefly reviewed here:

1. *Discuss the rationale with the family about why the skill is important to learn.* In order to motivate family members to actively participate in learning a particular skill, a clear rationale for its importance must first be established. The therapist can both provide an explanation for the skill and elicit reasons from the family by asking questions (e.g., "Why do you think it is important to express positive feelings to each other?"). Some rationales for the communication skills include the following: Active listening skills help

Table 2. Skills Taught in Communication Skills Training

Active listening
  Look at the speaker.
  Attend to what is said.
  Nod head, say "uh-huh."
  Ask clarifying questions.
  Check out what you heard.
Expressing positive feelings
  Look at the person with a pleasant facial expression.
  Say exactly what he or she did that pleased you.
  Tell the person how it made you feel.
Making positive requests
  Look at the person with a pleasant facial expression.
  Say exactly what you would like that person to do.
  Tell how it would make you feel.
Expressing negative feelings
  Look at the person with a serious facial expression: Speak firmly.
  Say exactly what the person did that upset you.
  Tell how it made you feel.
  Suggest how the person might prevent this from happening again in the future.

the listener attend to what is being said and convey interest and concern to the speaker. Expressing positive feelings about a specific behavior increases the chances that the behavior will occur again, and creates warm feelings between the parties. By making positive requests a person can avoid being perceived as coercive or demanding, and may improve compliance with the desired change. Expressing negative feelings constructively can be helpful by informing the person how his or her behavior effects the speaker, and how it could be changed to avoid creating the feeling in the future.

2. *Discuss each step of the skill with the family.* The therapist uses a blackboard, posters, and/or handouts to identify the specific steps and explain their role in clear communication. For example, when expressing a positive feeling, looking at specific persons lets them know that you are speaking to them. A pleasant facial expression conveys a nonverbal message that is congruent with the verbal one. Telling people exactly what they did enables them to pinpoint the behavior that pleased the other person. Describing the feeling the behavior caused precisely defines its impact on the speaker.

3. *Model the skill for the family to demonstrate its use.* The therapist strives to always model good communication skills in his or her interactions with family members. When the rationale and specific steps of the skill have been discussed, the therapist demonstrates for the family in a role-play how it is to be performed. After modeling the skills, the therapist asks the family members to identify which specific behaviors they observed, and the overall effectiveness of the communication. Modeling the skill for the family and eliciting specific feedback helps translate the abstract components into a "live" communication. This prepares the family to practice the skill themselves in a similar role-play. Severely dysfunctional families may benefit from extensive modeling of communication skills by the therapist early in treatment.

4. *Conduct a behavioral rehearsal (role-play) in which one family member uses the skill to communicate with another member.* Generally, it is preferable to first engage a more socially skilled family member in a role-play, so that less-skilled members are given additional opportunities to observe the desired behavior before they practice it themselves. The family member is asked to identify a recent situation in which the skill could have been used. The therapist then sets up the role-play with the family to reenact the original situation. The person practicing the role-play remains himself, while other family members are assigned roles as either themselves, another person, or observers of the interaction. The therapist is active and out of his or her seat in organizing the role-play by changing seating patterns, moving furniture, etc., to resemble the physical setting of the original situation. The therapist instructs (using a positive request) the person to try

the skill, while other members are to watch which steps of the skill were performed well. The role-play is stopped after the person spoken to has responded back. Role-plays are brief in duration (15–60 seconds), since succinct communication is encouraged between family members. This enables each person to practice the skill in several role-plays.

5. *If necessary, prompt and coach the family members as they rehearse the skill.* Some members have difficulty learning certain skills from instructions, modeling, and reinforcement alone, and require additional help during the role-play. Prompting is the therapist's use of gestures or signals to modify behavior during a role-play (e.g., the therapist points a thumb up to signal the family member to speak more loudly). Coaching involves giving verbal cues (e.g., "Good, keep up the eye contact" or "Tell him how it made you feel") and standing or kneeling close to the rehearsing person to give ongoing support and encouragement. Active support and coaching can be particularly useful with patients who have pronounced negative symptoms, since even very small improvements may be difficult for such patients. Coaching can also facilitate learning a skill for the first time, one that is different or awkward, or that the person is not used to communicating.

6. *Give positive and corrective feedback to the family member about his or her performance in the role-play.* The therapist first provides abundant positive reinforcement for good aspects of the role-play by asking other family members questions, such as "What did you like about the way your mother made a positive request to John to take out the garbage?" and pointing to the different steps of the skill on a blackboard or poster. In giving feedback, emphasis is placed on behavioral specificity, so that the participants know exactly what they did well (e.g., "You had good eye contact and pleasant tone of voice when you told John you would like him to take out the garbage," rather than "You did a nice job asking John to take out the garbage"). Special effort is made to identify some positive behavior to praise in even the most severely dysfunctional persons, and to teach family members to positively reinforce small improvements in social performance that occur slowly over time (i.e., shaping). After positive feedback, the therapist instigates a second role-play with the same person and situation, highlighting any steps they missed in the first role-play by requesting that they include them in the second. With less skilled family members it may be preferable for the therapist to request them to add only one behavior component per role-play. Feedback is given following the second role-play as with the first. Between two and four consecutive role-plays are recommended per family member when teaching communication skills. Family members who perform the skill well on the first role-play should nevertheless repeat it at least one more time for practice. After one person has improved over several role-plays, the therapist moves on to another person and proceeds to identify a new situation with this person around which to structure a role-play.

7. *Assign homework to practice the skill.* In order to ensure the transfer and generalization of skills taught in the session to the natural family environment, "homework" is given at the end of each session. Family members are given sheets on which to record social situations when they could have used a specific skill and whether they used the skill. At the beginning of each session the therapist checks the family members' homework and uses situations that occurred in the past week(s) to organize role-plays to practice the skill again. Noncompliance with homework is managed with a variety of strategies, including the therapist's expressing negative feelings and making positive requests, reviewing of the rationale for homework, problem solving with the family to remove obstacles to completing the homework, and requesting the family to do the homework at the beginning of the session.

Sometimes early in therapy family members express frequent, strong negative feelings to each other that are destructive to the learning process and risk alienating certain members. In such cases it is imperative that the therapist respond rapidly to block the negative affect, especially when it is directed at the patient, and attempt to build a cooperative spirit among the members. This can be accomplished by acknowledging the critical persons' concerns, assuring them that these will be addressed later in treatment (when appropriate), and praising the criticized person and the entire family for their willingness to work together learning how to cope with the illness. Highly critical families may also benefit from the therapist's prompting a "round of positive feelings" between the members at the beginning and/or end of the session.

The therapist monitors the acquisition and generalization of communication skills by examining family members' self-report from homework sheets, evaluating their performance in role-plays based on actual occurrences, and naturalistically observing their interactions during family sessions. When monitoring the interaction between family members, the therapist must correct common pitfalls to effective communication: coercive "should" statements, blaming others for feelings (e.g., "*You* made me feel bad" rather than "*I* felt bad when . . ."), *buts* that cancel out positives (e.g., "You look nice today, *but* why did you have to wear those shoes?!"), pseudomutual "we" statements, projected feeling statements, double-bind communications, vague ramblings, intrusive interruptions, and invalidation of others' feelings.

Most families require four to eight sessions to learn the core communication skills, although spot retraining is often required later in therapy as well. While four communication skills are routinely taught, families may benefit from learning supplementary communication skills, such as asking for a time-out to deal with stressful situations (Liberman, Cardin, McGill,

Table 3. Supplementary Communication Skills

Compromise and negotiation
    Look at the person.
    Explain your viewpoint.
    Listen to the other person's viewpoint.
    Repeat back what you heard.
    Suggest a compromise.
Requesting a time-out
    Indicate that the situation is stressful.
    Tell the person that it is interfering with constructive communication.
    Say that you must leave temporarily.
    State when you will return and be willing to problem-solve then.

Falloon, & Evans, 1987) or compromise and negotiation to facilitate problem solving (Table 3).

To illustrate the teaching of expressing positive feelings, a partial transcript of a family therapy session is presented. The patient was a 35-year-old Hispanic man ("Jesus") who participated in therapy with his wife ("Carla"). Jesus had a chronic course of schizophrenia over the past 15 years but had been able to achieve a moderate level of social functioning in the community by occasionally attending a day program and maintaining a family life with one child. The session was conducted in the family's home:

THERAPIST: Carla, can you think of something that Jesus did in the past week that made you feel good?

CARLA: Of course, when he ran. It's something I always want him to go back to doing.

THERAPIST: Let's reenact that scene so we can see how it happened.

CARLA: Okay. We were sitting right here. (Furniture is rearranged for role-play)

CARLA: (As Jesus enters the room) How are you doing? Hooray! (Claps hands) You did a good job!

JESUS: I'm so sore.

CARLA: Ah, you'll get over it.

JESUS: Yeah, I just have to relax a little.

CARLA: Okay.

JESUS: It felt good, though.

CARLA: Great.

THERAPIST: That was nicely done, Carla. Jesus, what did you notice Carla do to show that she appreciated what you did?

JESUS: She touched me.

THERAPIST: Right, she touched you. What else?

JESUS: She looked straight at me. And smiled a lot.

THERAPIST: Yes, she had a very nice expression on her face.

JESUS: And she sounded very caring.

THERAPIST: Yes, she also had a very pleasant tone of voice. Carla, I liked the way you were specific in telling Jesus what you liked. Did Carla follow all of the steps of expressing a positive feeling, Jesus? Did Carla look at you? (Therapist points to list of skills on easel)

JESUS: Yes, she looked at me.

THERAPIST: Did she tell you what it was that made her feel so good?

JESUS: Yes.

THERAPIST: Did she tell you how it made her feel?

JESUS: Ah, through her smiling.

THERAPIST: Yes, her nonverbal behavior.

You did a good job, Carla. I'd like you to do just one more thing next time, and that is to tell Jesus verbally how it made you feel when he ran. This makes the communication even more clear. Okay?

CARLA: Okay. (Role-play is set up again) Hi, how are you doing?

JESUS: Good, good.

CARLA: (Claps) You did a good job. Look, you're all wet. How was your running time?

JESUS: Alright. I did two miles today, but I'm sore.

CARLA: I'm glad you are running. You made me feel good, I'm proud that you ran just now.

JESUS: Yeah, that's good.

CARLA: So keep up the good work.

THERAPIST: Great, Carla, I really like the way you told Jesus that his running made you feel good.

CARLA: Okay.

PROBLEM-SOLVING TRAINING

Successful problem solving can be enhanced by increasing positive affect in the family (Isen, Daubman, & Nowicki, 1987). When family members have improved their communication skills, they are taught a structured approach to group problem solving. Problem-solving skills can facilitate the ability of the family to detect and lessen stressors impinging on the patient and other members, and to attain personal goals identified during assessments. Training in problem solving is accomplished by teaching a set of six sequential steps designed to minimize negative affect while maximizing successful resolution. Progress in these steps is recorded on problem-solving sheets by a "chairman" or "secretary" elected by the family. Families are taught to keep these problem-solving sheets in a notebook stored in a location accessible to all members (e.g., the living room), so that plans can be easily reviewed. The steps are briefly described below:

1. *Define the problem.* Family members are encouraged to express their opinions, listen to each other, and ask questions before agreeing on a definition of the problem. It is important that *all* family members agree on

the definition so everyone is motivated to work on resolving the problem. Establishing a definition that is satisfactory to all members may require some creativity. For example, the parents of one schizophrenic patient ("Bob") thought that his refusal to bathe was a problem, whereas the patient thought that their incessant shouting at him over bathing was the problem. The family was able to work together toward a successful resolution when they agreed on a definition of the problem as "Mom and Dad shout at Bob when he does not take baths regularly."

2. *List all possible solutions.* Family members "brainstorm" as many possible solutions as they can, and all ideas are acknowledged and recorded on the problem-solving sheet. When the family's efforts at generating solutions are stymied, the therapist can offer an outlandish suggestion to stimulate further brainstorming by family members. No solutions are evaluated at this time, and families are encouraged to identify a minimum of six solutions.

3. *Discuss the possible solutions.* Each solution is discussed in terms of its advantages and disadvantages for solving the problem or achieving the goal. Family members are taught to be brief and specific in their evaluation of solutions, and to avoid lengthy, heated debates. Families may be taught a simple system for summarizing the adequacy of each solution on the sheet, such as giving each one between zero (poor solution) and three "pluses" (very good solution).

4. *Agree on the best solution or combination of solutions.* Sometimes one solution is clearly outstanding, and the choice is obvious. At other times several alternatives may be suitable, or family members may need to compromise and negotiate to agree on solution(s).

5. *Plan how to carry out the chosen solutions.* In planning how to implement the agreed-upon solution, roles are assigned to family members for different parts of the task. One member coordinates the implementation. Family members determine what resources are needed, how they will be obtained, and who will obtain them. A date and time are chosen for when the solution will be implemented. Obstacles and possible problems are anticipated and solutions for overcoming them identified. Role-playing the implementation of the solution(s) can help ensure follow-through on the initial problem-solving effort.

6. *Review the implementation.* Families are requested to have at least one family problem-solving meeting per week outside of the therapy session. After a problem-solving session the family should meet again to discuss it and praise each other for progress made, and to determine how to overcome obstacles or consider other alternative solutions when the problem remains unsolved. The therapist helps family members understand that problem solving is an ongoing process that often requires repeated efforts over time to be successful.

Problem-solving training is taught by the therapist, who initially takes the role of the chairman and leads the family through the six sequential steps. Then, family members conduct their own problem-solving sessions, taking turns playing the role of the chairman, with the therapist intervening only to keep the family on task. Families are assigned to complete progressively more steps of problem solving at their own meetings between therapy sessions as homework assignments.

Progress in problem-solving skill is monitored by reports and problem-solving sheets completed at the family meetings, and by observing the family's skill during therapy sessions. In addition, problem-solving skill is routinely assessed with 10-minute assessments throughout treatment (see Assessment). The main goal of behavioral family therapy is for the family to regularly conduct their own problem-solving meetings with sufficient skill not to require the therapist's guidance.

Problem solving can be applied successfully to a wide range of problems, including division of household responsibilities, personal goals, drug abuse, medication compliance, and leisure and recreational activities. The approach can be useful in helping patients cope with persistent symptoms, such as depression, boredom, pervasive auditory hallucinations, and delusions of reference. To demonstrate how problem solving can be used to tackle the everyday problems patients experience, an example is provided.

CASE EXAMPLE

The patient was a 33-year-old chronic schizophrenic man ("Bill") who was hospitalized in the token economy unit of a clinical research unit. He was joined in family therapy sessions by his parents. His father volunteered to record the family problem-solving steps. The family agreed to work on the problem of Bill's spending too much time in his hospital room sleeping. This was a problem because Bill's sleeping precluded his participation in ward activities thought to be therapeutic. Moreover, the sleeping was costly since Bill had to purchase sleep time with tokens he could otherwise spend on other privileges. Family members generated several alternative solutions to the problem:

1. Reading a book.
2. Giving away his tokens, so he could not purchase sleep time.
3. Writing a letter.
4. Playing cards with Frank (a patient).
5. Playing the piano.
6. Playing a game with Cecil (a patient).
7. Talking to someone.

After all the solutions had been generated, the advantages and disadvantages of each solution were evaluated. An advantage of reading a book was the easy accessibility of a book, and a disadvantage of playing piano was that it required a fair amount of concentration. After each solution had been discussed, Bill selected playing games with Cecil or Frank, reading a book, or talking with someone as the best combination of solutions. To implement the plan, Bill needed to find where the games were stored, and to select a book or magazine to read. To prompt Bill to use the selected solutions, Bill's parents agreed to remind him of the solutions during their conversations on the phone. The following week progress on solving the problem was evaluated, and Bill indicated that the solutions had worked well for him.

Crises are also handled using the problem-solving approach, with the therapist stepping in to chair the session if the family is not yet sufficiently skillful. To demonstrate the use of problem solving in a crisis situation, a brief vignette is described.

Case Example

The family in treatment was very poor, had few resources, and lived in a crime- and drug-ridden neighborhood in the inner city. Four family members usually participated in the therapy sessions: Mother, two of her children—"Leroy," 27 the "identified patient" who has a schizoaffective disorder, and "Tamara," 31, who has schizophrenia, and Tamara's daughter "Sally" (15). Two months prior to the session Sally had given birth to her first child, "Lenore." The family had recently been under high stress following the grandmother's recent death from tuberculosis and the ongoing evaluation by the city health department of whether any other family members had also been infected.

When the therapist arrived at the home for the 17th family therapy session, it was immediately apparent that Tamara was extremely agitated. When her daughter's boyfriend (the father of Lenore) came into the apartment shortly after the therapist arrived, Tamara began to curse loudly at him and went after him with the globe of a hurricane lamp. Other family members were frightened and unsure of what to do. The therapist took control by first standing between Tamara and her daughter's boyfriend, politely requesting him to leave, and gently escorting him out of the apartment. Tamara appeared to be very paranoid, and the therapist began to problem-solve with the family, taking the role of the chairman. The problem was defined to everyone's satisfaction as "Tamara feels she might hurt somebody." The following solutions were generated:

1. Go to the community mental health center.
2. Go to the nearest hospital.
3. Take additional medication.
4. Leave the apartment.
5. Other family members leave the apartment.
6. Go to the psychiatric hospital where the therapist works.

After discussing each solution, the family agreed that going to the therapist's hospital was best, since they knew the treatment staff and Tamara needed immediate attention. To plan how to implement the solution, the following steps were determined:

1. Call the treatment team coordinator at the hospital.
2. Arrange for admission.
3. Arrange for transportation (a cab was called).
4. Have mother accompany Tamara.
5. Request treatment team coordinator to meet Tamara when she arrived at the hospital.

The family followed through on the solution as planned. Tamara was voluntarily admitted to the psychiatric hospital over the following 2 hours.

SPECIAL PROBLEMS

When families have acquired satisfactory problem-solving skills, some problems may remain that require special interventions. A wide range of behavioral techniques may be applied to treat these problems. Supplementary social skills training can be a useful adjunct treatment for patients with severe or situationally specific skills deficits (e.g., shyness with members of the opposite sex, assertiveness, anger problems). Self-monitoring, exposure, relaxation, and systematic desensitization can be used to treat anxiety problems that are not mediated by social skill deficiencies. Other strategies include contingency contracting for mutually desirable behavior changes, token economy programs for enhancing constructive daily activity, or cognitive-behavioral modification for depression. The entire family is usually involved in implementing and monitoring strategies for dealing with special problems. In some cases it may be desirable to refer family member(s) to another professional for concomitant treatment—such as problems in sexual functioning, alcoholism, or marital discord—depending on the therapist's areas of expertise.

To illustrate the use of behavioral family therapy with a schizophrenic patient, a case example is presented.

CASE EXAMPLE

Dave was the youngest of seven children and was raised by his father, a Baptist minister, and his mother, a homemaker, in a "protective" home environment. Dave began to develop his first psychiatric symptoms when he was 16 years old, after starting his junior year at a new high school. He had difficulty adapting to the new school and was frequently teased by his classmates, who called him "dumb." Gradually, Dave began to spend more and more time by himself, remaining in his room for hours listening to music, and interacting less with his family members and friends. Dave's parents' concern grew as his grades dropped from mediocre to poor, and he ceased playing the piano, which had formerly been his favorite activity. They attempted to talk to Dave about his problems at school, but he kept putting them off by saying that nothing was wrong, and they did not press him further.

After several months of increasing social withdrawal, Dave's behavior became grossly disorganized and bizarre. He began staying up nights, pacing, and talking excitedly about the FBI and the Mafia following him and interfering with his thoughts. Later he complained to his mother that voices were telling him to hurt himself and that he was receiving messages from the radio and TV. After an especially difficult day in which Dave became extremely agitated, started to throw food around the house, and attempted to climb the walls, his parents realized that he would not "snap out of it" and needed immediate medical attention, so they took him to a mental health clinic.

Dave was admitted to a local psychiatric hospital, where he was treated unsuccessfully with antipsychotic medications for a month, and was then transferred to a state hospital for longer-term treatment. Throughout much of his inpatient stay, Daves behavior alternated between aggressive, explosive outbursts, precipitated by delusions of having been raped or physically abused, to confusion in not being able to distinguish other patients from his family members, to apathy, depression, and social withdrawal. Eventually, he responded to electroconvulsive therapy (ECT) and was discharged after 6 months on maintenance chlorpromazine with a diagnosis of undifferentiated schizophrenia.

Dave returned home and completed high school. He did not have his second hospitalization until he was 21 years old and had begun attending music school. Although he was subsequently able to return to school and complete a 2-year associate's degree in music, the following 12 years were characterized by multiple hospitalizations, declining vocational and social functioning, and marked negative symptoms. He attended day treatment programs sporadically, and several relapses were precipitated by his discontinuing his medication.

When Dave was 33 years old and his parents were out of town for several weeks, he ran out of his antipsychotic medication and was not able to get his prescription refilled. He rapidly became psychotic and was involved in an altercation in which he was badly beaten by a security guard at a supermarket after leaving the store half naked, with some food he had not paid for. Dave was charged with simple assault and placed in a detention center, where he remained for 2 months until his family was able to get the charges dropped and arranged a transfer to a psychiatric hospital. Dave was admitted to a psychiatric hospital, where he was enrolled in an outpatient treatment program that combined low-dose fluphenazine decanoate with behavioral family therapy.

Following a 6-week hospitalization, Dave's positive symptoms were well-controlled, but he continued to have negative symptoms. His affect was flat, he had severe psychomotor retardation, he slept much of the time, and he interacted with few people outside his family. Dave began attending a day treatment program, he and his parents participated in monthly support groups, and they started behavioral family therapy sessions, which were conducted by a therapist who came to their house.

Before the family sessions began, each member was interviewed to identify specific goals for treatment and to assess their knowledge of schizophrenia. Despite more than 10 years' experience with repeated hospitalizations, no one in the family knew even the most elementary facts about the illness; they were unfamiliar with the symptoms, names, and side effects of medications, and they were ignorant of the effect of stress on the course of the illness. During the educational sessions, family members learned the early signs of schizophrenic relapse, which for Dave included suspiciousness, auditory hallucinations, and increased sleeping. On two occasions over the following 2 years, impending relapses were recognized and successfully avoided; Dave and his parents employed the family problem-solving skills that were taught in the family sessions.

In communication skills training special attention was given to improving Dave's nonverbal communication (eye contact, voice volume, tone), which was muted owing to his pronounced negative symptoms. Over the course of more than 25 sessions Dave engaged in numerous role-plays with his mother and father, rehearsing such skills as expressing positive and negative feelings. One skill that Dave found particularly difficult was making positive requests. In one family session he engaged in several role-plays with his parents portraying co-workers or a supervisor at his sheltered workshop, where he rehearsed requesting help on a job: "Chuck, could you show me how were supposed to assemble this? I'd really appreciate it." Dave's parents focused on increasing their verbal reinforcement to shape desired changes in his behavior by expressing positive feelings to him for small improvements. In one meeting Dave's father expressed his satisfaction with his participation in the sheltered workshop: "Son, Im really proud of you getting up so early every day to get to your program on time."

The family members learned quickly how to do cooperative problem solving following the structured sequence. However, extensive prompting was necessary to get the family to meet on their own for weekly problem-solving sessions, which they finally began after 10 months of treatment. A wide range of problems were addressed, including coping with auditory hallucinations, arriving late at the workshop, and feeling fatigued. One important goal for Dave was to begin practicing the piano again. After a period of 4 months and several problem-solving discussions, Dave increased his practicing from 0 times per week to an average of 3½ times per week. Dave began to accept invitations to play the piano, which he had formerly rejected, such as for the church choir and at parties. Coupled with his increase in playing the piano, Dave began again to arrange and write his own music, something he had not done for several years.

Thus, throughout the course of treatment Dave steadily improved. He gradually made the transition from a day hospital to a vocational workshop to prepare him for competitive employment. While Dave continued to have negative symptoms, they were reduced in severity. By the end of the first year of combined drug and family therapy, Dave's Brief Psychiatric Rating Scale scores declined from severe to mild for blunted affect, and from moderately severe to mild and very mild for psychomotor retardation and emotional withdrawal, respectively. Despite his residual symptoms, Dave's social adjustment continued to improve, enabling him to marry his girlfriend of several years. He was able to move out of his parents' home into an apartment with his wife, while continuing to attend his work program and remaining clinically stable. Much of the burden of care on his family was reduced by Dave's assuming more responsibility for managing his illness, such as attending follow-up medication appointments and a vocational program. In addition, he was able to transfer skills learned in family therapy to his relationship with his wife, such as having regular problem-solving meetings with her.

EVALUATION OF BEHAVIORAL FAMILY THERAPY

The effects of behavioral family therapy for schizophrenic patients have been examined in a well-controlled clinical outcome study conducted by Falloon and his colleagues (Falloon, 1975; Falloon et al., 1985). Thirty-six schizophrenic patients who had recently been discharged from a psychiatric hospital were randomly assigned to either 9 months of behavioral family therapy or equally intensive individual therapy. Family therapy was conducted in the home, whereas individual therapy was conducted at the clinic. The individual therapy utilized a goal-oriented behavioral approach that focused on improving the ability of patients to anticipate and cope with a range of environmental stressors. After the intensive therapy stage, patients and their families were provided with case management, crisis intervention services, and therapy on an "as-needed" basis for the remainder of the 2-year period. All patients were maintained on antipsychotic medications by psychiatrists who were unaware of the patients' treatment assignment. At the end of 2 years a thorough assessment was completed.

Results strongly favored the family over the individual treatment. After 9 months and at the 2-year follow-up, patients who received family treatment had significantly fewer hospitalizations, spent less time in the hospital, experienced fewer major exacerbations of schizophrenic symptoms and episodes of depression, and required fewer emergency crisis sessions than patients who received individual therapy. While few patients receiving individual therapy showed a complete remission of psychotic symptoms, over 75% receiving behavioral family therapy did show some improvement. Patients receiving the family intervention also improved more in their social and vocational adjustment. Over the 2-year period, family-treated patients spent an average of 12.6 months engaged in work or training activities, compared with only 7.2 months for individually treated patients.

Improvements in family functioning were also more evident in the family than in the individual treatments. The coping efforts of family members receiving family therapy were more effective than in families where the patient received individual therapy. Consistent with the improved prognoses of patients who returned to families engaged in family therapy, these families showed significant decreases in their level of tense and intrusive communications, compared with a slight worsening in communication for families of individually treated patients. Finally, the family-based treatment was more economical than the individual treatment.

This study provides empirical support that enhancing the coping effectiveness of family members and patient together may have a greater impact on the course of schizophrenia than attempts to directly modify only the patient's coping skills. The efficacy of behavior family therapy for schizophrenia is currently under examination in at least three different studies throughout the United States, including the NIMH Collaborative Study for Treatment Strategies in Schizophrenia. The extensive outcome research currently in progress on this treatment approach is likely to stimulate further interest and increase demand for its availability in the future.

NEED FOR COMPREHENSIVE TREATMENT

Behavioral family therapy can be optimally effective when it is embedded in a multifaceted treatment program. For the vast majority of patients, schizophrenia has a debilitating impact on a broad range of adaptive functioning; it becomes difficult, if not impossible, to attend to the most basic daily needs, such as housing, medical care, and necessary social services. While the goal of family therapy is to empower the family with skills to solve their own problems, mental health professionals must often make referrals to appropriate community resources.

Bellack and Mueser (1986) have proposed a model for the comprehensive treatment of schizophrenia that includes four components: *treatments* (e.g., medication, crisis intervention, family therapy), *rehabilitation* (e.g., job training), *social services* (e.g., income and housing), and *continuity of care*. The therapist must coordinate the different services involved in the patient's care, unless someone else is providing case management. As the family learns how to utilize the available resources, the role of the therapist as case manager is partially or completely relinquished. The teaching of family communication and problem-solving skills serves to bolster their collective ability to plan, coordinate, and implement treatment decisions bearing on the schizophrenic patient. The focus of behavioral family therapy on each member's attaining personal goals, in addition to the family's improved ability to manage the illness, ensures that the needs of individual family members will not be subjugated to those of the patient.

ACKNOWLEDGMENTS

Preparation of this paper was supported in part by NIMH grants MH39998 and MH38636.

REFERENCES

Anderson, C. M., Hogarty, G. E., & Reiss, D. J. (1980). Family treatment of adult schizophrenic patients: A psychoeducational approach. *Schizophrenia Bulletin, 6*, 490–505.

Bandura, A. (1969). *Principles of behavior modification.* New York: Holt, Rinehart & Winston.

Bateson, G., Jackson, D. D., Haley, J., & Weakland, J. (1956). Toward a theory of schizophrenia. *Behavioral Science, 1*, 251–264.

Bellack, A. S., & Mueser, K. T. (1986). A comprehensive treatment program for schizophrenia and chronic mental illness. *Community and Mental Health Journal, 22*, 175–189.

Bowen, M. (1961). The family as a unit of study and treatment. *American Journal of Orthopsychiatry, 31*, 40–60.

Brown, G. W., Birley, J. L. T., & Wing, J. K. (1972). Influence of family life on the course of schizophrenic disorders: A replication. *British Journal of Psychiatry, 121*, 241–258.

Brown, G. W., Carstairs, G. M., & Topping, G. (1958). The post hospital adjustment of chronic mental patients. *Lancet, 2*, 685–689.

Brown, G. W., Monck, E. M., Carstairs, G. M., & Wing, J. K. (1962). Influence of family life on the course of schizophrenic illness. *British Journal of Preventive and Social Medicine, 16*, 55–68.

Brown, G. W., & Rutter, M. (1966). The measurement of family activities and relationships. A methodological study. *Human Relations, 19*, 241–263.

Creer, C., & Wing, J. K. (1974). *Schizophrenia at home.* London: National Schizophrenia Fellowship.

Dearth, N., Labenski, B. J., Mott, M. E., & Pellegrini, L. M. (1986). *Families helping families: Living with schizophrenia.* New York: W. W. Norton.

Drake, R. E., Sederer, L. I. (1986). The adverse effects of intensive treatment of chronic schizophrenia. *Comprehensive Psychiatry, 27*, 313–326.

Evans, A. S., Bullard, D. M., & Solomon, M. H. (1961). The family as a potential resource in the rehabilitation of the chronic schizophrenic patient: A study of 60 patients and their families. *American Journal of Psychiatry, 117*, 1075–1083.

Falloon, I. R. H. (1975). *Family management of schizophrenia: A study of clinical, social, family, and economic benefits.* Baltimore: Johns Hopkins University Press.

Falloon, I. R. H., Boyd, J. L., & McGill, C. W. (1984). *Family care of schizophrenia.* New York: Guilford Press.

Falloon, I. R. H., Boyd, J. L., McGill, C. W., Ranzani, J., Moss, H. B., Gilderman, A. M., & Simpson, G. M. (1985). Family management in the prevention of morbidity of schizophrenia. Clinical outcome of a two year longitudinal study. *Archives of General Psychiatry, 42*, 887–896.

Falloon, I. R. H., & Liberman, R. P. (1983). Behavioral family interventions in the management of chronic schizophrenia. In W. R. McFarlane (Ed.), *Family therapy in schizophrenia.* New York: Guilford Press.

Farmer, A. E., McGuffin, P., & Gottesman, I. I. (1987). Twin concordance for DSM-III schizophrenia. *Archives of General Psychiatry, 44*, 634–641.

Fromm-Reichmann, F. (1948). Notes on the development of treatment of schizophrenics by psychoanalytic psychotherapy. *Psychiatry, 11*, 263–273.

Goldberg, H. H. (1982). Mental illness and family burden. *Hospital and Community Psychiatry, 33*, 557–559.

Goldstein, M. J. (1985). Family factors that antedate the onset of schizophrenia and related disorders: The results of a fifteen year prospective longitudinal study. *Acta Psychiatrica Scandinavica (Suppl. 319), 71*, 7–18.

Hatfield, A. B. (1978). Psychological costs of schizophrenia to the family. *Social Work, 23*, 355–359.

Hooley, J. M., Orley, J., & Teasdale, J. D. (1986). Levels of expressed emotion and relapse in depressed patients. *British Journal of Psychiatry, 148*, 642–647.

Isen, A. M., Daubman, K. A., & Nowicki, G. P. (1987). Positive affect facilitates creative problem solving. *Journal of Personality and Social Psychology, 52*, 1122–1131.

Karno, M., Jenkins, J. H., De La Selva, A., Santana, F., Telles, C., Lopez, S., & Mintz, J. (1987). Expressed emotion and schizophrenic outcome among Mexican-American families. *Journal of Nervous and Mental Disease, 175*, 143–151.

Kay, S. R., & Opler, L. A. (1987). The positive–negative dimension in schizophrenia: Its validity and significance. *Psychiatric Developments, 2*, 79–103.

Kuipers, L., & Bebbington, P. (1985). Relatives as a resource in the management of functional illness. *British Journal of Psychiatry, 147*, 465–470.

Leff, J., Kuipers, L., Berkowitz, R., Eberlein-Vries, R., & Sturgeon, D. (1982). A controlled trial of social intervention in the families of schizophrenic patients. *British Journal of Psychiatry, 141*, 121–134.

Leff, J., & Vaughn, C. J. (1985). *Expressed emotion in families*. New York: Guilford Press.

Lewine, R. R. J., Watt, N. F., Prentky, R. A., & Fryer, J. H. (1980). Childhood social competence in functionally disordered psychiatric patients and in normals. *Journal of Abnormal Psychology, 89*, 132–138.

Liberman, R. P. (1981). Managing resistance to behavioral family therapy. In A. S. Gurman (Ed.), *Questions and answers in the practice of family therapy* (Vol. 1). New York: Brunner/Mazel.

Liberman, R. P., Cardin, V., McGill, C. W., Falloon, I. R. H., & Evans, C. D. (1987). Behavioral family management of schizophrenia: Clinical outcome and costs. *Psychiatric Annals, 17*, 610–619.

Liberman, R. P., Falloon, I. R. H., & Aitchison, R. A. (1984). Multiple family therapy for schizophrenia: A behavioral, problem-solving approach. *Psychosocial Rehabilitation Journal, 4*, 60–77.

Liberman, R. P., Mueser, K. T., & Glynn, S. (1988). Modular behavioral strategies. In I. R. H. Falloon (Ed.), *Handbook of behavioral family therapy*. New York: Guilford.

Lidz, T., Fleck, S., & Cornelison, A. (Eds.). (1965). *Schizophrenia and the family*. New York: International Universities Press.

Massie, H. N., & Beels, C. C. (1972). The outcome of the family treatment of schizophrenia. *Schizophrenia Bulletin, 6*, 26–36.

McElroy, E. M. (1987). The beat of a different drummer. In A. B. Hatfield, & H. P. Lefly (Eds.), *Families of the mentally ill: Coping and adaptation*. New York: Guilford.

Miklowitz, D. J., Goldstein, M. J., & Falloon, I. R. H. (1983). Premorbid and symptomatic characteristics of schizophrenics from families with high and low expressed emotions. *Journal of Abnormal Psychology, 92*, 357–367.

Miklowitz, D. J., Goldstein, M. J., Falloon, I. R. H., & Doane, J. A. (1984). Interactional correlates of expressed emotion in the families of schizophrenics. *British Journal of Psychiatry, 144*, 482–487.

Nuechterlein, K. H., & Dawson, M. E. (1984). A heuristic vulnerability/stress model of schizophrenic episodes. *Schizophrenia Bulletin, 10*, 300–312.

Pogue-Geile, M. F., & Harrow, M. (1985). Negative symptoms in schizophrenia: Their longitudinal course and prognostic importance. *Schizophrenia Bulletin, 11*, 427–439.

Pollack, M., Woerner, M. B., Goodman, W., & Greenberg, I. M. (1966). Childhood development patterns of adult hospitalized schizophrenic and nonschizophrenic patients and their siblings. *American Journal of Orthopsychiatry, 36*, 510–517.

Prout, C. T., & White, M. A. (1956). The schizophrenic's sibling. *Journal of Nervous and Mental Disease, 123,* 162–170.

Rutter, M., & Brown, G. W. (1966). The reliability and validity of measures of family life and relationships in families containing a psychiatric patient. *Social Psychiatry, 1,* 38–53.

Singer, M. T., Wynne, L. C., & Toohey, M. L. (1978). Communication disorders and the families of schizophrenics. In L. C. Wynne, R. L. Cromwell, & S. Matthysse (Eds.), *The nature of schizophrenia.* New York: Wiley.

Spaniol, L. (1987). Coping strategies of family caregivers. In A. B. Hatfield & H. P. Lefley (Eds.), *Families of the mentally ill: Coping and adaption:* New York: Guilford Press.

Strachan, A. M., Goldstein, M. J., & Miklowitz, D. J. (1986). Do relatives express expressed emotion? In M. J. Goldstein, I. Hand, & K. Halweg (Eds.), *Treatment of schizophrenia: Family assessment and intervention.* Berlin: Springer-Verlag.

Strachan, A. M., Leff, J. P., Goldstein, M. J., Doane, J. A., & Burtt, C. (1986). Emotional attitudes and direct communication in the families of schizophrenics. A cross-national replication. *British Journal of Psychiatry, 149,* 279–287.

Sullivan, H. S. (1927). The onset of schizophrenia. *American Journal of Psychiatry, 7,* 105–134.

Terkelsen, K. G. (1983). Schizophrenia and the family: II. Adverse effects of family therapy. *Family Process, 22,* 191–200.

Tienari, P., Sorri, A., Lahti, I., Naarala, M., Wahlberg, K., Ronkko, T., Pohjola, J., & Moring, J. (1985). The Finnish adoptive family study of schizophrenia. *The Yale Journal of Biology and Medicine, 58,* 227–237.

Vaughn, C. E., & Leff, J. P. (1976). The influence of family and social factors on the course of psychiatric illness. *British Journal of Psychiatry, 129,* 125–137.

Waxler, N. E. (1974). Parent and child effects on cognitive performance: An experimental approach to the etiological and responsive theories of schizophrenia. *Family Process, 13,* 1–22.

Waxler, N. E., & Mishler, E. B. (1971). Parental interaction with schizophrenic children and well siblings. *Archives of General Psychiatry, 25,* 223–231.

Wynne, L., Ryckoff, I. M., Day, J., & Hirsch, S. (1958). Pseudomutuality in the family relations of schizophrenics. *Psychiatry, 21,* 205–220.

Wynne, L., & Singer, M. (1963). Thought disorder and family relations of schizophrenics. I. A research strategy. II. A classification of forms. *Archives of General Psychiatry, 9,* 191–206.

Zubin, J., & Spring, B. (1977). Vulnerability—A new view of schizophrenia. *Journal of Abnormal Psychology, 86,* 103–126.

10
Social Skills Training

RANDALL L. MORRISON AND JOHN T. WIXTED

Social dysfunction has been recognized as a key feature of schizophrenia since the disorder was first described. Deterioration of social relations is among the current defining diagnostic criteria specified in DSM-III-R (American Psychiatric Association, 1987), and social isolation or withdrawal and marked impairment in major role functioning are listed as predominant prodromal and residual symptoms. Although psychotic symptomatology may be the most salient and disturbing feature of schizophrenia, the importance of interpersonal dysfunction cannot be overemphasized. Evidence from several large-scale investigations indicates that poor premorbid functioning, especially in the area of social relationships, is prognostic of poor long-term outcome (Strauss, Klorman, & Kokes, 1977; Zigler & Phillips, 1961, 1962). Even when gross psychotic symptoms are pharmacologically controlled or in remission, schizophrenics can be expected to have marked difficulties in social interactions (Serban, 1975; Strauss, Carpenter, & Bartko, 1974). Because of these difficulties, schizophrenics frequently fail to become integrated into a natural social network that can assist them in coping with social demands and other life stressors (Gleser & Gottschalk, 1967; Marcella & Snyder, 1981; McClelland & Walt, 1968). Often, the schizophrenic's family is the only network to which he or she belongs. However, the interactional pattern of families of schizophrenics is frequently deviant and may provide additional stress, which the patient lacks the appropriate interpersonal skills to resolve. In fact, studies have consistently found that schizophrenics whose family relationships are characterized by hostile interactions are particularly

RANDALL L. MORRISON • Department of Psychiatry, Medical College of Pennsylvania at EPPI, 3200 Henry Avenue, Philadelphia, Pennsylvania 19129.   JOHN T. WIXTED • Department of Psychology, University of California, San Diego, La Jolla, California 92093.

likely to be rehospitalized within 9 months of discharge (Brown, Birley, & Wing, 1972; Vaughn & Leff, 1976).

On the basis of these findings, treatments aimed at teaching schizophrenic patients more effective social skills have become a standard component of many psychiatric programs (Bellack & Hersen, 1979). Indeed, the combined application of neuroleptic medication to control psychotic symptomatology and social skills training to remedy chronic interpersonal dysfunction is regarded as one of the most promising approaches to the overall treatment and management of schizophrenia (Schooler, 1986). Numerous applications of social skills training with chronically impaired patients have been reported during the past 15 years. However, there have recently been marked advances with regard to the identification of biological pathology associated with schizophrenia, diagnosis and subclassification of the disorder, and identification and description of other deficit symptoms. These developments have implications for psychosocial interventions with schizophrenics. The purpose of this chapter is to: (1) discuss social skills assessment and training procedures as they relate to the treatment of schizophrenia; (2) review empirical findings regarding the assessment of social dysfunction and outcome of social skills training with schizophrenics; and (3) relate findings regarding social skills and schizophrenia to other aspects of the disorder.

DEFINITION OF SOCIAL SKILL

Some degree of social incompetence is readily apparent in the behavior of many psychiatric patients. In a mental health setting, this condition is most often summarized by the appropriate, albeit vague, phrase "difficulty relating to others." Since the mid-1970s, a more precise account of the interpersonal deficits associated with disorders such as schizophrenia has been offered by the concept of social skill. Although no universally accepted definition exists, Hersen and Bellack (1976) define social skill as the ability to:

> . . . express both positive and negative feelings in the interpersonal context without suffering consequent loss of social reinforcement. Such skill is demonstrated in a large variety of interpersonal contexts and involves the coordinated delivery of appropriate verbal and nonverbal responses. In addition, the socially skilled individual is attuned to the realities of the situation and is aware when he is likely to be reinforced for his efforts. (p. 512)

As defined above, *social skill* is an aggregate term that encompasses a variety of interpersonal abilities; no one trait or behavioral characteristic fully exemplifies socially skilled performance. Moreover, according to the prevailing behavioral model of social skill, these abilities are acquired through learning and are not determined by inherent personality traits or dispositions. An individual who is interpersonally incompetent may never have learned the appropriate skills or, as might occur in the case of long-term hospitalization, may have lost them owing to prolonged disuse (Bellack & Hersen, 1979). An important implication of a learning-based view of social performance is that skill deficits will often be situation-specific. That is, an individual may have learned how to interact skillfully in some social situations but not in others.

An illness as disabling as schizophrenia is bound to interfere with the experiences that ordinarily shape interpersonal development. Social withdrawal and emotional detachment, for example, may emerge at a young age and effectively eliminate many learning opportunities. As the illness progresses, periodic hospitalizations can result in further isolation from the natural teaching community. The eventual effect of such limited social learning experience may be to render the patient incompetent in a variety of social contexts. As indicated above, the detrimental consequences of unskilled social behavior have been well established. The central tenet of social skills training is that deficits in social abilities can be defined, measured, and corrected by appropriate training procedures (Morrison & Bellack, 1984).

ASSESSMENT OF SOCIAL SKILL

PATIENT SELECTION

Any patient who exhibits difficulties in interpersonal interaction is a potential candidate for social skills training. Such patients can be identified through personal interview, interviews with significant others, direct observation of social interaction, or even chart review. Initially, the goal is to evaluate a patient's social behavior on a global level. Some issues to consider at this stage are the patient's ability to put people at ease during social encounters, initiate social contact, carry on casual conversations, and stand up for his or her rights. If, for example, a patient causes others to feel uncomfortable during social interaction by talking much too loudly, social skills training might be indicated. Before initiating such a program, however, efforts should be undertaken to ensure that the observed difficulty is indeed the result of a skills deficit. Interpersonal dysfunction can be caused by a variety of factors unrelated to the patient's learning history, and these should be given due consideration prior to embarking on skills training (cf. Carpenter, Heinrichs, & Alphs, 1985).

With regard to schizophrenic patients, the first issue to consider is whether the observed difficulties coincide with the exacerbation of psychotic symptomatology. Most patients will exhibit pronounced social impairment between psychotic episodes, but some may not. In the latter case, all of the patient's symptoms may respond satisfactorily to neuroleptic medication or may remit spontaneously with the passage of time. If the patient is not actively psychotic, the possibility that the observed social dysfunction is secondary to drug therapy should be considered. Akinesia and sedation are two common drug side effects that can severely impair social performance. Another possibility to be considered is that the patient's affective state is contributing to the symptom picture. Severe social anxiety or depression can both produce behavioral effects that are difficult to distinguish from skill deficits (Arkowitz, 1977; Weissman, Paykel, Siegel, & Klerman, 1971). Therefore, if an affective or anxiety disorder is suspected, treatments aimed at these problems should probably be given highest priority. It is worth noting, however, that social skills training is sometimes the treatment of choice for these disorders as well (Bellack, Hersen, & Himmelhoch, 1983; Shaw, 1979).

Recently, the implications of negative symptoms (e.g., blunted affect, poverty of speech) in schizophrenia have attracted widespread attention. While many symptoms contained within the negative symptom construct may be responsive to social skills training (Wixted, Morrison, & Bellack, 1988), others may be resistant to virtually all forms of treatment. Carpenter et al. (1985), for example, have suggested that a subset of negative symptoms, termed "primary" negative symptoms, may be a reflection of structural brain impairment (cf. Crow, 1980). If so, then social skills training may prove to be relatively ineffective. Unfortunately, the only method currently available to detect primary negative symptoms is to demonstrate that they are unresponsive to a full range of treatment interventions. We will further discuss the implications of negative symptoms for social skills training later in this chapter.

Still another factor to consider at this initial stage of patient selection is the situational variability of social skill. According to the behavioral model described earlier, skill deficits will tend to be situation-specific. Some patients, for example, may find it easy to assert their rights with peers but not with strangers. Others may have trouble thinking of something to say when interacting with opposite-sex partners but perform better when interacting with same-sex partners. To the extent that situational variability in social performance is evident, the presence of a skill deficit is implied. In addition to helping to establish the existence of a skill deficit, the identification of situational fluctuations in social performance permits the clinician to tailor training to the needs of individual patients.

In perhaps the majority of cases, many of the factors addressed above will be involved to some extent in the patient's social difficulties in addition to a skill deficit. In that case, social skills training is still a viable treatment option, but expectations for improvement must be correspondingly lowered. After the identification of patients who might benefit from a skills training program, a more exact assessment of skill deficits can be initiated.

AREAS OF SKILL DEFICITS

The deficits that a patient exhibits in different social situations must be defined in detail if training is to be successful. Vague descriptions of interpersonal difficulties suggest few if any behaviors to target for change. Table 1 lists the range of behavior that is usually evaluated in this regard. At the most elementary level, the components of social skill can be divided into various verbal, nonverbal, and social perceptual abilities. *Expressive elements* consist of the verbal and nonverbal response parameters involved in communicating a message to another individual. The most important of these is speech content. The words one chooses to use are of obvious importance in determining the received meaning of a spoken message. Thus, poverty of speech and/or poverty of content of speech (symptoms that are especially prominent in negative syndrome schizophrenics) can severely impair social performance.

Paralinguistic elements refer to the voice parameters that serve to qualify a verbal message. The same verbal statement can assume different

Table 1. Components of Social Skill

Expressive elements
  Speech content
  Paralinguistic elements
    Voice volume
    Pace
    Pitch
    Tone
  Nonverbal behavior
    Proxemics
    Kinesics
    Eye contact
    Facial expression
Receptive elements (social perception)
  Attention
  Decoding
  Knowledge of context factors and cultural mores
Interactive balance
  Response timing
  Turn-taking
  Social reinforcement

shades of meaning, depending on whether it was spoken with a flat or animated tone, with loud or soft voice volume, or in a slow or rapid manner. Psychiatric patients often exhibit deficits in this area, especially with respect to voice tonality. Most commonly, patients will speak in a monotone voice and will require direct training in the use of expressive tonality.

Nonverbal behavior refers to an individual's bodily positions and movements during social interaction. As with paralinguistic elements, these responses play an important role in that they can either strengthen or detract from a verbal message. Thus, for example, an assertive refusal of an unreasonable request is more likely to be effective when accompanied by direct eye contact and serious facial expression than when accompanied by downcast eyes and shuffling feet. Some common difficulties exhibited by schizophrenic patients in this regard include diminished facial responsiveness, minimal eye contact, and restricted bodily movements and gestures (kinesics).

Receptive elements refer to an individual's social perceptual abilities. Effective social interaction is dependent upon the ability to detect, interpret, and respond appropriately to what are often subtle interpersonal cues. Thus, for example, patients may need to be taught that conversational partners will sometimes indirectly signal that they are ready to end a conversation (e.g., by glancing at the door) and that steps taken to end the conversation at this point are appropriate. An important prerequisite of this ability, and one that can easily be taken for granted, is focused attention. Attentional deficits are common in schizophrenic patients (Cromwell, 1978; Kornetsky & Orzack, 1978; Wohlberg & Kornetsky, 1973), and they may be particularly severe in patients who exhibit negative symptoms (Andreasen, 1982; Green & Walker, 1984). Thus, many patients will require extensive training to attend to relevant interpersonal cues. In addition to simply attending to these cues, most patients will need to learn how to respond appropriately to them. Appropriate responses are determined both by transient contextual factors and by cultural mores.

A final category of social skill is *interactive balance*. Included in this category are response timing, turn-taking, and social reinforcement. Psychiatric patients may, for example, exhibit inappropriately long response latencies when they are asked a question, causing others to feel uncomfortable. They may also be ignorant of the give-and-take of conversational interaction and try to inject statements at inopportune moments. Social reinforcement refers to the cues one individual provides to another to indicate attention and interest (e.g., head nodding, "um-hm," occasional smiles). Schizophrenic patients often fail to emit such responses or do so infrequently.

The individual responses described above constitute many of the important components of social skill. They are defined on the most elementary level to permit detailed specification of any deficits that might exist. However, when considered on that level alone, a complete description of adequate behavior still does not capture the essence of skillful social performance. Competent social performance is characterized not only by the correct execution of individual response elements but also by the integration of those elements into a variety of high-level or complex behavioral repertoires. Conversation skills, assertive skills, heterosocial skills (e.g., dating behavior), and vocational skills are all examples of the complex repertoires that constitute skillful social behavior. Schizophrenic patients may exhibit deficits in all of these areas, and all have been the target of social skills training programs for these patients (Liberman, Mueser, Wallace, Jacobs, Eckman, & Massel, 1986). A detailed treatment manual for training psychiatric patients in the use of these skills has been developed by Beidel, Bellack, Turner, Hersen, and Luber (1981).

In order to train a patient in the use of complex behavioral skills, those skills must be reduced to less complex component responses. As an example, consider the training of basic conversational skills. Table 2 lists some of the behavioral skills required to carry on an ordinary conversation. Separate abilities are required for initiating, maintaining, and ending a conversation. However, even at that level of specificity, the moment-by-moment responses required of the patient are not specified. Table 3 provides an even more detailed description of the behavioral components of one aspect of conversation skills (initiating a conversation). Only when they are reduced to this level of detail can a patient be trained in the use of the molecular responses listed in Table 1 as they relate to conversational abilities. A similar procedure would be followed for training assertive, heterosocial, and job skills (Beidel et al., 1981).

Table 2. Conversational Skills

Initiating conversations
Initiating a brief conversation with an acquaintance
Initiating a brief conversation with a stranger
Social telephone calls
Maintaining conversations
Asking questions
Providing information
Social reinforcement
Social perception
Ending conversations
Timing
How to break off
Good-byes
Judging when the partner wants to leave

Table 3. Initiating a Conversation

---

1. Make contact, e.g., Smile and say, "Hello
   (*name*)."
2. Ask a general question, e.g., "How have you
   been?"
3. Ask a specific question or answer a question
   from the other person.
4. Give a reason for leaving and say good-bye,
   e.g., "I have an appointment . . ."

BEHAVIORAL OBSERVATION

The best way to determine whether a patient exhibits deficits in any of
the areas described above would be through extended observation of his or
her social behavior. To this end, clinical staff can be trained to attend specifically to relevant social responses. A nurse's observations of a patient's conversational abilities, for example, can be invaluable in the development of an
individualized skills training program. However, because the hospital environment does not provide a full range of social opportunities, additional
assessment methods will usually be necessary. Were it not for the time and
expense involved, a very complete social assessment would be provided by
direct observation of the patient's behavior in his or her natural environment. Fortunately, several more cost-effective methods have been developed in recent years. The most widely employed procedure in this regard is
the "role-play" test.

Role-Play Tests. A role-play test involves the brief enactment of a social
interaction as if the scene were really happening. In a typical test, a situation
is described to the patient, and the therapist, playing the role of another
individual in the situation, issues a verbal prompt. The patient is instructed
to respond to the prompt as realistically as possible, and the therapist extends the interaction for one or two more interchanges. For example, a
scene description read by the therapist might be as follows: "Imagine you
are home watching television when your roommate walks in and changes the
channel without asking. He says, 'Let's watch this channel for a while.'"
Following the patient's response, the therapist might continue: "You've
been watching your shows all day. This one is better anyway." Once again,
the patient would be asked to respond to the therapist's prompt.

Several role-play interactions can be videotaped for later scoring in
order to assess the patient's behavior in a variety of situations. Alternatively,
the clinician can simply evaluate the patient's role-play performance on an

ongoing basis, attending in particular to the skills listed in Table 1. Bellack (1979, 1983) has analyzed and reviewed the empirical evidence pertaining to the validity and utility of this assessment procedure. Although the data provide inconsistent support for this method, he nevertheless concludes that role-play tests may be the best option available for direct observational assessment.

The assessment procedures described in this section are designed to select appropriate patients for a skills training program, define their skill deficits as accurately as possible, and measure those deficits prior to and throughout training. The application of these procedures will help to prevent the inappropriate use of social skills training and will help to alert the therapist to ongoing progress or lack thereof. The following section describes the variety of methods employed in a skills training program.

SOCIAL SKILLS TRAINING PROCEDURES

Social skills training is an educative or reeducative process that is more analogous to motor skills training (e.g., teaching someone to play tennis) than to traditional psychotherapy. The therapist assumes the role of a teacher who instructs in the use of social skills and demonstrates how they are applied. In order to learn these skills, patients are required to practice newly acquired responses until they are able to perform them adequately. In general, an adequate level of performance is simply the minimal acceptable response and not the epitome of social skill.

Social skills training for psychiatric patients is generally conducted in a group format and proceeds in a highly structured fashion as described below. A typical group consists of approximately eight patients and meets three times a week for an hour. Fewer meetings would be unlikely to foster significant behavioral change, and more frequent sessions could exceed the learning capacity of many psychiatric patients (although Wallace, 1982, has used much more intensive training with good results). The duration of training will vary as a function of the syllabus. Usually, a minimum of 1 month must be devoted to a particular content area (e.g., assertiveness, job interview skills). The groups are best conducted by two therapists since it is difficult for one person to teach social skills and maintain control of the group on a continual basis. Moreover, the use of two therapists can greatly facilitate the demonstration, or modeling, of new social skills.

In order to organize and structure group activities, the therapist must identify a set of social situations that the patients typically encounter and that are relevant to their individual skill deficits. For example, initiating and maintaining conversations with other patients and requesting help from family members might be two situations around which to work on individual skills. Although the therapist will probably have to create most of these scenes, the patients in the group may be invited to describe situations in which they experience difficulty. The course of training generally proceeds from teaching the requisite skills for the least challenging social situation to the most challenging, using as many sessions as necessary at each level. The rationale for proceeding in this manner is that skills are more easily acquired under less threatening conditions, and the skills mastered at one level can serve as the basis for more complex skills to be learned later. Five techniques are generally employed to teach the patient a specific skill: instructions, modeling, rehearsal (role-playing), feedback and positive reinforcement, and homework.

INSTRUCTIONS

When presenting a new skill to be learned, the first step is to instruct the patient in its use and to provide a rationale for learning to use it. For example, when addressing the common negative symptom of blank facial expression, the therapist might say, "When listening to another person talk to you, an occasional nod and smile will let them know that you are listening and are interested in what they have to say." In keeping with the emphasis on training the minimally acceptable response, the instructions should be simple and straightforward and should not attempt to address subtle nuances of every skill.

MODELING

Although verbal instructions are helpful, one of the best ways to communicate essential information about a skill is to simply demonstrate or model its use. Immediately prior to demonstrating the skill, the therapist should draw attention to the most important response component (e.g., "Watch how I nod sometimes while I am listening"). A brief interaction can then be arranged using the cotherapist (if available) or another patient to assist in the demonstration. The enactment should be brief and to the point. Extended demonstrations are likely to exceed patients' attentional abilities or draw the patients' attention to extraneous behavior. The skill may have to be demonstrated repeatedly for some patients.

ROLE-PLAYING

After the skill has been demonstrated, the patient is asked to try to mimic the therapist's behavior in a brief role-play interaction. This is a most important component of social skills training because simply talking about and/or viewing skillful behavior is unlikely to impart those skills to the patient. Using the same scenario that was used to model the skill, each patient attempts to implement the skill in role-play with the therapist. Once the patients master the minimal components of the skill, the therapist can supervise further role-play and practice between the patients themselves. Although the learning abilities of individual patients will vary, in most cases extended practice and repetition will be necessary.

FEEDBACK AND SOCIAL REINFORCEMENT

In an effort to shape appropriate social skills, the therapist should provide feedback and positive reinforcement following every role-play. The feedback should be specific and focus initially on the positive aspects of the response under training. This principle is adhered to even when the patient's performance is grossly deficient. Only after the patient's attempt is appropriately praised are suggestions for change provided. For example, the therapist might say, "You did a very good job of looking at my eyes when you first started to speak. This time, try to do even more of that." A patient who experiences frequent feelings of success and who receives prodigious praise and encouragement from the therapist is far more likely to retain the motivation required to practice social skills to proficiency than one who receives only suggestions for improvement.

HOMEWORK

Role-play interaction provides an opportunity for the patient to learn and practice new skills, but additional practice between sessions is required in order for those skills to generalize to other settings. In this regard, patients are routinely given specific homework assignments to use the skills acquired in a particular session with other individuals prior to the next session. Specific assignments, such as "Ask your roommate to help you play cards tonight" are more likely to meet with compliance than vague assignments such as "Try requesting things from people." The assignment should be one that is likely to meet with success. Thus, the therapist should be reasonably certain that the patient is capable of carrying out the assignment and that it stands a good chance of receiving a favorable response. At the beginning of each session, the homework assignments from the preceding session are reviewed and any problems that have arisen are resolved before proceeding to a new skill.

SOCIAL PERCEPTION TRAINING

The mastery of individual response skills does not guarantee their effective use in social situations. In addition to training overt response skills, patients usually must be taught when and where to use them. These abilities require that the patient attend to and correctly interpret both interpersonal and contextual cues. For example, a patient who has just mastered the ability to initiate a conversation may also need to learn that it can be unwise to implement that skill with someone displaying an extremely unreceptive facial expression. Similarly, a patient who has learned to effectively refuse a request may need to learn that the skill can be put to good use when dealing with a saleperson, but not when dealing with a police officer.

Training in social perceptual abilities does not follow a separate structured sequence of activities but is instead integrated into the response training procedures described above. The objective is to train the patient to attend to and interpret interpersonal cues that signify the feelings and motives of other individuals and to contextual variables that determine the appropriateness of various responses. This can be accomplished during role-play interaction by introducing subtle variations in the therapist's behavior and inquiring into the possible meanings of those variations. For example, during role-plays involving casual conversation, the therapist can increasingly exhibit nonverbal cues indicating a lack of interest and a desire to leave (e.g., fidget, glance at watch, look at door). After each role-play, patients can be questioned about possible interpretations of, and acceptable responses to, such behavior. With respect to contextual cues, training is mainly achieved through didactic means. Thus, a portion of each session can be devoted to discussing the social rules that govern the acceptable use of the skills under consideration.

Wallace (1982) has developed a program specifically intended to improve the information-processing skills of schizophrenic patients. In this program, patients are taught to accurately receive and process incoming stimuli, and to subsequently send effective verbal and nonverbal responses. The distinctive component of this approach is its emphasis on interpersonal stimulus processing, or *problem solving*, during which patients are taught to generate various response options, weigh the value of those options, and devise an appropriate response implementation strategy. This approach has proven to be effective with many schizophrenic patients, and it appears to offer a practical means of addressing the information-processing deficits of negative schizophrenics.

EMPIRICAL EVALUATION OF SOCIAL SKILLS TRAINING

RESPONSE ACQUISITION

The ability of social skills training to effect change in a behavior has been empirically demonstrated in numerous single-case (Bellack, Hersen, &

Turner, 1976; Edelstein & Eisler, 1976; Hersen & Bellack, 1976; Hersen, Turner, Edelstein, & Pinkston, 1975) and group design studies (Bellack, Turner, Hersen, & Luber, 1984; Wallace & Liberman, 1985). For example, Bellack et al. (1976) exposed three chronic schizophrenics to several weeks of daily social skills training focusing on increasing eye contact, speech duration, and the use of gestures. A multiple-baseline procedure was employed in which treatment was applied to one skill at a time. When improvement in that skill was forthcoming, the focus of treatment was shifted to another skill, and so on. For all three subjects, the individual skills improved measurably upon the application of direct training.

Hersen and Bellack (1976) exposed two chronic schizophrenic patients to approximately 5 weeks of social skills training that concentrated on increasing eye contact, speech duration, and frequency of requests, and decreasing automatic compliance to the requests of others. A multiple-baseline design was employed and, as before, the results indicated that skills training *per se* was responsible for improvements in each of these areas for both patients. In addition, patients improved on overall ratings of assertiveness (both positive and negative assertion) in role-play interactions involving both males and females.

Wallace and Liberman (1985) compared the effectiveness of group social skills training to holistic health therapy (a common component of many inpatient and day hospital programs) for 28 male schizophrenic patients. Social skills training focused on improving patients' "receiving" skills (e.g., accurately perceiving problem situations), "processing" skills (e.g., considering several response alternatives), and "sending" skills (e.g., delivering appropriate verbal and nonverbal responses). Patients were randomly assigned to treatment condition, and both groups received daily sessions for 9 weeks. By the end of treatment, social skills training was shown to be substantially more effective than holistic therapy in improving patients' ability to correctly identify important social cues and to formulate effective responses.

GENERALIZATION AND MAINTENANCE

The extent to which the effects of social skills training generalize to nontraining environments, and persist following training, has raised a concern for some time. As early as 1976, Bellack and Hersen described the findings regarding generalization and maintenance with chronic psychiatric patients as "mixed." In a subsequent paper, Morrison and Bellack (1984) concluded that relatively little progress had been made in this area. In fact, it has only been relatively recently that investigators have considered generalization and maintenance in a methodologically sophisticated fashion. Early investigations evaluated outcome using the same laboratory role-play scenes that were used to assess pretreatment competence. Later, responses to novel role-play scenes were employed as a generalization measure (e.g., Bellack et al., 1976; Monti et al., 1979). Finally, investigators began to evaluate *in vivo* performance. Current findings indicate that generalization can be obtained if the skills training program includes procedures to specifically facilitate transfer to the natural environment (Baer, Wolf, & Risley, 1968). The procedure that has been used most widely has been *in vivo* practice. Liberman et al. (1984) have reported a series of controlled case reports in which the effects of intensive (20 hours per week) social skills training with three schizophrenic patients were augmented with *in vivo* homework assignments. Also, Finch and Wallace (1977) assigned homework to pairs of schizophrenic patients, to be completed together. This procedure was successful in increasing homework completion, and patients who received skills training and homework performed more skillfully than a matched nontreatment control group in spontaneously enacted situations occurring in the natural environment.

Similarly, investigators have become more sophisticated with regard to the evaluation and facilitation of maintenance of the effects of social skills training with chronic psychiatric patients. The results of earlier studies with follow-up assessments ranging from 8 weeks to 10 months posttreatment suggest that social skills training can produce durable improvements in social functioning (e.g., Bellack et al., 1976; Hersen & Bellack, 1976; Monti et al., 1979; Monti, Curran, Corriveau, Delancey, & Hagerman, 1980). However, most follow-up procedures have relied on either self-report or behavioral laboratory assessment procedures. Performance on these measures is an important indicator of whether the targeted responses remain in the patient's behavioral repertoire. However, it does not reflect the clinical significance of social skills training in terms of the patient's ongoing use of "new" skills in his or her interpersonal environment.

One of the more significant advances with regard to programming for both generalization and maintenance of social skills training effects is recent work by Janet St. Lawrence and her colleagues involving the social validation of target behaviors selected for social skills training (Hansen, St. Lawrence, & Christoff, 1985; Holmes, Hansen, & St. Lawrence, 1984). With this procedure, component behaviors for training, as well as performance criterion levels for the behaviors, are established from an assessment of the interpersonal skills of "normal" nonpsychiatric persons in the community. The rationale for this social validation approach is that training behaviors to criterion levels will permit the behaviors to more easily come under the control of environmental contingencies, thus facilitating both generalization and maintenance. Holmes et al. (1984) provided group social skills training that focused on specific conversational components and speech content to 10 chronic psychiatric patients enrolled in a partial hospitalization program. All of the patients had conversational difficulty. Results were evaluated using a multiple-baseline design, and demonstrated the effectiveness of the training procedures. Following training, the frequency of targeted component behaviors increased to socially validated criterion levels. Training effects generalized to unfamiliar, nonpsychiatric conversational partners and were maintained throughout a 7-month follow-up.

However, even these investigations by St. Lawrence and colleagues fail to fully address the overall *clinical* impact of social skills training. While their training techniques are effective in terms of patients' acquiring and maintaining new skills in their repertoires, and using these new skills during social interactions, the issue of whether these new skills provide a clinically meaningful difference has not been addressed. The purpose of any psychosocial intervention for schizophrenic patients is to facilitate better adjustment in the community and, ultimately, to prevent or postpone relapse. Unfortunately, the work by St. Lawrence and others did not address relapse. A frequent critique of social skills training has been that changes in social skills repertoires "do not often result in substantial differences in patients' quality if life" (Wallace et al., 1980, p. 60). Also, while considerable methodologic control was devoted toward the development and evaluation of the conversational skills treatment, this series of investigations involved a mixed diagnostic group of patients. Therefore, the findings may not be applicable to a carefully diagnosed sample of schizophrenics.

Bellack et al. (1984) used a 12-week day hospital program supplemented by comprehensive social skills training to treat a group of 44 chronic schizophrenic patients. The performance of these patients was assessed using a battery of self-report and behavioral measures and was compared to the performance of 20 chronic schizophrenic patients who received only day hospital treatment. Results indicated that both patient groups had improved at posttreatment. However, during the 6-month posttreatment period, patients who had received social skills training either continued to improve or maintained their gains on most measures, while the patients receiving day hospital treatment alone either maintained gains or lost them. Finally, almost half of the patients in both groups were hospitalized at least once during the year following treatment. Thus, the findings suggest that social skills training did little to forestall relapse with these patients.

Subsequent findings reported by Liberman, Mueser, and Wallace (1986) indicate that schizophrenics who received intensive (12 hours per week) social skills training as inpatients evidenced better functioning and had spent less time hospitalized and had fewer symptomatic relapses 2 years after treatment than a comparable patient group that had received holistic health treatment during the index inpatient hospitalization. Thus, these results support the efficacy of social skills training in the treatment of schizophrenia. That the findings reported by Bellack et al. (1984) and Liberman et al. (1986) are so discordant with regard to the prevention of relapse may be attributable to differences in the skills training protocols and/or to characteristics of the patients themselves. With regard to treatment, the skills training procedures utilized by Liberman et al. were much more intensive. This factor should receive further consideration in relationship to treatment outcome.

Data reported by Hogarty et al. (1986) attest to the importance of possible interactions between social skills training and specific patient characteristics. These investigators examined the effects of social skills training, family psychoeducation, and maintenance medication in the aftercare treatment of schizophrenic and schizoaffective patients. Both social skills training and family treatment, administered in conjunction with medication, resulted in a significant reduction in first-year relapse rates relative to control subjects (maintenance neuroleptic treatment). Furthermore, combined treatment (social skills training and family psychoeducation) reduced first-year relapse to 0% (among 17 subjects receiving combined treatment). Finally, the effects of social skills training were apparently somewhat mitigated among patients discharged in a psychotic state. Three patients in the social skills training condition experienced a Type II relapse, defined by the authors as a "severe clinical exacerbation of persistent psychotic symptoms" (p. 636).

While these findings suggest an important symptomologic parameter that may relate to outcome of social skills training, additional parameters must be examined. For example, further knowledge is needed about relapse in schizophrenia, in order to evaluate what specific changes in skill/behavior may occur prior to, and thus perhaps be influential in the occurrence of, relapse. In essence, it is important to evaluate the relationship of social skills deficits to other aspects of schizophrenic symptomatology. It is becoming increasingly apparent that neither the skills deficit model nor social skills training as typically practiced is sufficient to account for the complexities of interpersonal behavior. As we noted earlier, a number of factors relating to schizophrenic symptomatology can have an impact on the social functioning of these patients. Skills other than motoric response components must be considered. A comprehensive perspective on the interpersonal functioning of schizophrenics requires consideration of such diverse factors as social perception, cognitive and problem-solving abilities, family and social networks, and medication effects, as well as an understanding of the potential impact of the natural course of the disorder. Two of the most significant factors that have recently been receiving considerable attention are negative symptoms and attentional/cognitive impairment. We will discuss potential relationships between these symptoms and social skills in the next section.

THE RELATIONSHIP OF SOCIAL DYSFUNCTION TO ATTENTIONAL IMPAIRMENTS AND NEGATIVE SCHIZOPHRENIC SYMPTOMS

It is now apparent that schizophrenia involves a wide range of basic cognitive and information-processing impairments. These include attentional impairments (Cromwell, 1978; Kornetsky & Orzack, 1978; Wohlberg & Kornetsky, 1973), distractibility (Oltmanns & Neale, 1975; Oltmanns, Ohayon, & Neale, 1978), and slowed information processing (Davidson & Neale, 1974; Rochester, 1978). In addition, the impact of deficit symptoms of schizophrenia (e.g., anergia, apathy) that constitute the negative syndrome of the disorder has recently been emphasized (e.g., Andreasen & Olsen, 1982). These factors have potentially significant implications for the assessment and treatment of social dysfunction.

ATTENTION AND PERCEPTION

Information-processing deficits could prevent schizophrenics from accurately perceiving interpersonal cues, which would in turn prohibit them from emitting a response that was appropriate within the context of those cues. In fact, it has been suggested that the deficits in interpersonal and role functioning that characterize schizophrenics may be secondary to impaired information processing (Nuechterlein & Dawson, 1984). However, few empirical studies have specifically addressed this relationship.

Recently, increasing attention has been focused on affect recognition as a particular aspect of information processing that may relate to the impaired interpersonal functioning of schizophrenics. One of the most consistently reported findings in the literature on schizophrenia during the past 10 years has been that patients have problems in the perception of affect (Feinberg, Rifkin, Schaffer, & Walker, 1986). In particular, schizophrenics' difficulties in decoding facial expressions of affect have been widely reported (e.g., Feinberg et al., 1986; Novic, Luchins, & Perline, 1984; Walker, McGuire, & Bettes, 1984). The mechanisms underlying these difficulties are unclear. There is some suggestion that the facial affect recognition deficits of at least a subgroup of schizophrenics could be mediated by right hemisphere lesions. There is extensive evidence indicating that the perception of affect is primarily mediated by the right hemisphere (Bradshaw & Nettleton, 1981). Also, right-brain-damaged patients evidence affect recognition deficits similar to those exhibited by schizophrenics (e.g., Cicone, Wapner, & Gardner, 1980). There is also some suggestion that paranoid schizophrenics may be particularly likely to exhibit right-hemisphere-mediated facial affect recognition deficits (Morrison, Bellack, & Mueser, 1988). However, on the basis of their findings that emotion recognition deficits were greater in adult than in child schizophrenics, Walker et al. (1984) suggested that the deficits may be, at least partially, a consequence of social withdrawal.

A number of issues should be addressed in developing remediative techniques for affect recognition deficits in schizophrenics. First, the possibility that, in at least a subset of patients, these deficits may be mediated by a right hemisphere lesion and/or atypical preferred information-processing strategies (e.g., Walker & McGuire, 1982) should be considered. As a result, there may be a limitation on the extent of recoverability of affect recognition skills. For example, such behavioral deficits as impaired conceptual abilities and visual-spatial deficits have been recalcitrant to treatment among brain-damaged adults (Goldstein & Ruthven, 1983). However, the degree of recoverability of function is often related to the extent of the loss of function and/or severity of the lesion. Moreover, data indicate that while the normal process of facial affect recognition may be disrupted among right-hemisphere-damaged patients, these patients may be able to make relevant distinctions between affective states by using alternative mechanisms (Etcoff, 1984). Thus, even if the affect recognition deficits of some schizophrenics are organically mediated, there may be appropriate rehabilitative techniques available. The particular mechanisms that Etcoff observed right-brain-damaged patients utilizing included:

> . . . scanning for physical landmarks on the face, and recalling and mentally imagining situations where particular expressions are commonly seen. The use of these strategies can lead to accuracy or inaccuracy in decoding facial emotion depending on the extent to which the subject scans the face for the appropriate landmarks, the subject's knowledge of the correlation between particular landmarks and particular emotional states, the extent of the subject's knowledge of situations which generate particular emotions, the quality and quantity of the subject's stored associations between particular expressions and particular situations, and, finally, the extent to which the subject thinks to use any of the above in a task. (p. 410)

Similar strategies may be appropriate for affect recognition training with schizophrenics.

Alternatively, affect recognition deficits among schizophrenics may be secondary to their more general attentional and/or information-processing impairments. That is, the deficit in affect recognition may be due to an inability to attend to interpersonal partners' affective cues, rather than to a specific problem *decoding* those cues. If affect recognition impairments are secondary to attentional impairments or general visuopatial difficulties, they might be alleviated by interventions that improve the general level of attentional or processing skill, as with neuroleptics (Braff & Saccuzzo, 1982). Finally, affect recognition deficits that stem from social withdrawal and/or lack of practice would presumably be responsive to a training approach emphasizing repeated practice and performance feedback as typically characterizes skills training based on the behavioral model. Wallace and his colleagues have reported preliminary findings on training procedures of this sort (Wallace, 1982). Training involves question-and-answer sessions based on videotaped social vignettes that are presented to the patient. After viewing a vignette, the patient is questioned about his or her perception of situational parameters, and processing of response options to the situation (e.g., Who are the people talking in the scene? What did the first speaker say? What is the problem in the situation? What is the best solution to the problem?).

Also, Marlowe and Marcotte (1984) have reported on the development of a training curriculum that was intended to help psychiatric patients learn to identify nonverbal cues of emotion. However, they did not report outcome data pertaining to the use of this training program. While these efforts appear promising, much further work is needed in the training of affect recognition skills in schizophrenics, and the evaluation of the generalization and maintenance of training effects.

NEGATIVE SYNDROME SCHIZOPHRENIA

Recently, considerable attention has been focused on the subtyping of schizophrenic patients into groups exhibiting primarily negative symptoms versus nonnegative syndrome patients. This contemporary interest was fueled by Strauss et al. (1974), who proposed a tripartite framework that distinguished between positive symptoms, negative symptoms, and "disorders in relating." Positive symptoms comprise the manifest psychotic features of the disorder that clearly exceed the boundaries of normal experience. Hallucinations and delusions are the most commonly cited examples. Negative symptoms, on the other hand, are characterized by the loss or absence of normal functioning and include such phenomena as blunting of affect, apathy, and thought blocking. Negative symptoms have commanded considerable recent attention because they have been hypothesized to be inflexible, indicative of intellectual impairment, prognostic of poor outcome, and resistant to neuroleptic therapy (Crow, 1980, 1985; Owens & Johnstone, 1980).

The third symptom category described by Strauss and others, disorders in relating, comprises the social and interpersonal deficits of schizophrenics. However, most researchers have subsequently adopted a dichotomous view of schizophrenic symptoms (negative vs. positive). While some have incorporated the Strauss et al. third category into their definition of negative symptoms (e.g., Andreasen, 1982), others have rejected the notion that impaired social competence is a direct result of the schizophrenic disease process (e.g., Crow, 1980). As a consequence of these differing perspectives, definitions of the negative symptom complex vary widely among investigators.

This disagreement notwithstanding, patients who exhibit negative symptoms (however defined) have been consistently found to be more socially impaired than other schizophrenic patients. For example, Andreasen and Olsen (1982), using a broad-based definition of negative symptoms that included a measure of social withdrawal, reported that negative syndrome patients had poorer premorbid adjustment and greater social impairments than those who exhibited primarily positive symptoms or a mixture of both positive and negative symptoms. Pogue-Geile and Harrow (1984) employed a narrower definition of negative symptoms that did not contain a measure of social functioning, and reported virtually the same findings regarding social impairment. Thus, whether or not deficits in social functioning are considered to constitute the negative syndrome, negative schizophrenics appear to be among the most socially impaired psychiatric patients.

As the severity of the negative syndrome has become evident, interest in the development of effective treatment strategies for negative schizophrenics has accelerated (Crow, 1985; Pogue-Geile & Harrow, 1985). Current opinion varies widely with regard to the merits of neuroleptic medication for treating these patients, perhaps owing to the multiple definitions that the negative symptom construct has received). After reviewing a series of recent investigations, Meltzer, Sommers, and Luchins (1986) and Schooler (1986) conclude that antipsychotic drugs can be effective in the treatment of negative symptoms, especially if the patient is treated during the early stages of the illness. However, Schooler (1986) has further observed that neuroleptics provide only a partial response to the treatment needs of negative schizophrenics, and that the combined use of pharmacological and psychosocial therapies may be the most efficacious treatment approach. Because of the marked social dysfunction exhibited by these patients, social skills training may be a critical treatment component. Although the etiology of social impairment in negative schizophrenia is unclear, one possibility is that the chronic nature of negative symptoms consistently interferes with the experiences required to learn effective social behavior. Positive symptoms, which tend to be more transient and episodic, may interfere with these experiences on a more intermittent basis and may therefore be less socially damaging. According to this view, social skills training may be particularly appropriate for negative schizophrenics who require explicit training (or retraining) in behavior normally shaped (and/or maintained) by the social environment.

However, an alternate perspective on the relationship between negative symptoms and social dysfunction is provided in the data reported by Pogue-Geile and Harrow (1985). In their study, negative and positive symptoms were investigated longitudinally in a group of young schizophrenic patients at two follow-up assessments approximately 2.5 and 5 years after hospital discharge. Among their findings was that negative symptoms were more frequent at follow-up among schizophrenics who had poor educational achievement and poor social functioning prior to the index hospitalization. These data suggest that poor social functioning may be prognostically significant for the development of negative symptoms. Pogue-Geile and Harrow posit that both negative symptoms and general role-functioning deficits are influenced by some shared factors and thus tend to occur concurrently. However, the prognostic significance of poor social functioning should not be minimized. It may be the case that social skills training, if initiated early enough in the course of the disorder, could become a secondary prevention intervention against the subsequent development of negative symptoms.

A final issue with regard to social skills training with negative syndrome patients has to do with the possible adverse impact of aspects of the negative syndrome on patients' ability to benefit from treatment. A number of investigators has reported an association between negative symptoms and intellectual deficits (Andreasen & Olsen, 1982; Owens & Johnstone, 1980; Pogue-Geile & Harrow, 1985). Owing to these deficits, negative schizophrenics may have only limited capacity to benefit from structured learning therapies such as social skills training. Therefore, it is critical that the difficulty and complexity of the skills training protocol be carefully matched to the needs and capacities of the patients in treatment. A second, equally limiting aspect of the syndrome complex may be the amotivational state of the negative schizophrenic patient. While in some cases the patient's energy and interest levels may improve as a result of neuroleptics, many negative schizophrenics will show little interest in participating in treatment. Successful skills training will depend as much upon the therapist's ability to have an impact on the patient's motivation to participate as upon the specific skill curriculum on which training is based.

CONCLUSION

Social skills training is one of the predominant psychosocial treatments for schizophrenia. While current training technology has been shown to be effective, in order to maximize treatment outcome, future social skills training programs should be carefully matched to specific subtypes of schizophrenic symptomatology, and integrated with pharmacological interventions. The specific impact of social skills training on the functioning of negative syndrome patients should be evaluated. Also, the role of information-processing deficits in social dysfunction requires further evaluation. Finally, social skills training techniques need to be further expanded to better address skills such as social perception and problem solving. These advances will undoubtedly serve to increase the importance of social skills training in the treatment of schizophrenia.

ACKNOWLEDGMENT

Preparation of this paper was supported in part by a research grant (MH38636-04) from the National Institute of Mental Health.

REFERENCES

American Psychiatric Association. (1987). *Diagnostic and statistical manual of mental disorders* (3rd ed., rev.). Washington, DC: Author.

Andreasen, N. C. (1982). Negative symptoms in schizophrenia: Definition and reliability. *Archives of General Psychiatry, 39*, 784–788.

Andreasen, N. C., & Olsen, S. (1982). Negative vs. positive schizophrenia: Definition and validation. *Archives of General Psychiatry, 39*, 789–794.

Arkowitz, H. (1977). Measurement and modification of minimal dating behavior. In M. Hersen, R. M. Eisler, & P. M. Miller (Eds.), *Progress in behavior modification* (Vol. 5). New York: Academic Press.

Baer, D. M., Wolf, M. M., & Risley, T. R. (1968). Some current dimensions of applied behavior analysis. *Journal of Applied Behavior Analysis, 1*, 91–97.

Beidel, D. C., Bellack, A. S., Turner, S. M., Hersen, M., & Luber, R. F. (1981). Social skills training for chronic psychiatric patients: A treatment manual. *JSAS Catalog of Selected Documents in Psychology, 11*, 36 (MS. 2257).

Bellack, A. S. (1979). A critical appraisal of strategies for assessing social skill. *Behavioral Assessment, 1*, 157–176.

Bellack, A. S. (1983). Recurrent problems in the behavioral assessment of social skill. *Behaviour Research and Therapy, 21*, 29–42.

Bellack, A. S., & Hersen, M. (Eds.). (1979). *Research and practice in social skills training*. New York: Plenum Press.

Bellack, A. S., Hersen, M., & Himmelhoch, J. M. (1983). A comparison of social skills training, pharmacotherapy, and psychotherapy for depression. *Behaviour Research and Therapy, 21*, 101–107.

Bellack, A. S., Hersen, M., & Turner, S. M. (1976). Generalization effects of social skills training in chronic schizophrenics: An experimental analysis. *Behaviour Research and Therapy, 14*, 391–398.

Bellack, A. S., Turner, S. M., Hersen, M., & Luber, R. F. (1984). An examination of the efficacy of social skills training for chronic schizophrenic patients. *Hospital and Community Psychiatry, 35*, 1023–1028.

Bradshaw, J. L., & Nettleton, N. C. (1981). The nature of hemispheric specialization in man. *Behavioral and Brain Sciences, 4*, 51–91.

Braff, D., & Saccuzzo, D. (1982). Effect of antipsychotic medication on speed of information processing in schizophrenic patients. *American Journal of Psychiatry, 193*, 1127–1130.

Brown, G. W., Birley, J. L. T., & Wing, J. K. (1972). Influence of family life on the course of schizophrenic disorders: A replication. *British Journal of Psychiatry, 121*, 241–258.

Carpenter, W. T., Heinrichs, D. W., & Alphs, L. D. (1985). Treatment of negative symptoms. *Schizophrenia Bulletin, 11*, 440–452.

Cicone, M., Wapner, W., & Gardner, H. (1980). Sensitivity to emotional expressions and situations in organic patients. *Cortex, 16*, 145–158.

Cromwell, R. L. (1978). Attention and information processing: A foundation for understanding schizophrenia? In L. C. Wynne, R. L. Cromwell, & S. Matthysse (Eds.), *The nature of schizophrenia: New approaches to research and treatment.* New York: Wiley.

Crow, T. J. (1980). Molecular pathology of schizophrenia: More than one dimension of pathology? *British Medical Journal, 289*, 66–68.

Crow, T. J. (1985). The two-syndrome concept: Origins and current status. *Schizophrenia Bulletin, 11*, 471–485.

Davidson, G. S., & Neale, J. M. (1974). The effects of signal-noise similarity on visual information processing of schizophrenics. *Journal of Abnormal Psychology, 83*, 683–686.

Edelstein, B. A., & Eisler, R. M. (1976). Effects of modeling and modeling with instructions and feedback on the behavioral components of social skills. *Behavior Therapy, 7*, 382–389.

Etcoff, N. L. (1984). Perceptual and conceptual organization of facial emotions: Hemispheric differences. *Brain and Cognition, 3*, 385–412.

Feinberg, T. E., Rifkin, A., Schaffer, C., & Walker, E. (1986). Facial discrimination and emotional recognition in schizophrenia and affective disorders. *Archives of General Psychiatry, 43*, 276–279.

Finch, B. E., & Wallace, C. J. (1977). Successful interpersonal skills training with schizophrenic patients. *Journal of Consulting and Clinical Psychology, 45*, 885–890.

Gleser, G. C., & Gottschalk, L. A. (1967). Personality characteristics of chronic schizophrenics in relationship to sex and current functioning. *Journal of Clinical Psychology, 23*, 349–354.

Goldstein, G., & Ruthven, L. (1983). *Rehabilitation of the brain-damaged adult.* New York: Plenum Press.

Green, M., & Walker, E. (1984). Susceptibility to backward masking in positive versus negative symptom schizophrenia. *American Journal of Psychiatry, 141*, 1273–1275.

Hansen, D. J., St. Lawrence, J. S., & Christoff, K. A. (1985). Effects of interpersonal problem-solving training with chronic aftercare patients on problem-solving component skills and effectiveness of solutions. *Journal of Consulting and Clinical Psychology, 53*, 167–174.

Hersen, M., & Bellack, A. S. (1976). A multiple-baseline analysis of social skills training in chronic schizophrenics. *Journal of Applied Behavior Analysis, 9*, 239–245.

Hersen, M., Turner, S. M., Edelstein, B. A., & Pinkston, S. G. (1975). Effects of phenothiazines and social skills training in a withdrawn schizophrenic. *Journal of Clinical Psychology, 34*, 588–594.

Hogarty, G. E., Anderson, C. M., Reiss, D. J., Kornblith, S. J., Greenwald, D. P., Javna, C. D., & Madonia, M. J. (1986). Family psychoeducation, social skills training, and maintenance chemotherapy in the aftercare treatment of schizophrenia. *Archives of General Psychiatry, 43*, 633–642.

Holmes, M. R., Hansen, D. G., & St. Lawrence, J. S. (1984). Conversational skills training with aftercare patients in the community: Social validation and generalization. *Behavior Therapy, 15*, 84–100.

Kornetsky, C., & Orzack, M. H. (1978). Physiologic and behavioral correlates of attention dysfunction in schizophrenic patients. In L. C. Wynne, R. L. Cromwell, & S. Matthysse (Eds.), *The nature of schizophrenia: New approaches to research and treatment*. New York: Wiley.

Liberman, R. P., Lillie, F., Falloon, I. R. F., Harpin, R. E., Hutchinson, W., & Stoute, B. (1984). Social skills training with relapsing schizophrenics: An experimental analysis. *Behavior Modification, 8,* 155–179.

Liberman, R. P., Mueser, K. T., & Wallace, C. J. (1986). Social skills training for schizophrenic individuals at risk for relapse. *American Journal of Psychiatry, 143,* 523–526.

Liberman, R. P., Mueser, K. T., Wallace, C. J., Jacobs, H. E., Eckman, T., & Massel, H. K. (1986). Training skills in the psychiatrically disabled: Learning coping and competence. *Schizophrenia Bulletin, 12,* 631–646.

Marcella, A. J., & Snyder, K. K. (1981). Stress, social supports, and schizophrenic disorders: Toward an interactional model. *Schizophrenia Bulletin, 7,* 152–163.

Marlowe, H. A., Jr., & Marcotte, A. (1984). Non-verbal decoding. *Journal of Psychosocial Nursing, 22,* 8–15.

McClelland, D. C., & Walt, N. F. (1968). Sex role alienation in schizophrenia. *Journal of Abnormal Psychology, 12,* 217–220.

Meltzer, H. Y., Sommers, A. A., & Luchins, D. J. (1986). The effect of neuroleptics and other psychotropic drugs on the negative symptoms of schizophrenia. *Journal of Clinical Psychopharmacology, 6,* 329–338.

Monti, P. M., Curran, J. P., Corriveau, D. P., Delancey, A., & Hagerman, S. (1980). Effects of social skills training groups and sensitivity groups with psychiatric patients. *Journal of Consulting and Clinical Psychology, 48,* 241–248.

Monti, P. M., Fink, E., Norman, W., Curran, J. P., Hayes, S., & Caldwell, A. (1979). The effects of social skills training groups and social skills bibliotherapy with psychiatric patients. *Journal of Consulting and Clinical Psychology, 47,* 189–191.

Morrison,, R. L., & Bellack, A. S. (1984). Social skills training. In A. S. Bellack (Ed.), *Schizophrenia: Treatment, management, and rehabilitation* (pp. 247–279). New York: Grune & Stratton.

Morrison, R. L., Bellack, A. S., & Mueser, K. T. (1988). Deficits in facial-affect recognition and schizophrenia. *Schizophrenia Bulletin, 14,* 67–83.

Morrison, R. L., Bellack, A. S., & Mueser, K. T. (in press). Facial affect recognition and schizophrenia. *Schizophrenia Bulletin.*

Novic, J., Luchins, D. J., & Perline, R. (1984). Facial affect recognition in schizophrenia: Is there a differential deficit? *British Journal of Psychiatry, 144,* 533–537.

Nuechterlein, K. H., & Dawson, M. W. (1984). A heuristic vulnerability/stress model of schizophrenic episodes. *Schizophrenia Bulletin, 10,* 300–312.

Oltmanns, T. F., & Neale, J. M. (1975). Schizophrenic performance when distractors are present: Attentional deficit or differential task difficulty? *Journal of Abnormal Psychology, 84,* 205–209.

Oltmanns, T. F., Ohayon, J., & Neale, J. M. (1978). The effect of antipsychotic medication and diagnostic criteria on distractibility in schizophrenia. In L. C. Wynne, R. L. Cromwell, & S. Matthysse (Eds.), *The nature of schizophrenia: New approaches to research and treatment*. New York: Wiley.

Owens, D. G. C., & Johnstone, E. C. (1980). The disabilities of chronic schizophrenia: The nature and the factors contributing to their development. *British Journal of Psychiatry, 136,* 384–395.

Pogue-Geile, M. F., & Harrow, M. (1984). Negative and positive symptoms in schizophrenia and depression: A followup. *Schizophrenia Bulletin, 10,* 371–387.

Pogue-Geile, M. F., & Harrow, M. (1985). Negative symptoms in schizophrenia: Their longitudinal course and prognostic importance. *Schizophrenia Bulletin, 11*, 427–439.

Rochester, S. R. (1978). Are language disorders in acute schizophrenia actually information-processing problems. In L. C. Wynne, R. L. Cromwell, & S. Matthysse (Eds.), *The nature of schizophrenia: New approaches to research and treatment.* New York: Wiley.

Schooler, N. R. (1986). The efficacy of antipsychotic drugs and family therapy in the maintenance treatment of schizophrenia. *Journal of Clinical Psychopharmacology, 6,* 11s–19s.

Serban, G. (1975). Functioning ability in schizophrenia and normal subjects. Short-term prediction for rehospitalization of schizophrenics. *Comprehensive Psychiatry, 16,* 447–456.

Shaw, P. (1979). A comparison of three behavior therapies in the treatment of social phobia. *British Journal of Psychiatry, 134,* 620–623.

Strauss, J. S., Carpenter, W. T., & Bartko, J. J. (1974). The diagnosis and understanding of schizophrenia. Part III. Speculation on the processes that underlie schizophrenic symptoms and signs. *Schizophrenia Bulletin, 1,* 61–69.

Strauss, J. S., Klorman, R., & Kokes, R. F. (1977). Premorbid adjustment in schizophrenia. Part V: The implications of findings for understanding, research, and application. *Schizophrenia Bulletin, 3,* 240–244.

Vaughn, C. E., & Leff, J. P. (1976). The influence of family and social factors on the course of psychiatric illness: A comparison of schizophrenic and depressed neurotic patients. *British Journal of Psychiatry, 129,* 125–137.

Walker, E., & McGuire, M. (1982). Intra- and interhemispheric information processing in schizophrenia. *Psychological Bulletin, 92,* 701–725.

Walker, E., McGuire, M., & Bettes, B. (1984). Recognition and identification of facial stimuli by schizophrenics and patients with affective disorders. *British Journal of Psychiatry, 23,* 37–44.

Wallace, C. J. (1982). The social skills training project of the Mental Health Clinical Research Center for the study of schizophrenia. In J. P. Curran & P. M. Monti (Eds.), *Social skills training: A practical handbook for assessment and treatment* (pp. 57–89). New York: Guilford Press.

Wallace, C. J., & Liberman, R. P. (1985). Social skills training for patients with schizophrenia: A controlled clinical trial. *Psychiatry Research, 15,* 239–247.

Wallace, C. J., Nelson, C. J., Liberman, R. P., Aitchison, R. A., Lukoff, D., Elder, J. P., & Ferris, C. (1980). A review and critique of social skills training with schizophrenic patients. *Schizophrenia Bulletin, 6,* 42–63.

Weissman, M. M., Paykel, E. S., Siegel, R., & Klerman, G. L. (1971). The social role performance of depressed women: Comparisons with a normal group. *American Journal of Orthopsychiatry, 41,* 390–405.

Wixted, J. T., Morrison, R. L., & Bellack, A. S. (1988). Social skills training in the treatment of negative symptoms. *International Journal of Mental Health, 17,* 3–21.

Wohlberg, G., & Kornetsky, C. (1973). Sustained attention in remitted schizophrenics. *Archives of General Psychiatry, 28,* 533.

Zigler, E., & Phillips, L. (1961). Social competence and outcome in psychiatric disorders. *Journal of Abnormal and Social Psychology, 63,* 264–271.

Zigler, E. & Phillips, L. (1962). Social competence and the process-reactive distinction in psychopathology. *Journal of Abnormal and Social Psychology, 65,* 215–222.

11

Psychotherapy

C. Wesley Dingman and Thomas H. McGlashan

INTRODUCTION: THE RATIONALE FOR A BROADLY CONCEIVED PSYCHOTHERAPY

Schizophrenia is heterogeneous with respect to its symptoms, course, and outcome. So, too, are the individuals afflicted with it, with respect to their vulnerabilities, assets, and needs. For these reasons, our overall guiding principle in the therapy and management of this disorder is that no single treatment can be definitive or preferred. Instead, as illustrated by the variety of therapeutic interventions described in this volume, the treatment of schizophrenia requires a broad approach using multiple modalities.

Central to any array of treatments being offered to persons with schizophrenia lies their relationship with a professional clinician. In the context of such a continually available relationship, the afflicted individuals can develop trust and derive the support and understanding that will carry them through the exacerbations and remissions of the illness. This relationship between clinician and patient is what we mean by psychotherapy. Our goal in this chapter is to describe this relationship and to explicate some of the more important perspectives and techniques available to those engaging in such work.

A generation of empirical research has failed to demonstrate the efficacy of psychotherapy as the primary, and certainly as the only, treatment of schizophrenia. These data have been reviewed recently (Gomes-Schwartz, 1984). Basically, most studies have tested a fairly narrowly conceived form of

C. Wesley Dingman and Thomas H. McGlashan • Chestnut Lodge Hospital, 500 West Montgomery Avenue, Rockville, Maryland 20850.

psychoanalytically oriented dynamic psychotherapy, referred to in this chapter as investigative psychotherapy. Clearly, the findings do not support the *carte blanche* application of this form of psychotherapy and call for a reformulation of psychotherapeutic techniques. Accordingly, we are proposing a much broader concept of psychotherapy, one that uses a variety of strategies applied flexibly depending upon the individual patient and his or her type and phase of schizophrenia. We conceive of psychotherapy as a continuous relationship between patient and doctor/therapist which is primarily clinical in nature but which is informed and guided by psychotherapeutic principles.

If *disease* is viewed as an objective biologic process that may be understood in current scientific terms, then *illness* might be conceived of as the subjective human response to disease. That is, the illness is the particular, and often idiosyncratic, grouping of discomforts, complaints, anxieties, and changes in mood that are expressed by the person afflicted with the disease (Rogers, 1974). Rogers (1974) points out that physicians can cure only a few *diseases*, and they may be able to modify the course of several more, but they should always be prepared to treat most, if not all, *illnesses* within their particular area of training. He proclaims that physicians "need to become much better managers of illness" (especially the chronic and fatal illnesses), rather than to consider themselves solely as eradicators of disease.

Grandiosity and impatience, spawned by much of current training and practice, which emphasizes the rapidly effective and often technologically sophisticated cure of many diseases, often lead us to neglect treating patients suffering from those many other illnesses, either chronic or fatal, that do not similarly respond. We are prone to lose sight of the fact that our therapeutic expertise should be directed as much to the patient experiencing the illness as to the disease itself, and that appropriate treatment may not always be synonymous with cure (Charon, 1986; Rogers, 1974). Unquestionably, schizophrenia is among those many disorders that are not usually cured by any of our currently available interventions. In fact, despite our well-intentioned efforts, the course and outcome of schizophrenia is frequently chronic (McGlashan, 1988). Thus, until such time as cure can be reasonably expected as a result of some as yet undiscovered intervention(s), the more rational goals of our therapeutic efforts should properly be to lessen the severity and frequency of the illness's manifestations, and to facilitate the patient's maximal development of constructive adaptations (Ginzberg, 1987). These goals are complex and often call for periods of specialized treatment in different facilities by a variety of highly trained technicians. Such a melange of interventions, however necessary and indicated, runs the risk of aggravating the patient's fright, confusion, and despair. For this reason alone the patient needs a trusted and persevering therapist to help him or her manage this chronic, devastating illness and its treatment over time.

THE NATURE OF THE DISEASE

Our approach to the individual psychotherapy of this disorder is based on certain assumptions regarding the nature of schizophrenia. We hold that schizophrenia is a catastrophic de-integration of mental processes, the etiology of which remains largely unknown. On the one hand, genetics certainly plays a role in determining vulnerability to schizophrenia in many cases (Gottesman, McGuffin, & Farmer, 1987). On the other hand, subsequent biochemical and psychosocial events, both salutary and detrimental, may affect its onset, severity, course, and outcome. It is this interaction between the individual's disease process and other biologic and psychosocial variables (Engel, 1980) that determines the specific and overt responses and symptoms that we diagnose as a schizophrenic illness.

The above interaction has come to be known as the vulnerability-stress model of schizophrenia (McGlashan, 1986). This biopsychosocial paradigm accepts that the role of nurture (if any) in etiology will remain obscure until we first fully understand the biological implications of the genetically determined vulnerability to schizophrenia. It shifts emphasis from the possible role of psychosocial factors in etiology to their role as stressors or protectors in determining the vicissitudes of each individual's illness. Many aspects of this vulnerability are undoubtedly genetic, while other biologic factors that enhance vulnerability may be acquired during development through uterine, birth, and postnatal complications. In addition, there may be psychosocial factors that either induce (Wynne, 1978) or diminish vulnerability.

The current collection of specific deficits that appear to be associated with enhanced vulnerability is extensive. Some have been demonstrated, and more have been postulated (Nuechterlein & Dawson, 1984). A modest and cursory list includes: (1) deficits in the processing of complex information, in maintaining a steady focus of attention, in distinguishing between relevant and irrelevant stimuli, and in forming stable abstractions; (2) dysfunctions in psychophysiology, suggesting deficits in sensory inhibition and poor control over autonomic responsivity, especially to aversive stimuli; (3) impairments in social competence, such as eye contact, assertiveness, or conversational capacity; and (4) general coping deficits, such as overevaluating threat, underappraising internal resources, or extensive use of primitive defenses such as projection and denial.

Following this model, the vicissitudes of a schizophrenic illness are determined by the level of the individual's vulnerabilities on the one hand, and the potency of the environmental stressors on the other. In a highly vulnerable individual, sufficient stress can precipitate transient, intermediate (prodromal) states of dysfunction that amplify existing perceptual, cognitive, affective-autonomic, and social coping deficits. These, in turn, interact negatively with the existing stressors and magnify their effect in a progressive deterioration that ultimately becomes manifested as a full-blown clinical syndrome.

Although there remains controversy regarding the origins of the classical symptoms of schizophrenia (Munich, 1987), we feel that they fall into two main categories. The first category of symptoms seems to be primary to the disease process. Examples are disordered attention, perceptual distortions and hallucinations, intense affect poorly modulated to context, and disordered thought. The second category of symptoms are those that seem to represent the individual's compensatory defensive and adaptive responses to these primary defects and their experienced effects. Examples are denial, social withdrawal, preoccupation with fantasies having bizarre sexual, violent, grandiose, or apocalyptic themes, defensive irritability, feelings of entitlement, bizarre rituals, dependence, ideas of reference, paranoid and grandiose delusions, and assaultiveness (see also Anscombe, 1987). We believe that the primitiveness of these psychic defenses is a reflection both of the destructiveness of this illness to the ego and the sense of self-continuity (Pao, 1979) and of the fact that this disease compromises the very organ (the brain) that is most responsible for developing appropriate psychobiological adaptations. Both categories of symptoms, primary and secondary, contribute in turn to panic and anxiety, to a pervasive sense of helplessness and guilt, and, as a result of a highly defect-ridden self-image, to an extraordinarily low self-esteem.

THE NATURE OF THE PATIENT

Patients suffering from schizophrenia bring to the therapist some general characteristics that set the stage for many of the processes and events described below. These general characteristics stem from the psychopathology, primitive defenses, and inadequate adaptations that are relatively common to such patients, as noted above. They can be summarized (McGlashan, 1983) as: (1) a bitter antipathy toward reality, with intolerance of frustration; (2) poor control over the contents of awareness, with resulting hatred of uncertainty leading to premature, unrealistic perceptual and cognitive closure to master disorganization; (3) lack of awareness of needs, wants, and affects, and inability to feel or experience pleasure; (4) the absence of a sense of self or self-cohesion and identity, except as someone alien and absolutely different from others; (5) a conviction that the illness is static and unchangeable; (6) an experience of total passivity (things happen *to* one);

and (7) marked ambivalence in relationships, characterized by endless oscillations between merger and isolation driven by loneliness on the one hand, and terror of closeness on the other. Also, the patient, despite great emptiness, usually anticipates a joyless and often frightening relationship with the therapist—a large hurdle that must be overcome before much constructive work can be accomplished.

Despite these difficulties, we learn repeatedly in our work with patients suffering from schizophrenia that their own basic goals and desires are very human and culturally congruent. To be a normal man or woman, to have a job or profession, to have a family and friends, to experience some measure of joy are, like our own, their verbalized desires. Severe conflicts, which often become a focus in psychotherapy, are thus generated by the great discordance between these goals and the patient's compensatory defensive and adaptive responses to the illness. Repeated frustration and defeat in overcoming the illness and in achieving these goals, especially when early life experiences and successes generate high expectations, often precipitates hopelessness, depression, and even suicide (Dingman & McGlashan, 1986; Drake, Gates, Cotton, & Whitaker, 1984; Roy, Schreiber, Mazonson, & Pickar, 1986). Thus, our psychotherapeutic interventions are based on the assumption that, underlying the bizarre and often confusing set of overt symptoms, there exists a core of humanness that can be reached and engaged sufficiently to develop a working alliance.

In our view, many of the patient's psychological conflicts, which become revealed and elaborated during the course of therapy, are not very different in kind from those struggled with by other individuals (including the therapist) from the same cultural background. However, the magnitude of these conflicts is often immensely exaggerated by the schizophrenic illness, and the volitional, perceptual, and cognitive structures by which a patient tries to cope with these conflicts have frequently suffered severely from the underlying pathology.

Extraordinary resistance to change is another hallmark of people with severe schizophrenic illness, and the reasons for this often perplex us in the face of the patients' yearnings to live a fuller, more rewarding life, and the strikingly joyless and restricted existence they actually sustain. However, psychotherapeutic experience helps us appreciate that their defenses, psychotic and otherwise, are needed in order to *survive at all* (Benedetti, 1980) in the face of overwhelming terror or "organismic panic" (Pao, 1979). In addition, the learning of new behaviors and mental constructs, a prerequisite for adaptive and constructive change, may be impaired by the primary psychopathology of schizophrenia (Anscombe, 1987; Holzman, 1987). Seen in this light, the patient's massive and often unyielding resistance becomes more understandable, and such a perspective should temper the use of premature interpretations that aim at the early removal of these defenses.

THE ELEMENTS OF PSYCHOTHERAPY

Psychotherapy, as we conceptualize and practice it, includes three major interpersonal transactions: (1) relationship building, (2) administration and triage, and (3) "psychotherapy" *per se,* both supportive and investigative. Relationship building constitutes the prerequisite step of establishing a meaningful affective bond and working alliance with the patient through understanding. Administration refers to the therapist as the pivotal agent of triage, orchestrating the entire system of health and rehabilitation as it pertains to the patient's specific needs. Psychotherapy means using the relationship between therapist and patient for treatment. It cannot be divorced from the first two transactions, although attempts have frequently been made to do so. Psychotherapies can assume many forms, although we somewhat arbitrarily subdivide them here into supportive and investigative modes, supportive when the doctor–patient relationship is used prosthetically and investigative when the relationship is used to modify relatedness itself.

ESTABLISHING THE RELATIONSHIP

Establishing a relationship with a patient suffering from schizophrenia is often unusually difficult because of the patient's intense and overwhelming ambivalence about human attachments and his or her resulting active destruction of, or passive withdrawal from, relatedness. Treatment, of necessity, often begins with a prolonged preparatory period of sitting with the patient to resume human contact and to foster a relationship characterized by sufficient trust to allow the more formal work of therapy to proceed (Huszonek, 1987; McGlashan, 1983).

The key to establishing an understanding and affective relationship with schizophrenic patients lies in being open to learning from these patients what the illness means to them. It requires being persistent, consistent, and straightforward with the patients, counting on the likelihood that they often simply want understanding rather than definitive help (Cohen, personal communication, 1987). Indeed, because the psychotic experience is not one that is likely to be shared by most psychotherapists, there is a primary need for them to learn from their patients just what such an experience can be like. Apropos of this, we recommend to therapists embarking on the treatment of such persons that they read many of the first-person accounts that have been published (see, for example, Anonymous, 1986; Bockes, 1985; Houghton, 1982).

The therapist tries to tease forth or elucidate the patient's feelings or thoughts in the here and now, the principle goals being to organize the latter's emotional and interpersonal communication, to provide tolerance of life experience as it is, and to guide the patient into sharper conceptualizations and the use of shared meanings, metaphors, and syntax (McGlashan, 1983). Such strategies are particularly relevant to schizophrenic patients since they are uniquely inhibited or deficient in their capacity to express feelings, to identify needs, or to understand the internal origin or signal value of affect. Their affective organization often seems to correspond to preverbal physiologic tension states with little cognitive or psychological elaboration, such that the patient is unable to know who is feeling or what is being felt. Emotions are experienced as immediate, and often overwhelming, concrete reality without subtle differentiations, leading to global defenses against all affect, and rendering the patient apparently dead to all feeling. Breakthroughs of affect are then experienced as uncontrolled flooding with anger, despair, hopelessness, panic, or excitement.

Among the component technical strategies of this stage are listening, treating psychotic symptoms and content as signals, acknowledging and labeling feelings, narrowing the focus, elaborating concrete detail, and demanding facts (McGlashan, 1983). Equally important, the therapist must be able to tolerate the elucidated experiences, or "bear" the thoughts and feelings which have been acknowledged and which may contain highly negative feelings about the therapist. This has often been referred to as empathy and containment. It encompasses the therapist's capacity to identify with the experience of the patient, including that which the patient disavows or cannot articulate, and not become overwhelmed or unduly frightened. It also involves sensing when the patient is ready to be reacquainted with these dissociated aspects of his or her psychological experience.

Establishing an understanding, affective relationship means accepting patients as they are and fostering harmony by empathizing without interpreting. From a psychodynamic perspective, it may be viewed as a process of mobilizing an omnipotent, idealizing transference. Having no inner soothing resources of their own, psychotic patients construct an omnipotent delusional world to deny their sense of helplessness and vulnerability. This defensive construct may then be projected onto the therapist. Patients take the latter's calmness as evidence of strength. By accepting (i.e., not challenging or interpreting) such projections, the therapist "colludes" in this and creates a therapeutically expedient protective *folie à deux* until such time as the patient is ready to entertain less idealized transferences. Thus, idealization of the therapist by the patient, even when carried to delusional extremes, is preferable to psychotic nonrelatedness (Levick & Tepp, 1985) and helps to foster the development of a therapeutic alliance. With time, this will be followed, first by de-idealization, and then by more reality tempered re-idealizations (Levick & Tepp, 1985).

ADMINISTRATION AND TRIAGE

As noted, unidimensional therapies are rarely successful with schizophrenic patients. The disease is frequently chronic. It varies in presentation. It may wax and wane in intensity. It may change symptomatically. Because of this, different treatment approaches are potentially effective at different times in the course of the illness. We will not specify these further since they constitute the other chapters of this book. Our point here is that multiple treatment modalities require some *one* to orchestrate them. That person can be the patient's psychotherapist (Carpenter, 1986; McGlashan, 1986). In fact, we feel the patient's psychotherapist may be the *ideal* person to perform this triage function since he or she may be the person most trusted by the patient and the person with whom the patient has formed the most stable and viable working alliance. Every treatment for the schizophrenic patient, whatever the modality, works best in the context of a relatively low level of denial: on the part of the patient, on the part of the family, and on the part of the individual therapist. It is our experience that this prerequisite can best be achieved though an ongoing, consistent, empathic, and supportive psychotherapeutic relationship.

The following technical strategies are common to this aspect of the work (McGlashan, 1986): (1) *Evaluation*—a thorough evaluation of the patient precedes any decision about treatment. Especially important is ruling out problems with other treatment implications. (2) *Continuous reevaluation*—the dynamic and fluid nature of schizophrenia (as with many other chronic illnesses) demands periodic reassessment of course and prognosis, phase of illness, and target problems. As these change, so do treatment goals. Supportive techniques and psychotropic medications, for example, may be therapeutic during the acute phase of illness, but then foster deficit functioning later on. (3) *Timing*—the phasic natural history of schizophrenia dictates that attention be paid to *when* certain treatments are indicated. According to Hogarty (1984) for example, little if anything should be expected of the patient for the first 6 to 12 months following an acute episode in order to minimize stress and forestall relapse. Once the patient is asymptomatic and shows the first signs of revitalization, rehabilitation efforts may be introduced slowly. Higher levels of nonsheltered social and/or instrumental functioning may be attempted 1 to 2 years later, but only upon completion and consolidation of earlier gains. (4) *Titration*—treatments should be applied with graded increases in complexity and intensity. There is evidence that early, active, and ambitious psychosocial treatments may be toxic for certain patients (Drake & Sederer, 1986; Liberman, 1982). This does not endorse a treatment strategy of withdrawal and neglect but highlights the importance of tailoring and titrating treatment interventions. (5) *Integration with psychopharmacology*—practitioners of the psychotherapies must regard psychoactive drugs as frequently necessary and useful and formulate integrated strategies aimed at optimizing the risk-to-benefit ratios of both the psychotherapy and the medication. The psychotherapeutic relationship, for example, is especially crucial for low-dose or targeted drug strategies (see, for example, Heinrichs, Cohen, & Carpenter, 1985). The heightened risk of relapse common to these approaches, and the high risk of noncompliance with medications in general, places a premium on a viable working alliance for the early identification of prodromal states. Such an alliance often exists only with the patient's psychotherapist.

PSYCHOTHERAPY

By psychotherapy we mean using the doctor–patient relationship for mutative purposes. In the tradition of treating schizophrenia with psychotherapy, this relationship has usually been structured in two ways: as either supportive or investigative in its goals and strategies (McGlashan, 1983). Unfortunately, the history of the psychotherapy of schizophrenia is filled with the detritus of conflict between the supportive and investigative camps. Investigative psychotherapists often maintained that supportive or "nurturing" techniques were intrusive and infantilizing, that they fostered splitting or dependency and stifled mastery and autonomy. Supportive psychotherapists retorted that investigative techniques made unrealistic demands upon the patient's ego and financial resources, encouraged regression, and further damaged self-esteem.

In the privacy of the consulting room, however, conflict usually gave way to a liberal sampling of the adversary's armamentarium. Supportive management, if successful, sometimes resulted in the patient's wish for more analytic or investigative work. Investigative psychotherapy, on the other hand, frequently evolved into a supportive relationship, especially for patients with a severe long-term illness. Some therapists considered a supportive nurturing relationship to be a prerequisite to investigative psychotherapy with patients suffering from schizophrenia; others maintained that investigation itself was supportive. Most practitioners, especially in more recent times, have advocated a middle position of maintaining a level of support without which the patient cannot thrive at all. Although much overlap exists in practice, the theoretical and technical distinctions between supportive and investigative psychotherapy nevertheless remain heuristically useful, largely because the patient with schizophrenia presents a melange of difficulties demanding a diversity of techniques.

Setting: Length, Frequency, and Location of Sessions

A proper setting or milieu with flexible parameters is vital for the conduct of both forms of psychotherapy. For example, some degree of versatility in the length and frequency of sessions may be useful. Early in the course of work with a highly disturbed patient, during the development of a relationship, short (even less than 30 minutes) and more frequent sessions (up to once a day in some cases) may be better tolerated than rigidly scheduled 50-minute sessions and may more easily facilitate the development of trust. Sensitivity to the patient's fear of attachment as well as to his or her difficulty correctly perceiving the therapist's intent is helpful in guiding decisions regarding these parameters during the delicate early phases (Huszonek, 1987). Similar adaptability during subsequent crises and exacerbations of illness is also recommended. In these parameters, as in all aspects of the therapeutic relationship, trust and self-esteem are enhanced by allowing the patient some degree of control.

The location of sessions, while usually in the therapist's office, may also vary depending on the patient's clinical state and needs of the moment. Sessions may be held in the patient's home, be held in a hospital ward, or take place on a walk, especially with an agitated or paranoid patient who becomes frightened at being closed up in a small room with the therapist. Sessions may also be dedicated to an outing arranged to accomplish some specific task that the patient is too frightened or inexperienced to accomplish alone. The therapist might also accompany the patient during some aspect of the daily activities, such as eating, playing, or working in a prevocational training setting (Huszonek, 1987). Although tasks such as shopping, applying for SSI, or starting a bank account can often be accomplished by the patient with the help of other persons in the patient's social and/or therapeutic network, there are occasions when the therapist is the only person whom the patient trusts sufficiently to allow this type of support during early and tentative forays back into the community, especially after a severe regression and prolonged hospitalization.

Therapeutic "Attitudes"

A large part of the technique of psychotherapy consists of the therapist's attitudes about the interpersonal interaction. This constitutes a nonspecific but necessary background for all specific technical strategies, whether supportive or investigative.

The interventions of the therapist should generally reflect a nonjudgmental attitude and be designed to enhance the possibility of a positive, supportive relationship. For example, uses of the third person (Burnham, personal communication, 1974) (e.g., statements like "sometimes people feel . . .") are less likely to be perceived as a personal attack or criticism. They also reflect an attitude on the part of the therapist that the patient is a bona fide member of the human race. Similarly, acknowledging that the patient has much to teach the therapist helps rekindle a sense of being valued. The purpose of such techniques is to minimize the likelihood of eliciting defensiveness and withdrawal in patients who are already highly sensitized to being labeled as defective and strange. Furthermore, patients are frequently plagued by excessive and unrelenting guilt stemming from repeated academic or vocational failure, from harboring ego-dystonic sexual or aggressive fantasies, from primitive and intense longings to be cared for, and from a sense of self as evil. They are often convinced that their illness is a punishment for some past sin or egregious mistake. Verbal interventions that reflect a feeling that the patients are somehow etiologically responsible for their illness and its resulting social, academic, and vocational failures only aggravates guilt and reinforces the need for defensive denial, projection, and distortion.

Most important, the therapist needs to be versatile and maintain a willingness to shift the nature of his or her interventions in the face of the patient's often unexpected shifts in mental status and clinical state. Nevertheless, this flexibility works best against a background of consistency in one's general therapeutic attitude toward the patient, that is, an attitude reflecting that one regards the patient with basic human respect, that one ultimately stands for the patient's autonomy, that one respects the patient's need for privacy, and that one is generally optimistic while at the same time not harboring rescue fantasies or feelings of omnipotence with respect to one's therapeutic capacities (McGlashan 1983; Winston, Pinsker, & McCullough, 1986).

Thompson (1980) suggested that the therapist keep in mind that the major problem faced by schizophrenic patients is not difficulty expressing anger or rage but difficulty expressing warmth and tenderness. He exhorted therapists to find some healthy area in the patient's psyche to begin working with and to nourish and encourage to grow. He felt that therapists should ask clarifying questions, beginning with "how," "what," "when," or "where," but not with probing questions prefaced with "why," which can often be perceived as pejorative and accusing. Finally, Thompson suggested that the therapist let the patient get well at his or her own pace, and be aware that the giving up of symptoms like hallucinations or strongly held delusions may be very difficult, "like relinquishing old friends."

Supportive Techniques

The short- and long-term goals of supportive psychotherapy are relatively modest (McGlashan, 1982). They include relief from immediate crises, reduction of symptoms to premorbid levels, reestablishment of psychic homeostasis through a strengthening of defenses, sealing over of the psychotic experience and conflicts in order to achieve social recovery without the demand for personality change, circumscribed fostering of pragmatic adaptations, and mobilization of the healthy aspects of the patient to enable his or her optimal functioning despite continuing deficits.

The overall attitude of supportive psychotherapy is one of pragmatism and management, in which the therapist loans his or her healthier ego to help the patient interpret and adapt to reality. As such, the therapist often defines reality, offers direct reassurance, gives advice about current problems in living, urges modification of expectations, and actively organizes the environment for patients who cannot do so for themselves. For purposes of administration and triage, the therapist often acts as a liaison and maintains close contacts with important others, intervening when indicated, as an advocate for the patient with family, employers, or social agencies.

In the one-to-one supportive psychotherapeutic interaction, many elements of the psychosis, particularly symptoms, are ignored as a source of deeper meanings. Psychopathology is interpreted as an unwanted intrusion of inappropriate thoughts and feelings. The flow and pace of the therapy sessions are structured and drugs are used early and in sufficient dosage to mobilize the patient and combat regression. The therapist sides with the patient's defensiveness, and some denial, suppression, repression, and displacement are fostered so as to decrease anxiety and to achieve a suppression of overt symptoms. The therapist fosters positive transference but does not interpret it as such. That is, positive feelings are treated as real, and negative feelings are neither interpreted nor encouraged. The basic content and emphasis is on teaching and relearning as opposed to exploration and insight. The therapist may become very active in helping the patient learn new ways of adapting, and at appropriate times, will encourage or prescribe additional therapeutic interventions described in other chapters of this volume.

These basically supportive approaches to the therapy of persons with schizophrenia have their origins in the work of Federn (1952) and have been well described recently by Huszonek (1987) and by Winston et al. (1986). Among their technical suggestions they advocate that the therapist's style of communication be conversational, friendly in tone, and signifying to the patient both respect and commitment. The therapist should be willing at times to offer the patient nourishment (coffee, cookies, or fruit) to foster a benign parental image. The therapist should support the patient's self-esteem whenever realistically possible. This may often be accomplished by simply stating, "I agree with you." Similarly, the therapist should be willing to offer advice, preferably in the form of alternatives and based not on his or her own values but upon empathy with the patient's needs of the moment. The rationale for such advice should be made explicit. The therapist should be ready to apply problem-solving skills and knowledge of individual and social behavior to the patient's problems. This may prove educational for the patient and help to foster identification with the therapist. A certain amount of appropriate and timely self-disclosure by the therapist may also enable patients with severe ego deficits to build more stable, cohesive self- and object representations through identification. Finally, while the object of supportive therapy is not the analysis of defenses, it is correct to discourage use of maladaptive defenses with immediate and/or obvious destructive consequences.

Investigative Techniques

In contrast to supportive psychotherapy, the goals of investigative psychotherapy are generally more ambitious and include insight, some degree of personality change, and resumption of emotional growth (McGlashan, 1982).

In the one-to-one investigative psychotherapeutic mode, the doctor–patient transaction is scrutinized to elucidate and understand patients' characteristic patterns of relating with others, both in their current situation and in the context of their life histories. The basic attitude is analytic: The therapist reacts to the patient's feelings as intrapsychic phenomena that are interesting and worthy of understanding (Giovacchini, 1969). The therapist generally does not act as an alter ego; the patient's wants, problems with family, experiences with reality, needs for reassurance, wishes for direction are all explored first rather than responded to directly and concretely.

In the one-to-one investigative transaction, the patient's psychosis and symptoms are considered meaningful parts of the patient which he or she has defensively disclaimed and disavowed. Therefore, psychopathology and some regression is tolerated and treated as a source of information. The flow and pace of the sessions are less structured. Although neuroleptics are a frequent adjunct, they may be used more sparingly in many cases or not at all as part of a targeted drug strategy (Carpenter & Heinrichs, 1983). An effort is made to explore, but tolerate, the patient's shifting equilibrium between anxiety and defensiveness. Sources of anxiety in the therapeutic relationship are identified and linked with characteristic defenses mobilized to handle this anxiety. The therapist may confront the ways in which patients contribute to their own misery and difficulty with relationships in an effort to help such patients reclaim self-control. The therapist does not attempt to manipulate transference but interprets it as such.

Investigative psychotherapy is not for every schizophrenic patient. Indeed, empirical research fails to support its across-the-board application to schizophrenia, as already noted. Our first duty is to do no harm (Crown, 1983), and it is worth reminding ourselves that intensive investigative psychotherapy can be countertherapeutic. Assiduous efforts at "uncovering" in patients who have little ego strength and who lack sources of support for their self-esteem can be dangerous and lead to further regression and disorganization. Similarly, active confrontation of primitive defenses and psychotic denial rarely lead to positive changes but may enhance the patient's sense of isolation, alienation, and defectiveness, the ultimate result being further withdrawal from the therapist. Too much opaqueness and distance, just like too much interest and closeness, can be frightening and confusing (McGlashan, 1983). Hospitalized patients, in particular, may be vulnerable to the regressive effects of intensive, exploratory techniques (Drake & Sederer, 1986).

In general, during the active symptomatic phases, investigative psychotherapy may deepen regression or prolong relapse by its demand for responsible participation, for relinquishing defensive constructs, and for examining intolerably painful issues. Instead, supportive and structured interventions are indicated. Later, during phases of stabilization, when the patient has plateaued psychopathologically and defensively, investigative strategies may be called for, especially if the patient remits to a troublesome defect state or to a personality disorder replete with self-defeating patterns. At such points, the last two phases of classical psychodynamic technique (integrating the patient's experiences into an expanded perspective of the self, and working through) may be relevant (McGlashan, 1983).

Investigative psychotherapy might have a place in the treatment of schizophrenia, but we would reserve such intensive approaches for those patients (1) who have developed and are maintaining a reasonably secure sense of self, (2) who use a minimum of denial, (3) who have established a consistent working relationship with their therapist, (4) who exhibit an ability to make constructive and adaptive use of trials of such techniques, and (5) who demonstrate some of the following characteristics: an ego-dystonic illness that is painful, the presence of good premorbid features, and the presence of some capacity for self-observation, curiosity, frustration tolerance, concern, and humor.

Special Situations—Suicide, Paranoia, and Assaultiveness

An important objective of the individual therapy of persons suffering from schizophrenia is the prevention of suicide, estimated to be about 10% of all deaths in this patient population (Tsuang, 1978). Fortunately, there are some established premorbid, psychodynamic, and illness course factors that help one predict who is at greatest risk. Among these are being male, having relatively high premorbid educational and social achievements, being aware of the damaging effects of one's illness, having multiple hospitalizations, having high internalized standards of performance, and experiencing a deteriorating course (Dingman & McGlashan, 1986; Drake et al., 1984; Roy et al., 1986). Addressing the psychodynamic factors that may lead to suicide, Cotton, Drake, and Gates (1985) have enumerated what they believe are the therapeutic responsibilities of the psychotherapist for effective suicide prevention. These involve: (1) sharing the burden of despair, (2) continually assessing the level of self-esteem, (3) appreciating the protective functions of some of the psychotic symptoms, (4) differentiating inability to function from unwillingness to function, (5) monitoring familial relationships, and (6) dealing adequately with the loss, even a temporary loss, of the therapist.

The severely paranoid patient represents another special problem. A conservative and supportive approach, especially in the early phases of treatment, is necessary if there is to be some chance of developing a working alliance (McGlashan, 1983). Because such patients often enter treatment feeling coerced and exhibiting great mistrust and hostility, they are best greeted by the therapist with a removed but matter-of-fact attitude. A high degree of professionalism and reliability, and no evident desire to be liked by the patient, will enhance the possibility of success in establishing some trust. The reality of the patient's delusions should neither be accepted nor argued, and observations should be offered as hypotheses. The therapist should keep in mind that paranoia and paranoid delusions often evolve as projective defenses against overwhelming feelings of guilt and/or a sense of oneself as evil. As such, these defenses may be life-saving for the patient until such time as he or she develops sufficient self-esteem and trust to relinquish them. Attempts to modify or diminish these paranoid defenses should be made only after a reasonable working alliance has been established, and should be undertaken without ambitious expectations on the part of the therapist.

Finally, the assaultive patient (who is often paranoid as well) requires great care and some experience in order for one-to-one interactions to be safe. The maintenance of mutual respect, firmness, and an undistorted awareness of one's own anxiety are all strongly recommended. Limit setting, ranging from verbal remonstrances, to meeting in the presence of readily available help, to the use of restraints, to timely termination of a volatile session, can be instituted as the situation dictates (McGlashan, 1983). Very frequently, the open and candid admission by the therapist to a highly threatening patient that he or she is frightened will defuse the patient's need to be defensively attacking.

In all of these situations, it is important that the therapist acknowledge his or her own difficulties in becoming comfortable with the patient. Should these difficulties prove insurmountable, the therapist should seek supervision or consider a change of therapist. It is highly unrealistic to expect oneself to be both comfortable and effective with all patients.

THE THERAPIST

What should be the attributes of those who attempt to work with patients suffering from schizophrenia? The optimal psychotherapist is never easy to define because in the long run it is often the individual characteristics and needs of the patient that determine what and how the therapist presents. Nevertheless, the foregoing discussions about the therapist's roles and strategies suggest certain key parameters, such as versatility and interest in understanding another person's experience relatively free of theoretical bias (Benedetti, 1980; Thompson, 1980). Therapists should be resistant to polarized thinking and premature closure yet be willing to act when necessary despite inadequate information. Other attributes frequently mentioned are a capacity to tolerate intense affects, bizarre communications (Heydt, personal communication, 1978), and symbiotic demands as well as liberal amounts of ambiguity and confusion (Huszonek, 1987; McGlashan, 1983). It is essential that the therapist view patients as human beings afflicted with an illness against which they are struggling rather than as culpable misfits who bear some perverse responsibility for their plight. A willingness to recognize and be comfortable with one's similarities with patients also appears to be crucial.

It is important also that the therapist be well trained and up to date in the clinical neurosciences (Detre, 1987) in order to assess the significance of any neurobiological signs and symptoms, whether or not he or she is actually prescribing medical treatments. Obviously the therapist need not be a physician (Carpenter, 1986), although there may be advantages in some cases when this is so. Among these are the ability to explore, evaluate, and answer many of the patient's questions and concerns (both rational and delusional) regarding the physical and institutional aspects of both the disease and its treatment. Additionally, this relationship, if continuous and trusting, offers the therapist and the patient the opportunity of developing a shared strategy for recognizing and intervening rapidly at the earliest signs of an impending relapse (Heinrichs et al., 1985).

Finally, personal analysis or therapy, and satisfaction in life apart from one's work with such patients, all help to buffer the therapist from the frustrations and setbacks that characterize such work (McGlashan, 1983). We would also recommend during the first years of work with these patients that one obtain supervision from two or three experienced therapists, each of whom might, by espousing somewhat different points of view and approaches to the treatment of schizophrenia, help to add a flexible repertoire to the therapist's developing clinical perspectives.

SUMMARY

Our difficulties relinquishing dualistic thinking regarding the mind and the body (Eisenberg, 1986) play themselves out in the dialogues and controversies over the appropriate treatment of schizophrenia. Those who hypothesize that this ailment is a mental derangement resulting from chaotic interpersonal interactions in early life find support in those (few) patients who make spectacular recoveries, apparently with the help of psychotherapy alone. Those who envision the disease as a purely neurophysiologic affliction of the brain point proudly to the many patients whose symptoms are dramatically altered by neuroleptic drugs. However, given the decidedly incomplete results of most of our current attempts at the treatment of schizophrenia, it would seem rational at the present time to offer the patient a reasonably individualized array of interventions that address the individual's deficits and develop his or her demonstrated assets.

Ideally, this individualized set of therapies would be selected and coordinated by the one person most familiar with the patient and to whom the patient responds with some level of trust. We suggest that the person best suited to such a role is the patient's individual therapist, a person with the requisite training and experience who perseveres with the patient throughout the exacerbations and remissions of the illness, and shares with him or her both the defeats and successes of the other therapies over the long haul. This, we believe, is fundamental to the proper practice of therapy, where "listening and recognizing" (Charon, 1986) are primary to all other interventions.

What does the psychotherapeutic relationship have to offer that is different from other treatments of schizophrenia? To our minds, the following are its most unique aspects: (1) a provision for the patient of at least one person dedicated to understanding the patient and to sharing his or her struggles to adapt, and to being *with* the patient irrespective of the latter's variable mental state and level of functioning; (2) the prospect of a sufficiently safe interpersonal encounter dedicated to the development of constructive identifications and adaptations, and to help the patient comprehend both inner and outer realities (a psychoeducational function in part); and (3) the coordination and integration of the many therapeutic modalities and interventions available, a task that requires repeated psychosocial and neurobiological assessment during the course of the patient's illness.

The prescribed form that such a clinical relationship should take continues to evolve (Carpenter, 1986). Even within most current therapeutic relationships, the form and character of the interventions change over time and are often heavily influenced by the patient's clinical state and by the patient's dynamic and phase-dependent input into the dyad. In this context, the old and classical distinction between investigative and supportive techniques becomes largely trivial, as it perhaps should be if the therapist is to be truly responsive to the individual needs of the patient and to the idiosyncratic facets of this heterogeneous group of ailments.

REFERENCES

Anonymous. (1986). "Can we talk?" The schizophrenic patient in psychotherapy. *American Journal of Psychiatry, 143,* 68–70.

Anscombe, R. (1987). The disorder of consciousness in schizophrenia. *Schizophrenia Bulletin, 13,* 241–260.

Benedetti, G. (1980). Individual psychotherapy of schizophrenia. *Schizophrenia Bulletin, 6,* 633–638.

Bockes, Z. (1985). First person account: "Freedom" means knowing you have a choice. *Schizophrenia Bulletin, 11,* 487–489.

Carpenter, W. T., Jr. (1986). Thoughts on the treatment of schizophrenia. *Schizophrenia Bulletin, 12,* 527–539.

Carpenter, W. T., Jr., & Heinrichs, D. W. (1983). Early intervention, time-limited, targeted pharmacotherapy of schizophrenia. *Schizophrenia Bulletin, 9,* 533–542.

Charon, R. (1986). To listen, to recognize. *Pharos, Fall,* 10–13.

Cotton, P. G., Drake, R. E., & Gates, C. (1985). Critical treatment issues in suicide among schizophrenics. *Hospital and Community Psychiatry, 36,* 534–536.

Crown, S. (1983). Contraindications and dangers of psychotherapy. *British Journal of Psychiatry, 143,* 436–441.

Detre, T. (1987). The future of psychiatry. *American Journal of Psychiatry, 144,* 621–625.

Dingman, C. W., & McGlashan, T. H. (1986). Discriminating characteristics of suicides. Chestnut Lodge follow-up sample including patients with affective disorder, schizophrenia and schizoaffective disorder. *Acta Psychiatrica Scandinavica, 74,* 91–97.

Drake, R. E., Gates, C., Cotton, P. G., & Whitaker, A. (1984). Suicide among schizophrenics: Who is at risk? *Journal of Nervous and Mental Disease, 172,* 613–617.

Drake, R. E., & Sederer, L. I. (1986). Inpatient psychosocial treatment of chronic schizophrenia: Negative effects and current guidelines. *Hospital and Community Psychiatry, 37,* 897–901.

Eisenberg, L. (1986). Mindlessness and brainlessness in psychiatry. *British Journal of Psychiatry, 148*, 497–508.

Engel, G. L. (1980). The clinical application of the biopsychosocial model. *American Journal of Psychiatry, 137*, 535–544.

Federn, P. (1952). *Ego psychology and the psychoses.* New York: Basic Books.

Ginzberg, E. (1987). Psychiatry before the year 2000: The long view. *Hospital and Community Psychiatry, 38*, 725–728.

Giovacchini, P. L. (1969). The influence of interpretation upon schizophrenic patients. *International Journal of Psychoanalysis, 50*, 179–186.

Gomes-Schwartz, B. (1984). Individual psychotherapy of schizophrenia. In A. S. Bellack (Ed.), *Schizophrenia: Treatment, Management, and Rehabilitation* (pp. 307–335). Orlando: Grune & Stratton, Inc.

Gottesman, I. I., McGuffin, P., & Farmer, A. E. (1987). Clinical genetics as clues to the "real" genetics of schizophrenia. *Schizophrenia Bulletin, 13*, 23–47.

Heinrichs, D. W., Cohen, B. P., & Carpenter, W. T. Jr. (1985). Early insight and the management of schizophrenic decompensation. *Journal of Nervous and Mental Disease, 173*, 133–138.

Hogarty, G. E. (1984). Depot neuroleptics: The relevance of psychosocial factors—A United States perspective. *Journal of Clinical Psychiatry, 45*, 36–42.

Holzman, P. S. (1987). Recent studies of psychophysiology in schizophrenia. *Schizophrenia Bulletin, 13*, 49–75.

Houghton, J. H. (1982). First person account: Maintaining mental health in a turbulent world. *Schizophrenia Bulletin, 8*, 548–552.

Huszonek, J. J. (1987). Establishing therapeutic contact with schizophrenics: A supervisory approach. *American Journal of Psychotherapy, 16*, 185–193.

Levick, S. E., & Tepp, A. V. (1985). The role of the idealizing transference in the treatment of psychotic patients. *Journal of Nervous and Mental Disease, 173*, 292–297.

Liberman, R. P. (1982). Social factors in the etiology of the schizophrenic disorders. In L. Grinspoon (Ed.), *Psychiatry update: The American Psychiatry Association annual review* (Vol. 1). Washington, DC: American Psychiatric Press.

McGlashan, T. H. (1982). DSM-III schizophrenia and individual psychotherapy. *Journal of Nervous and Mental Disease, 170*, 752–757.

McGlashan, T. H. (1983). Intensive individual psychotherapy of schizophrenia: A review of techniques. *Archives of General Psychiatry, 40*, 909–920.

McGlashan, T. H. (1986). Schizophrenia: Psychosocial treatments and the role of psychosocial factors in its etiology and pathogenesis, *Annual Review of Psychiatry, 5*, 96–111.

McGlashan, T. H. (1988). Selective review of recent North American follow-up studies of schizophrenia. *Schizophrenia Bulletin, 14*(4).

Munich, R. L. (1987). Conceptual trends and issues in the psychotherapy of schizophrenia. *American Journal of Psychotherapy, 16*, 23–37.

Nuechterlein, K. H., & Dawson, M. E. (1984). Vulnerability and stress factors in the developmental course of schizophrenic disorders. *Schizophrenia Bulletin, 10*, 158–159.

Pao, P. N. (1979). *Schizophrenic disorders: Theory and treatment from a psychodynamic point of view.* New York: International Universities Press.

Rogers, D. E. (1974). The doctor himself must become the treatment. *Pharos, October,* 124–129.

Roy, A., Schreiber, J., Mazonson, A., & Pickar, D. (1986). Suicidal behavior in chronic schizophrenic patients: A follow-up study. *Canadian Journal of Psychiatry, 31*, 737–740.

Thompson, S. V. (1980, October 3). *Some considerations regarding psychoanalytically oriented psychotherapy.* Paper delivered at the 26th Annual Chestnut Lodge Symposium.

Tsuang, M. (1978). Suicide in schizophrenics, manics, depressives and surgical controls. A comparison with general population suicide mortality. *Archives of General Psychiatry, 35,* 153–155.

Winston, A., Pinsker, H., & McCullough, L. (1986). A review of supportive psychotherapy. *Hospital and Community Psychiatry, 37,* 1105–1114.

Wynne, L. C. (1978). From symptoms to vulnerability and beyond: An overview. In L. C. Wynne, R. L. Cromwell, & S. Matthysse (Eds.), *The nature of schizophrenia: New approaches to research and treatment* (pp. 698–714). New York: Wiley.

12

Social Problem-Solving Interventions in the Treatment of Schizophrenia

JANET S. ST. LAWRENCE

Schizophrenic diagnoses implicitly reflect ineffective interpersonal behavior and its consequences (Tisdelle & St. Lawrence, 1986). Competent social functioning involves the use of "identifiable, learned behaviors that individuals use in interpersonal situations to obtain or maintain reinforcement from others in their environment" (Kelly, 1982, p. 3). These global definitions of social competence subsume qualitatively different skills such as assertion, conversational skill, and interpersonal problem-solving adequacy. Competence levels for each skill subset may not correlate within individuals or be consistent across situations (Kelly, 1982). Thus, social competency is a multidimensional construct that needs to be further subdivided into specific behavioral skill units and components. Interpersonal problem solving is one subset of social competence with emotional and behavioral relevance for schizophrenia.

Social problem-solving interventions became a widely researched clinical tool during the mid-1970s. As a result, assessment and training of problem-solving skills became a popular focus for cognitive-behavioral interventions.

JANET S. ST. LAWRENCE • Department of Psychology, Jackson State University, Jackson, Mississippi 39217, and University of Mississippi Medical Center, 2500 North State Street, Jackson, Mississippi 39216.

DEFINITION

Problem solving is an overt or covert process that makes available a variety of potentially effective responses for dealing with a problematic situation and increases the probability of selecting an effective response from among various alternatives (D'Zurilla & Goldfried, 1971). More recently, social problem solving has been defined as a cognitive-affective-behavioral process through which an individual or group identifies or discovers effective means of coping with problems encountered in everyday living (D'Zurilla, 1986; D'Zurilla & Nezu, 1982). Other terms, such as *interpersonal problem solving, personal problem solving,* and *applied problem solving,* are used interchangeably with the term *social problem solving.*

SOCIAL PROBLEM-SOLVING AND ADJUSTMENT

A series of studies by Zigler, Phillips, and their associates in the early 1960s revealed that postdischarge adjustments of schizophrenic patients were positively associated with premorbid social competence and that more severe symptomatology was exhibited by those who displayed greater premorbid social deficits (Levine & Zigler, 1973; Phillips & Zigler, 1961, 1964; Zigler & Phillips, 1961, 1962). The research to date suggests that problem-solving skills are deficient in persons who receive schizophrenic diagnoses and that impaired problem-solving skill has detrimental consequences for overall adjustment (Coche & Flick, 1975; Goldsmith & McFall, 1975; Spivack & Shure, 1974).

Peer evaluation studies indicate that poor problem-solvers are more likely to be disliked by others than are effective problem-solvers (e.g., Spivack & Shure, 1974). This makes intuitive sense since ineffective problem resolution is likely to lead to interactions that are characterized by negative expectations, social rejection, and poor conflict resolution. In addition, reduced positive reinforcement, withdrawal, hostility, and negative self-labeling are also more likely when problems are not addressed effectively (Combs & Slaby, 1977). A cyclical interaction can follow when the negative behavioral feedback leads to even more inept future problem solving. Ineffectual social behavior may also be strengthened when inadequate problem solutions are inadvertently reinforced (Patterson, Littman, & Bricker, 1967; Solomon & Wahler, 1973). For example, an aggressive solution may successfully secure peer submission or attention from others, but it is a less desirable strategy than compromise or negotiation. The ability to reason through and implement effective responses to social problems should result in higher-quality interpersonal relationships than would responses that are emotionally triggered, pursue self-gratifying goals, or do not consider inter-personal consequences.

Several authors suggest that knowledge and use of effective interpersonal problem solving may be central, or even prerequisite, to mental health and behavioral adjustment (Foster & Ritchey, 1979; Jahoda, 1958; Spivack & Shure, 1974). D'Zurilla and Goldfried (1971) stated that ineffective coping in problematic situations, along with its personal and social consequences, is sufficient to lead to behavioral and emotional disorders requiring psychological intervention. Several lines of research confirm their assertions. Empirical evidence confirms that social ineffectiveness seriously impedes adjustment (Combs & Slaby, 1977; Krasnor & Rubin, 1981), and correlational evidence suggests that socially ineffective children are more likely to have later life-adjustment problems (Combs & Slaby, 1977; Roff, Sells, & Golden, 1972; Ullmann, 1957).

When schizophrenics' social problem-solving competencies are contrasted with nonpatients' problem-resolution skills, significant differences have repeatedly emerged. Platt and Spivack (1972a) found that psychiatric inpatients exhibited fewer problem-solving skills than hospital employees and that the patients' solutions were often irrelevant to the actual problem at hand. Later research by the same authors further confirmed psychiatric patients' deficient problem-solving content (Platt & Spivack, 1974). Adult schizophrenic patients tend to respond with immediate action but overlook the mediating stages of thinking and planning that characterize control groups' problem-solving efforts. Additional evidence suggests that schizophrenic patients are less able than controls to provide relevant solutions or appropriate means for resolving interpersonal problems (Platt & Spivack, 1972b). Problem-solving ability is also positively associated with higher levels of premorbid social competence (Platt & Spivack, 1972b; Platt & Siegel, 1976). Poor problem-solvers also displayed more clearly schizophrenic patterns on the Minnesota Multiphasic Personality Inventory (MMPI), leading Platt and his colleagues to characterize poor problem-solvers as socially inadequate individuals (Platt & Spivack, 1972b; Platt & Siegel, 1976).

Schizophrenic patients typically have poorer social networks and fewer intimate relationships than do nonpatients to aid them in times of stress (Froland, Brodsky, Olson, & Stewart, 1979). Mitchell (1982) studied 35 outpatient schizophrenic adults and their families and reported that interpersonal problem solving was positive and significantly related to the number of friendships and degree of family support. Mitchell concluded that clinical interventions to increase schizophrenics' problem-solving skill may actively shape positive social support networks and ensure more stable functioning in the community.

When effective and ineffective social problem-solvers are compared, specific abilities distinguish good from poor problem-solvers. Three significant skills that are deficient among chronic schizophrenics are: (1) ability to plan step-by-step ways to achieve a social goal, often referred to as means–end thinking; (2) inability to generate alternative solutions to social problems; and (3) ability to accurately predict the result of a particular course of action.

The relevance of proposed solutions to the actual problem also appears to be a distinguishing feature that differentiates schizophrenic adults from nonpatient controls. Schizophrenic populations tend to produce less relevant, more impulsive, and more aggressive means than do more socially competent populations. Even the ability to select an appropriate goal in a relatively unstructured social interaction appears to be problematic for schizophrenic adults (Renshaw & Asher, 1982). Considering all of the implications for long-term adjustment, clinical interventions to assist chronic schizophrenics in identifying and resolving interpersonal difficulties appear to represent both justifiable and ethical treatment.

However, the specific means to accomplish this clinical goal are less clear-cut. Although the relevance of social problem-solving skills was identified nearly two decades ago, the conceptual underpinnings for clinical problem-solving interventions remain poorly articulated. Assessment strategies are unstandardized and interventions tend to be unvalidated. A variety of studies have established a relationship between inept social problem-solving skills and schizophrenic behavior and have documented that schizophrenic individuals are deficient in problem-solving abilities when compared with normal control groups. Yet methodological flaws in the literature have left many questions unanswered. Inadequate population descriptions are common, as well as failures to validate either a treatment group's deficiencies or the control group's "normalcy" (Tisdelle & St. Lawrence, 1986). As a result, the adequacy of research group classifications is sometimes unclear. Many treatment outcome studies employ raters who are not blind to the experimental conditions, introducing obvious problems with potential measurement bias. Another problem is the use of differing criteria for problem-solving adequacy. For example, many studies measure only one or two of the components that have been identified as being relevant in the overall problem-solving process. The result is that outcome data may not generalize to more global social problem-solving effectiveness. In addition, problems with the measurement devices themselves remain unresolved.

Important conceptual differences have yet to be resolved. Concepts such as "social inadequacy" and "emotional disturbance" are not well defined, making it difficult to compare results across studies or to generalize findings across populations. Another conceptual issue involves distinguishing verbal problem-solving solutions from behavioral competence in implementing a solution (D'Zurilla & Nezu, 1982). Taken together, inadequate conceptual underpinnings, imprecise definitions, and assessment problems introduce some doubt as to whether results attributed to improved problem solving may be confounded by mediating variables such as anxiety, conversational ability, assertiveness, or verbal fluency (Tisdelle & St. Lawrence, 1986).

Most of the literature establishing a link between problem solving and life adjustment is based upon correlational research and cannot establish any causal relationship between the two. Poor problem-solving skills may lead to maladjustment. Equally plausible is the possibility that some other factor, such as cognitive deficiency or thought disorder, results in both maladjustment and poor problem solving. Thus, causal relationships have not been established and remain speculative. However, evidence of positive outcome effects from problem-solving interventions with schizophrenics does suggest a convincing relationship between problem solving and social functioning that has important treatment implications.

Some of the problem-solving literature focuses on the cognitive styles that people use to solve impersonal intellectual tasks, such as puzzles, anagrams, or arithmetic problems (Sarason, 1981; Spivack & Shure, 1974), despite evidence that causal thinking about impersonal events is not the same as causal thinking about social events (Gotlib & Asarnow, 1979; Spivack & Shure, 1974). Thus, a distinction must be drawn between the skills needed to solve impersonal tasks and the behaviors needed to deal effectively with interpersonal difficulties. Social problems may require handling interpersonal conflict, seeking help, planning a course of action leading toward a particular social outcome, and considering the future implications of various alternatives. Social problem solving may also need to be differentiated from emotional problem solving, such as coping with one's negative emotions. Emotional problem solving correlates with IQ but has not reliably differentiated clinical from nonclinical populations (Platt & Spivack, 1974; Siegel & Platt, 1976). This suggests that when the therapeutic goal is to improve interpersonal adjustment, assessment and treatment should focus on social problem solving rather than on impersonal or intellectual tasks.

ASSESSMENT OF SOCIAL PROBLEM-SOLVING SKILLS

Problem-solving skills are traditionally evaluated through self-report (verbal) assessment and/or behavioral (observational) assessment. Verbal assessment strategies may employ questionnaires, paper-and-pencil inventories, interviews, or verbal problem-solving tests based on actual or hypothesized problem situations. Observational assessment usually involves direct observation of the person in a problematic situation. The problematic situation may be contrived in an experimental setting or occur naturally in the environment.

Cognitive/Verbal Assessment. The Means-Ends Problem-Solving task (MEPS; Platt & Spivack, 1975) is widely utilized as a measure of interpersonal problem-solving skill. The MEPS consists of six hypothetical situations that present the beginning and end of a story. The outcome goal is clearly indicated and the subject is asked how the specified end can be achieved. Thus, the instrument measures step-by-step means to reach a terminal goal. Responses may be elicited in written or verbal form and are typically judged and scored according to some *a priori* criteria.

Psychometric properties for the MEPS have not been established nor have normative data been forthcoming. Specific strategies for use of the MEPS vary from study to study and the sampled content areas are narrow, making generalization difficult (Krasnor & Rubin, 1981). The relationship of MEPS scores to actual behavioral performance or observed indices of problem resolution have not been demonstrated, and the unstandardized use of the MEPS makes it difficult to establish the method's validity. Investigators frequently modify the measure to suit their particular needs by adapting scene content to be more relevant to the specific population under study. The frequency with which this is done suggests that clinical researchers believe it is beneficial to employ a more personalized assessment approach and that a universal measure may not be the optimal assessment strategy.

Three other verbal/cognitive assessment strategies have been reported, although these are less frequently encountered in the research literature. The Problem Solving Self-Evaluation Test (PSET; Bedell, Archer, & Marlowe, 1980) is a Likert-type questionnaire collecting self-rated probabilities of actually performing problem-solving behaviors in a difficult situation. The Problem-Solving Knowledge and Information Test (PKIT) by the same authors (Bedell et al., 1980) is a multiple-choice test of knowledge about the problem-solving process.

The Problem-Solving Inventory (PSI; Heppner & Petersen, 1982) is a 35-item Likert scale that measures the respondent's self-appraisal of problem-solving skill. The measure has good reliability (Heppner & Peterson, 1982), distinguishes individuals who have completed problem-solving training from those who have not (Dixon, Heppner, Petersen, & Ronning, 1979; Heppner, Baumgardner, Larson, & Petty, 1983), and has some limited data suggesting that PSI performance is related to actual problem-solving performance (Heppner, Hibel, Neale, Weinstein, & Rabinowitz, 1982; Heppner & Peterson, 1982).

If the goal of assessment is to reflect individual differences in problem resolution, skill in implementing the hierarchical components of problem solving, and situationally relevant changes in problem-solving behavior, then the particular social situations that are problematic for the particular group to handle should be identified. Schizophrenic adults are not all deficient in the same social situations, despite their shared diagnostic label. Even when two individuals exhibit similar terminal behavior, the observed behavior may result from deficiencies at different stages in the problem-solving process. Identifying the precise troublesome situations and the specific skill deficits is desirable if researchers are to avoid vague, abstract, or hypothetical assessment. It is possible that relevant, as opposed to hypothetical, situations may also foster generalization after training since there will be fewer abstract associations intervening between the clinical training and situations that are actually encountered in daily life (Kelly, 1982).

Individualized assessment creates a further assessment problem in deciding just how the problem situations are to be identified. Often, this is done intuitively, with little empirical support to document any relationship between the assessment situations and patients' actual difficulties in their daily lives. Although more objective determinations of the specific and problematic assessment situations is desirable, it is a step rarely encountered in the literature. In addition, a totally individualized approach to assessment may not be practical in many applied settings because of the time and cost constraints that would be incurred.

Hansen, St. Lawrence, and Christoff (1985) introduced a strategy to identify problematic situations that should be practical in most applied settings. Their subjects were chronic schizophrenic patients receiving day treatment in a community mental health center's partial hospitalization program. Patients' self reports of troublesome situations were collected over time, as were staff descriptions of situations they overheard and which were difficult for the patients to resolve appropriately. Over time, 57 problem situations accumulated that had actually been difficult for at least one of the schizophrenic patients in the treatment program. In order to establish which situations were most relevant and problematic for the patients as a whole, the situations were each presented individually to each patient. After each situation was read, the patient was then asked, "Have you ever been in a situation like this?" and "Would it be hard for you to figure out what to do in this situation?" Dichotomous yes or no responses were recorded for each question. The number of participants who responded "yes" was divided by the total number of responses (yes plus no) to establish a relevancy index and a difficulty index for each situation. Twenty-two of the original pool of situations received relevance and difficulty indexes greater than .50, indicating that the situation had actually happened to, or been problematic for, at least half the patients in the program. Those 22 situations were retained and used for assessment and training during a problem-solving intervention with the chronic schizophrenic patients.

Such a strategy offers a workable compromise between truly individualized assessment and the practical realities that must be considered in applied settings. The above procedure ensured that each situation was personally relevant and difficult for at least half of the program's participants. In addition, it offered an alternative to the impractical time and cost constraints a truly individualized assessment would have imposed.

Behavioral Assessment. The problem-solving literature generally assumes a relationship between verbal/cognitive performance and actual behavior (Tisdelle & St. Lawrence, 1987). Whether self-report or ancillary measures reflect *actual* problem-solving skill in troublesome situations should be the most important evidence of improved competency. Unfortunately, this step is rarely taken. As a result, conclusions about treatment efficacy are frequently based on self-report measures and/or indirect adjustment indices, with little evidence documenting changes in behavioral performance. This lack of behaviorally specific assessment is one of the most neglected assessment issues in the problem-solving literature, although recommendations for improvement are frequently encountered (Tisdelle & St. Lawrence, 1986, 1988). Krasnor and Rubin (1981) suggest that behavioral assessment should involve observation of actual problems as they arise in a person's daily social interactions. While such an assessment method would provide evidence of *in vivo* competency and effectiveness, the time and effort required, as well as problems inherent in uncontrolled observations and intrusiveness of the observations, pose significant obstacles.

Evans and Nelson (1977) recommended a "simulated situation" method as a feasible compromise. In this procedure, contrived situations are arranged with experimental confederates to evoke problem-solving behavior. Such analogue strategies offer a cost-effective compromise between naturalistic observation and structured assessment. However, identifying relevant situations that can be readily contrived and will accurately reflect *in vivo* problem solving presents procedural difficulties. Contrived performance opportunities may or may not reflect generalization to the natural environment, and the external validity of such analogue assessment methods should be verified. Given the practical limitations of *in vivo* assessment, however, contrived analogue situations would seem to offer a viable alternative if their external validity can be verified. At present, the assumption that contrived performances reflect naturalistic behavior has not been empirically confirmed in the problem-solving literature. At best, it should be regarded as indirect assessment evidence until psychometric support is forthcoming (D'Zurilla, 1986).

Several studies have attempted to employ some form of behavioral assessment. For example, one study simulated a grocery store and required the schizophrenic subjects to purchase food while the cashier precipitated a "problem" by overcharging them at the cash register (Edelstein, Couture, Cray, Dickens, & Lusebrink, 1980). This stimulated situation may confound problem solving with assertiveness since both skills would seem necessary in resolving the "problem."

Measurement problems plague the problem-solving literature. Behavioral measures are rarely employed, and even when behavioral measures have been introduced, their presumed relevance to problem solving is unclear. The specific situations employed for behavioral assessment are often confounded by other social skills, such as assertion or job interviewing skill. For example, Sarason and Sarason (1981) used a job interview paradigm to assess participants' postintervention performance. Yet grooming, assertiveness, conversational skill, and job qualifications also influence job interview ratings, and the participants were not rated on the specific problem-solving behaviors that were trained in the interpersonal problem-solving program. Similar lapses are common in the literature. For example, Ollendick and Hersen (1979) employed a problem-solving intervention based on instruction, modeling, rehearsal, and feedback. However, the assessment measures evaluated assertive responses to simulated role-play situations. Scene content in the role-play situations included responding to a compliment—a situation which may not have emerged as a "problem" during training and which may not have been perceived by the participants as a social problem-solving dilemma relevant to their newly learned skills.

SOCIAL PROBLEM-SOLVING INTERVENTIONS WITH SCHIZOPHRENIC PATIENTS

Specific intervention strategies for training social problem-solving skills vary from study to study. Common treatment methods include verbal instruction and rationale, modeling, feedback, reinforcement, behavior rehearsal, and/or group discussions. Early reports of problem-solving interventions with chronic schizophrenic patients attempted to improve patients' overall social adequacy (Siegel & Spivack, 1976a,b). The training consisted of 14 exercises involving didactic presentations, slides, and audiotape cassettes. Although Siegel and Spivack conducted two pilot studies using the program and indicate that patients responded favorably, no objective outcome data were reported.

A series of studies by Coche and his colleagues provided more empirical evidence of the effectiveness of social problem solving with schizophrenic patients. In the first (Coche & Flick, 1975), attention control and no-treatment control groups were compared with a sample who completed problem-solving training. Patients in the problem-solving group improved more on the MEPS than did patients in either control group. Later, Coche and Douglass (1977) replicated the study, adding two other self-report measures of personal adjustment to the MEPS. Similar groups were used for the comparison, but this replication produced no significant differences between any of the three groups on the MEPS after training. Coche and Douglass (1977) noted that attrition may have created a ceiling effect, since the problem-solving group was considerably higher on the dependent measures at pretreatment after data for the noncompleters were deleted, and this may well have affected the results. The intervention group did show more improvement on the adjustment indices than either of the two control groups.

A later study compared a problem-solving intervention against "interactive group therapy" on measures such as self-esteem, self-confidence, psychopathology, and nurses' ratings of improvement on three target behaviors (Coche, Cooper, & Petermann, 1984). No significant group differences emerged, although there is some suggestion that patients' sex may have been a mediating factor. Men showed more improvement from the problem-solving training, while women showed more improvement from the interactive therapy group.

Three treatment approaches with different conceptual underpinnings are encountered in the problem-solving literature: (1) skills training approaches that sequentially target specific component behaviors for intervention, (2) social learning approaches, or (3) cognitive modification programs that emphasize self-instructional training.

COMPONENT SKILL INTERVENTIONS

Component skill approaches identify sequential component skills that facilitate successful resolution of interpersonal problems and teach a step-by-step problem-resolution strategy (D'Zurilla & Goldfried, 1971; Krasnor, 1982; Sarason, 1981; Siegel & Platt, 1976). Skills components commonly include: (1) identifying the problem, (2) specifying the desired outcome goal, (3) generating alternative solutions, (4) comparing the consequences of alternative solutions, (5) selecting an alternative, (6) implementing the selected method, and (7) evaluating success of the chosen method.

An exemplary study using the skills component approach was conducted by Goldsmith and McFall (1975). An interpersonal skills training program was developed for adult male schizophrenic patients and the authors attempted to assess actual behavior during an interpersonal problem. Through extensive interviews and judges' ratings, several problematic situations were identified for assessment and training. Although such a procedure was not new (Goldfried & D'Zurilla, 1969), it transcended the usual reliance on clinical intuition to identify performance deficits, and the study is a model effort in the problem-solving literature. By including an assessment-only control group and a pseudotherapy control group, the authors controlled for attention and for exposure to the assessment situations. The intervention was relatively brief, consisting of only three individually administered sessions, and during the intervention subjects also received training in assertion and conversational skill in addition to interpersonal problem solving. As a result, it is difficult to disengage which particular aspect of the intervention led to posttreatment change or to what degree each contributed to overall improvement. After the training, all subjects were assessed in a conversational situation, and the skills training group proved to be more skillful. The results provide only preliminary evidence of generalization to actual behavior since similar measures were not taken before the intervention, and the task evaluated conversational skills rather than problem-solving skills.

Edelstein et al.(1980) trained schizophrenic patients in problem-solving components using separate "modules" and assessed progress with a multiple-baseline design across the problem-solving skill components. Analogue situations assessed generalization at baseline and after each module was completed. Patients who were initially deficient in problem-solving skills were better able to identify problems and choose more effective alternatives following training. Improvement was maintained when novel problem situations were presented and during *in vivo* problem simulations. The results are confounded since subjects were prompted during the analogue assessment task if they did not spontaneously recognize the problem. Subjects were also aware of being assessed, introducing the possibility of measurement reactivity. The repeated assessmen of a single problem situation also introduces the possibility that change may have reflected practice effects.

Few studies report any long-term follow-up documenting whether outcome changes maintain over time. While research with other populations suggests good skill maintenance following problem-solving training (Chaney, O'Leary, & Marlatt, 1978), specific evidence from schizophrenic populations is also needed since unique features may influence maintenance in different clinical subgroups. Hansen et al. (1985) reported a 1- and 4-month follow-up after problem-solving training with a small group of chronic schizophrenic patients. The 4-month follow-up data suggested some regression toward baseline over time. More rigorous long-term follow-ups are needed to document the degree and duration of problem-solving change with schizophrenic patients.

SOCIAL LEARNING INTERVENTIONS

Social learning approaches to problem solving emphasize exposure to models as a means for producing changes in social problem-solving effectiveness. In reality, many of the articles both include a component skill emphasis and incorporate social learning principles, making it difficult to differentiate between the two approaches. In addition, most of the problem-solving literature employing social learning approaches deals with nonschizophrenic populations. Sarason and Sarason (1981) evaluated a modeling approach using three groups of high school students: One group observed a live model exhibiting social and cognitive problem-solving skills, another group saw the same models on videotape, and a control group participated in classroom discussion. Skill deficits were identified through interviews with significant adults rather than the common practice of selecting situations on the basis of their presumed relevance for the population. Following intervention, the experimental groups generated more effective problem-solving means and identified more alternative solutions than did the control group participants.

Hansen et al. (1985) extended the social learning and component skills paradigm to chronic schizophrenic aftercare patients and found measurable and significant improvement in problem-solving competency followed intervention. Subjects were seven chronic schizophrenic patients in a partial hospitalization program at a regional mental health center. All participants had received schizophrenic diagnoses and were stabilized on antipsychotic medication. Problem situations were identified through patient observation and staff reports. This process has been described in a previous section and need not be repeated here. Five problem-solving components were targeted for training (problem identification, goal definition, evaluation of alternatives, selection of a best solution, and solution evaluation), and the participants' responses to each problem situation were audiotape-recorded and later rated for the occurrence or nonoccurrence of each component. Solutions were also rated for effectiveness, the raters' subjective evaluations of the solution's overall quality, and how well the raters believed the solution would resolve the problem.

Training was conducted in a group format twice weekly at the partial hospitalization program. The skill components were targeted sequentially, and training consisted of instruction and skill rationale, modeling, behavior rehearsal, feedback, and verbal reinforcement for improvement. Each session began with the therapist's providing instructions and a rationale for the component, then modeling the skill before participants practiced its use. Corrective feedback and praise were provided by the therapist. Immediately after each training session, participants were individually assessed on four trained situations and two situations randomly selected each time from a pool of generalization situations.

During the baseline period, each of the five component skills remained consistently near zero on both the trained and unfamiliar generalization situations. During baseline, subjects were almost never able to identify the core problem or define a desired outcome goal. Furthermore, the schizophrenic subjects rarely evaluated the effectiveness of their chosen solutions or examined any other alternative. Not surprisingly, since the participants did not evaluate alternatives, they did not select a "best" solution. Each component skill improved rapidly following the introduction of training, and improvement generalized to the untrained situations. Change always occurred at the precise time when the training specifically focused on a skill, demonstrating that the participants' behavior change was a direct result of their training. Statistical analyses supported the clinical significance of the change. Ratings of the participants' overall effectiveness also improved over time, with the largest increase taking place during the solution evaluation phase. Statistical analyses also confirmed the significant improvements in the participants' overall effectiveness in resolving problems over the course of the intervention and through a 1- and 4-month follow-up period.

Only a limited number of studies have attempted to isolate the ingredients responsible for change in social learning approaches to problem-solving interventions. Since most have used other populations—in particular, children—their results cannot be generalized to adult schizophrenics. Mc-Clure, Chimsky, and Larcen (1978) attempted to tease out confounding treatment effects by comparing modeling alone against modeling in combination with role-play and discussion. There was a trend for role-playing to produce more effective problem solving, but no one treatment component was unequivocally supported. However, in this study, subjects were normal elementary school students. A range of programs may be effective with adjusted populations, while maladjusted groups may require more circumscribed intervention strategies. A study by Ollendick and Hersen (1979) suggests that skills training approaches that include rehearsal, feedback, reinforcement, and *in vivo* practice are effective when they are combined with modeling to increase problem-solving effectiveness. Further systematic research is needed with adult schizophrenic populations to articulate the ingredients for change and the optimal combination of intervention components.

SELF-INSTRUCTIONAL INTERVENTIONS

Several authors discuss the role of internalized language as a mediating factor in motor behavior, abstract thought, and problem solving (Luria, 1961; Vygotsky, 1962). Several investigators adopted verbal mediation theory into cognitive behavioral programs (e.g., Kendall, 1977; Robin, Schneider, & Dolnick, 1976). These programs have typically been conducted with elementary school children rather than with schizophrenic adults (cf. Ault, 1973; Drake, 1970) and with nonsocial tasks such as maze performance (e.g., Kendall & Finch, 1978; Meichenbaum & Goodman, 1971) rather than with social problem solving. Evidence generated from schizophrenic samples suggests that performance on such impersonal cognitive problem-solving tasks is not highly correlated with interpersonal problem-solving skill (Platt & Spivack, 1974; Shure, Spivack, & Jaeger, 1971; Spivack & Shure, 1974). In addition, self-instructional programs that focus on impersonal problem solving have generally not demonstrated any generalization to overall adjustment measures. This raises some question as to whether self-instructional methods are the most appropriate strategy with adult schizophrenic patients, although their efficacy has not been evaluated. Although normal children have benefited from self-instructional training (e.g., Bornstein & Quevillon, 1976), their effectiveness with problem children has not been demonstrated. As yet, research simply does not affirm the efficacy of self-instructional methods for improved social problem solving in impaired clinical samples. As a result, it is premature to draw any conclusion regarding the potential usefulness of self-instructional methods for training problem-solving skills with adult schizophrenics.

SOCIAL VALIDATION OF PROBLEM-SOLVING INTERVENTIONS

A neglected aspect of problem-solving assessment is whether such training produces outcome effects that are comparable to the skills of nonclinical populations. Social validation is rarely attempted, despite its importance in determining treatment efficacy (Urbain & Kendall, 1980). If the aim of clinical treatment is to teach schizophrenic persons more adaptive living skills, such social validation efforts are critical. Such a social validation approach was used to train conversational skills among schizophrenics (Holmes, Hansen, & St. Lawrence, 1984), although only one published outcome study assessed problem-solving competencies in the community at large and then compared

whether schizophrenic patients approximated the performance levels of normal individuals after training (Hansen et al., 1985). More frequently, statistical significance is the sole outcome criterion in problem-solving research.

SUMMARY AND CONCLUSION

The theoretical and conceptual underpinnings of problem-solving training are not well delineated despite their relevance for assessment, treatment, generalization, and maintenance. Although there is empirical support for the problem-solving components (D'Zurilla & Nezu, 1982), the relative contribution of each sequential step to overall behavioral competence or problem-solving effectiveness remains speculative. More careful evaluation of the efficiency, even necessity, of each sequential problem-solving stage could be helpful in clarifying the nature of effective problem solving. At present, the specific sequence popularly employed in the literature is only assumed to be the most efficacious strategy, and empirical verification is still needed.

Problem solving in real life rarely proceeds according to the neatly ordered stages that characterize the research literature (D'Zurilla & Nezu, 1982). In contrast to experimentally contrived problem situations, problems that arise in the natural environment are often more ambiguous than most experimental situations. The available information and environmental cues for identifying outcome goals often are considerably more subtle than most research investigations reflect. Given the vague parameters of *in vivo* problems and the complex nature of human information processing, problem-solving stages may well overlap and interact with impressions formed in one stage serving to modify later stages. Thus, effective problem solving may be considerably more complex and multifaceted than the literature implies.

McFall (1982) identified a conceptual model of social interaction that can be adapted to illustrate the complexity of social problem solving. His first stage, "decoding," addresses the perception and interpretation of incoming stimuli. This phase corresponds to the problem recognition stage, influenced by sensory skills and attentional factors, as well as subjective interpretation and environmental cues. The "decision" stage that follows involves searching among alternatives, evaluating the potential outcome from each, and eventually selecting an appropriate response. This corresponds to the cognitive steps in the problem-solving process. "Encoding," McFall's final stage, requires that cognitive decisions be translated into behavioral performance. This aspect is often neglected in the problem-solving literature and a host of factors may influence performance, such as fatigue, practice, behavioral repertoire, attitudes, social anxiety, frustration tolerance, and memory. To date, the problem-solving literature focuses almost exclusively on the second stage in McFall's theory, learning the cognitive rules for more effective problem solving.

However, problem-solving knowledge by itself cannot fully account for terminal behavior and may or may not be the primary mediating factor influencing performance. Given the complexity of social interactions and the ambiguity of most social problems, emphasizing only the problem-solving steps may be too narrow and constricted a focus. Populations that are deficient in problem-solving competency are often deficient in other social skills as well, such as conversational ability or assertion (Conger & Keane, 1981; Holmes et al., 1984; Kelly & Lamparski, 1985). No single intervention in isolation is likely to produce social competence in a population as socially impaired as schizophrenic patients.

Another theoretical question is whether more direct behavioral interventions (such as assertion training or relaxation training, for example) may also lead to the acquisition of problem-solving skills through different, and more behavioral, mechanisms. Although cognitive processes play a role in social behavior, it does not necessarily follow that cognitive treatment strategies are the most effective or efficient means to produce changes in social problem-solving effectiveness. In other words, the different labels attached to specific interventions may mask underlying similarities in the cognitive end point each produces. Cognitive "rules" can be taught through a variety of techniques, but these techniques have not been evaluated against one other (Rathjen, Rathjen, & Hiniker, 1978). For example, the literature reflects an emerging support for direct behavioral treatments, rather than cognitively based treatment for phobic behavior (Mavissakalian & Barlow, 1981); participant modeling over covert modeling (O'Brien, 1981; Rimm & Lefebvre, 1981); in vivo rather than imaginal flooding (Emmelkamp & Wessels, 1975); and in vivo rather than imaginal desensitization (Barlow, Leitenberg, Agras, & Wimcze, 1969). Thus, problem-solving research may do well to examine the most effective and efficient means to achieve the desired cognitive and behavioral outcome goals. Research comparing direct behavioral approaches with cognitively oriented problem-solving interventions would prove helpful in this regard.

Generalization and maintenance issues have rarely been addressed in the problem-solving literature. Only rarely is generalization from trained to untrained problems, to behavior within sessions, or to in vivo behavior addressed. The problem-solving literature seems to reflect an underlying assumption that cognitive/verbal problem-solving skills will automatically generalize into behavior. As noted by Urbain and Kendall (1980), "a major hypothesis based on the social cognitive problem-solving model is that training at the level of the cognitive processes that presumably mediate competence across a broad range of situations will 'build in' generalization as an integral part of treatment" (p. 110). This hypothesis awaits empirical support.

Current assessment strategies reflect a narrow focus, and even the data analytic methods may be constricted. Researchers may be blinded to the process or function of cognition when descriptions of thought content or frequency counts of cognitive categories are attended to in isolation. Sequential analysis of thought patterns could potentially reveal rich information with important theoretical and treatment implications. For example, Notarius (1981) noted that males high or low in heterosocial anxiety report comparable levels of positive, negative, and neutral self-statements. However, high anxious subjects display negative thoughts followed by other negative thoughts, while low anxious subjects counter those negative cognitions with positive thoughts. Schwartz and Gottman (1976) successfully discriminated assertive from unassertive individuals on the basis of time series analysis, and Glass (1981) reported that the type of self-statement that followed an assertive response differentiated high- from low-guilt subjects. Thus, the pattern or sequence of self-statements may be a factor worthy of attention. More elaborate study of the cognitive sequence during problem-solving efforts may be a promising and innovative approach for further research.

The problem-solving literature has largely ignored how differences in situational parameters may influence problem-solving effectiveness. D'Zurilla and Nezu (1982) identified five classes of social problem-solving situations: threat of punishment, loss of reinforcement, frustration or prevention of goal attainment, interpersonal conflict, and personal conflict. Situational contexts have been shown to be vitally important in assertive responding and to produce differences in responding (St. Lawrence, Hansen, Cutts, Tisdelle, & Irish, 1985). As yet, the problem-solving literature has not addressed whether response demands in social problem-solving may also be influenced by situational differences. Given the substantial empirical support for situational specificity in other subsets of social competence, this is an issue that warrants careful evaluation in the problem-solving literature.

Problem-solving training may be most helpful when it is used adjunctively as part of a broad spectrum intervention remedying social deficits. On a theoretical level, problem-solving training may produce incremental benefits in generalization or maintenance following therapeutic change (Tisdelle & St. Lawrence, 1986). Cognitive skills training approaches are often advocated for this purpose, and self-regulatory training, in particular, has been promoted as a maintenance strategy (Mahoney & Mahoney, 1976). However, there has been little empirical support (Leventhal & Cleary, 1980). Kirschenbaum and Tomarken (1982) reviewed the self-regulatory literature and concluded that "part of self-regulatory failure is inadequate planning of activities, misrecognition of potentially problematic situations, and underestimation of the riskiness of certain situations" (p. 144). Recognizing a problem, planning how to cope, and learning to evaluate the consequences of alternative solutions are part and parcel of problem-solving training. Empirical evaluations of programs that incorporate problem solving may produce useful information as to whether including a problem-solving component improves maintenance. A study examining the effectiveness of problem solving in preventing smoking relapse found significantly fewer relapses in smokers who also received the problem-solving training (Karol & Richards, 1978, reported in D'Zurilla & Nezu, 1982).

At the present time, very few problem-solving studies compare subjects with unimpaired peer groups (Hansen et al., 1985). The usual procedure of comparing a treatment group with other maladjusted individuals may not result in a meaningful evaluation of social problem solving. Even when statistically significant improvements are documented, they do not ensure that subjects were rendered normal responders (Tisdelle & St. Lawrence, 1986). Comparisons with adjusted populations can better establish social validation for social problem-solving training.

In conclusion, although social problem solving appears to be useful and effective intervention with schizophrenic patients, considerable effort needs to be directed toward perfecting assessment strategies, disentangling the relative contributions of each component stage to problem-solving effectiveness, and resolving the many ambiguities in the problem-solving literature.

REFERENCES

Ault, R. L. (1973). Problem-solving strategies of reflective, impulsive, fast-accurate, and slow-accurate children. *Child Development, 44,* 259–266.

Barlow, D. H. Leitenberg, H., Agras, W. S., & Wincze, J. P. (1969). The transfer gap in systematic desensitization: An analogue study. *Behaviour Research and Therapy, 7,* 191–197.

Bedell, J. R., Archer, R. P., & Marlowe, H. A., Jr. (1980). A description and evaluation of a problem solving skills training program. In D. Upper & S. M. Ross (Eds.), *Behavioral group therapy: An annual review.* Champaign, IL: Research Press.

Bornstein, P. H., & Quevillon, R. P. (1976). The effects of a self-instructional package on overactive preschool boys. *Journal of Applied Behavior Analysis, 9,* 179–188.

Chaney, E. F., O'Leary, M. R., & Marlatt, G. A. (1978). Skill training with alcoholics. *Journal of Consulting and Clinical Psychology, 46,* 1092–1104.

Coche, E., Cooper, J. B., & Petermann, K.J. (1984). Differential outcomes of cognitive and interactive group therapies. *Small Group Behavior, 15,* 497–509.

Coche, E., & Douglass, A. A. (1977). Therapeutic effects of problem-solving training and play reading groups. *Journal of Clinical Psychology, 33,* 820–827.

Coche, E., & Flick, A. (1975). Problem-solving training groups for hospitalized psychiatric patients. *Journal of Psychology, 91,* 19–29.

Combs, M. L., & Slaby, D. A. (1977). Social skills training with children. In B. B. Lahey & A. E. Kazdin (Eds.), *Advances in clinical child psychology* (Vol. 1, pp. 161–201). New York: Plenum Press.

Conger, J. C., & Keane, S. P. (1981). Social skills interventions in the treatment of isolated and withdrawn children. *Psychological Bulletin, 90,* 478–495.

Dixon, D. N., Heppner, P. P., Petersen, C.H., & Ronning, R. R. (1979). Problem-solving workshop training. *Journal of Counseling Psychology, 26,* 133–139.

Drake, D. M. (1970). Perceptual correlates of impulsive and reflective behavior. *Developmental Psychology, 2,* 202–214.

D'Zurilla, T. J. (1986). *Problem-solving therapy: A social competence approach to clinical intervention.* New York: Springer.

D'Zurilla, T., & Goldfried, M. (1971). Problem-solving and behavior modification. *Journal of Abnormal Psychology, 78,* 104–126.

D'Zurilla, T., & Nezu, A. (1982). Social problem-solving in adults. In P. C. Kendall (Ed.), *Advances in cognitive behavioral research and therapy* (Vol. 1, pp. 201–274). New York: Academic Press.

Edelstein, B. A., Couture, E., Cray, M., Dickens, P., & Lusebrink, N. (1980). Group training of problem-solving with psychiatric patients. In D. Upper & S. M. Ross (Eds.), *Behavioral group therapy 1980: An annual review* (pp. 85–102). Champaign, IL: Research Press.

Emmelkamp, P. M. G., & Wessels, H. (1975). Flooding in imagination vs. flooding in vivo: A comparison with agoraphobics. *Behaviour Research and Therapy, 13,* 7–15.

Evans, I., & Nelson, R. (1977). Assessment of child behavior problems. In A. Ciminero, K. Calhoun, & H. Adams (Eds.), *Handbook of behavioral assessment* (pp. 601–681). New York: Wiley.

Foster, S., & Ritchey, W. (1979). Issues in the assessment of social competence in children. *Journal of Applied Behavior Analysis, 12,* 625–638.

Froland, C., Brodsky, G., Olson, M., & Stewart, L. (1979). Social support and social adjustment: Implications for mental health professionals. *Community Mental Health, 15,* 32–93.

Goldfried, M. R., & D'Zurilla, T. J. (1969). A behavior-analytic model for assessing competence. In C. D. Spielberger (Ed.), *Current topics in clinical and community psychology.* New York: Academic Press.

Goldsmith, J. G., & McFall, R. M. (1975). Development and evaluation of an interpersonal skill training program for psychiatric inpatients. *Journal of Abnormal Psychology, 84,* 51–58.

Gotlib, I., & Asarnow, R. F. (1970). Interpersonal and impersonal problem-solving skills in mildly and clinically depressed university students. *Journal of Consulting and Clinical Psychology, 47,* 86–95.

Hansen, D. J., St. Lawrence, J. S., & Christoff, J. S. (1985). Effects of interpersonal problem-solving training with chronic aftercare patients on problem-solving component skills and effectiveness of solutions. *Journal of Consulting and Clinical Psychology, 53,* 167–174.

Heppner, P. P., Baumgardner, A., Larson, L. M., & Petty, R. E. (1983). *Problem-solving training for college students with problem-solving deficits.* Paper presented to the American Psychological Association, Anaheim.

Heppner, P. P., Hibel, J. H., Neal, G. W., Weinstein, C. L., & Rabinowitz, F. E. (1982). Personal problem solving: A descriptive study of individual differences. *Journal of Counseling Psychology, 29,* 580–590.

Heppner, P. P., & Petersen, C. H. (1982). The development and implications of a personal problem solving inventory. *Journal of Counseling Psychology, 29,* 66–75.

Holmes, M. R., Hansen, D. J., & St. Lawrence, J. S. (1984). Conversational skills training with aftercare patients in the community: Social validation and generalization. *Behavior Therapy, 15,* 84–100.

Jahoda, M. (1958). *Current concepts of positive mental health.* New York: Basic Books.

Kelly, J. A. (1982). *Social skills training: A practical guide for interventions.* New York: Springer.

Kelly, J. A., & Lamparski, D. M. (1985). Outpatient treatment of schizophrenics: Social skills and problem-solving training. In M. Hersen & A. S. Bellack (Eds.), *Handbook of clinical and behavior therapy with adults* (pp. 485–500). New York: Plenum Press.

Kendall, P. C. (1977). On the efficacious use of verbal self-instructional procedures with children. *Cognitive Therapy and Research, 1,* 331–341.

Kendall, P. C., & Finch, A. J., Jr. (1978). A cognitive-behavioral treatment for impulsivity: A group comparison study. *Journal of Consulting and Clinical Psychology, 46,* 110–118.

Kirschenbaum, D. S., & Tomarken, A. J. (1982). On facing the generalization problem: The study of self-regulatory failure. In P. C. Kendall (Ed.), *Advances in cognitive-behavioral research and therapy* (Vol. 1, pp. 119–200). New York: Academic Press.

Krasnor, L. R., & Rubin, K. H. (1981). Assessment of social problem-solving skills in young children. In T. Merluzzi & M. Genest (Eds.), *Cognitive assessment* (pp. 452–474). New York: Guilford Press.

Leventhal, H., & Cleary, P. D. (1980). The smoking problem: A review of the research and theory in behavioral risk modification. *Psychological Bulletin, 88,* 370–405.

Levine, J., & Zigler, E. (1973). The essential-reactive distinction in alcoholism: A developmental approach. *Journal of Abnormal Psychology, 81,* 242–249.

Luria, A. R. (1961). *The role of speech in the regulation of normal and abnormal behavior.* New York: Liveright.

Mahoney, M. J., & Mahoney, K. (1976). *Permanent weight control.* New York: Norton.

Mavissakalian, M., & Barlow, D. H. (1981). Phobia: An overview. In M. Mavissakalian & D. H. Barlow (Eds.), *Phobia: Psychological and pharmacological treatment* (pp. 1–33). New York: Guilford Press.

McClure, L. F., Chinsky, J. M., & Larcen, S. W. (1978). Enhancing social problem-solving performance in an elementary school setting. *Journal of Educational Psychology, 70,* 304–313.

McFall, R. (1982). Review and reformulation of the concept of social skills. *Behavioral Assessment, 4,* 1–33.

Meichenbaum, D. H., & Goodman, J. (1971). Training impulsive children to talk to themselves. *Journal of Abnormal Psychology, 77,* 115–126.

Mitchell, R. E. (1982). Social networks and psychiatric clients: The personal and environmental context. *American Journal of Community Psychology, 10,* 387–401.

Notarius, C. I. (1981). Assessing sequential dependency in cognitive performance data. In T. V. Merluzzi, C. R. Glass, & M. Ginest (Eds.), *Cognitive assessment* (pp. 343–357). New York: Guilford Press.

O'Brien, G. T. (1981). Clinical treatment of specific phobias. In M. Mavissakalian & D. H. Barlow (Eds.), *Phobia: Psychological and pharmacological treatment* (pp. 63–102). New York: Guilford Press.

Ollendick, T. H., & Hersen, M. (1979). Social skills training for juvenile delinquents. *Behaviour Research and Therapy, 17,* 347–354.

Patterson, G. R., Littman, R. A., & Bricker, W. (1967). Assertive behavior in children. *Monographs of the Society for Research in Child Development, 32,* 1–43.

Phillips, L., & Zigler, E. (1961). Social competence: The action-thought parameter and vicariousness in normal and pathological behaviors. *Journal of Abnormal and Social Psychology, 63,* 137–146.

Phillips, L., & Zigler, E. (1964). Role orientation, the action-thought dimension and outcome in psychiatric disorder. *Journal of Abnormal and Social Psychology, 68,* 381–389.

Platt, J. J., & Siegel, J. M. (1976). MMPI characteristics of good and poor social problem solvers among psychiatric patients. *Journal of Community Psychology, 94,* 245–251.

Platt, J. J., & Spivack, G. (1972a). Problem-solving thinking of psychiatric patients. *Journal of Consulting and Clinical Psychology, 39,* 148–151.

Platt, J. J., & Spivack, G. (1972b). Social competence and effective problem-solving thinking in psychiatric patients. *Journal of Clinical Psychology, 28,* 3–5.

Platt, J. J., & Spivack, G. (1974). Means of solving real-life problems: 1. Psychiatric patients versus controls and cross-cultural comparisons of normal females. *Journal of Community Psychology, 2,* 45–48.

Platt, J. J., & Spivack, G. (1977). *Manual for Means-Ends Problem-Solving Procedure.* Philadelphia: Department of Mental Health Sciences, Hahnemann Community Health/ Mental Retardation Center.

Rathjen, D. P., Rathjen, E. D., & Hiniker, A. (1978). A cognitive analysis of social performance: Implications for assessment and treatment. In J. P. Foreyt & D. P. Rathjen (Eds.). *Cognitive behavior therapy: Research and application* (pp. 61–107). New York: Plenum Press.

Renshaw, P. D., & Asher, S. R. (1982). Social competence and peer status: The distinction between goals and strategies. In K. H. Rubin & H. S. Ross (Eds.), *Peer relationships and social skills in childhood* (pp. 375–395). New York: Springer-Verlag.

Rimm, D. C., & Lefebvre, R. C. (1981). Phobic disorders. In S. M. Turner, K. S. Calhoun, & H. E. Adams (Eds.), *Handbook of clinical behavior therapy* (pp. 12–40). New York: Wiley.

Robin, A., Schneider, M., & Dolnick, M. (1976). The turtle technique: An extended case study of self control in the classroom. *Psychology in the Schools, 13,* 449–453.

Roff, M., Sells, B., & Golden, M. (1972). *Social adjustment and personality development in children.* Minneapolis: University of Minnesota Press.

Sarason, B. R. (1981). Dimensions of social competence: Contributions from a variety of research areas. In J. D. Wine & M. D. Smye (Eds.), *Social competence* (pp. 100–122). New York: Guilford Press.

Sarason, I. G., & Sarason, B. R. (1981). Teaching cognitive and social skills to high school students. *Journal of Consulting and Clinical Psychology, 49,* 908–918.

Schwartz, R. M., & Gottman, J. M. (1976). Toward a task analysis of assertive behavior. *Journal of Consulting and Clinical Psychology, 44,* 910–920.

Shure, M. B., Spivack, G., & Jaeger, M. A. (1971). Problem-solving thinking and adjustment among disadvantaged preschool children. *Child Development, 42,* 1791–1803.

Siegel, J. M., & Platt, J. J. (1976). Emotional and social real-life problem-solving thinking in adolescent and adult psychiatric patients. *Journal of Clinical Psychology, 32,* 230–232.

Siegel, J. M., & Spivack, G. (1976a). Problem solving therapy: The description of a new program for chronic psychiatric patients. *Psychotherapy: Theory, Research, and Practice, 13,* 368–373.

Siegel, J. M., & Spivack, G. (1976b). A new therapy program for chronic patients. *Behavior Therapy, 7,* 129–130.

Solomon, R. W., & Wahler, R. G. (1973). Peer reinforcement of classroom problem behavior. *Journal of Applied Behavior Analysis, 6,* 49–56.

Spivack, G., & Shure, M. (1974). *Social adjustment of young children.* San Francisco: Jossey-Bass.

St. Lawrence, J. S., Hansen, D. J., Cutts, T. F., Tisdelle, D. A., & Irish, J. D. (1985). Situational context: Effects on perceptions of assertive and unassertive behavior. *Behavior Therapy, 16,* 51–62.

Tisdelle, D. A., & St. Lawrence, J. S. (1986). Interpersonal problem-solving competency: Review and critique of the literature. *Clinical Psychology Review, 6,* 337–356.

Tisdelle, D. A., & St. Lawrence, J. S. (1988). Interpersonal problem-solving skills training with conduct-disordered inpatient adolescents: Social validation and generalization to in-vivo behavior. *Behavior Therapy, 19,* 171–182.

Ullmann, C. A. (1957). Teachers, peers, and tests as predictors of adjustment. *Journal of Educational Psychology, 47,* 257–267.

Urbain, E. S., & Kendall, P. C. (1980). Review of social cognitive problem-solving interventions with children. *Psychological Bulletin, 88,* 109–143.

Vygotsky, L. (1962). *Thought and language.* New York: Wiley.

Zigler, E., & Phillips, L. (1961). Social competence and outcome in psychiatric disorder. *Journal of Abnormal and Social Psychology, 63,* 264–271.

Zigler, E., & Phillips, L. (1962). Social competence and the process-reactive distinction in psychopathology. *Journal of Abnormal and Social Psychology, 65,* 215–222.

13

The Young Chronic Patient

MAXINE HARRIS

In the past several years both researchers and clinicians have delineated the concept of the young adult chronic patient (Bachrach, 1982; Pepper, Kirshner, & Ryglewicz, 1981; Schwartz & Goldfinger, 1981) in an attempt to anticipate and define the service needs of a subgroup of chronic patients in the postdeinstitutionalization era. Authors have focused on patients' functional disabilities (Pepper & Ryglewicz, 1984), their tendency to drift from place to place and from experience to experience (Lamb, 1982), their pervasive use of drugs and alcohol (Bergman & Harris, 1985; Safer, 1987), and their misuse and occasional abuse of the service delivery system (Pepper, Ryglewicz, & Kirshner, 1982; Schwartz & Goldfinger, 1981).

While initially it may have been convenient to think of young adult chronic patients as representing a discrete service entity, it has become increasingly clear that the members of this subgroup are in fact quite heterogeneous both in their clinical presentations (Schacter & Goldberg, 1982; Sheets, Prevost, & Reihman, 1982) and in their treatment needs (Harris & Bergman, 1987a). Consequently, we now need a more complicated approach to understanding these patients beyond a mere description of population demographics.

The question has been asked, "Are we dealing with a new clinical entity when we treat young adult chronic patients?" Pepper et al. (1982), among others (Gralnick, 1984), has maintained that we are not. In terms of psychopathology, today's young patients are no different from chronically mentally ill patients who presented for treatment 20 years ago. Why then do they

---

MAXINE HARRIS • Community Connections, 1512 Pennsylvania Avenue, S.E., Washington, DC 20003.

pose such problems for our treatment system? The answer lies only partially with the patients themselves. We must also examine the confluence of social, economic, and cultural factors that converge to produce the treatment milieu of the 1980s.

First, we must begin by understanding the unique psychological deficits that characterize chronic patients, since it is with the limitations brought on by these deficits that patients must process and integrate any future psychological or social events. The first set of demands that must be met by chronic patients are those imposed by the developmental phase of young adulthood. Unfortunately, the onset of psychiatric symptoms often coincides with the onset of young adulthood, a developmental phase whose tasks are often awesome even for individuals who do not suffer from major psychological impairment. Second, young chronic patients must confront their illnesses and their developmental struggles in a treatment climate that supports community-based care and greater freedom and autonomy for the individual. Third, they must survive in a community that is economically competitive and socially fragmented. Finally, they must make their way in a culture that is more narcissistic and self-orientated than that of past generations.

Young adult chronic patients exist not because pathology has changed but because a variety of factors have converged in a particular way at a particular time. We can speculate that if any of these factors were absent, the result would be a different clinical phenomenon. Bert Pepper and his colleagues in Rockland County, New York (1984), who are credited with originating the term *young adult chronic patient*, also maintain that these patients exist as the result of a complex interaction of factors. The problems of young adulthood, the stresses of community life, and the present conditions of the service system all contribute to the phenomenon of the young adult chronic patient.

THE PATIENT

Chronically mentally ill adults, whether they are young adult chronic patients or older institutionalized patients, experience a constellation of psychological deficits that make coping difficult under even the best of circumstances. Chronic mental illness, almost by definition, entails a span of ego deficits, ranging from impaired reality testing and poor judgment to difficulty controlling impulses and modulating affect (Harris & Bergman, 1987b; Pepper et al., 1982; Schwartz & Goldfinger, 1981). Additionally, chronic patients are especially vulnerable to stress, making their precarious peace with the world vulnerable to disruption by events that might not appear stressful to a less disabled individual.

Not surprisingly many chronically mentally ill patients do not possess a stable sense of either themselves or other people (Harris & Bergman, 1987b). They may experience themselves as being discontinuous across situations and may be unable to utilize past experiences to plan future endeavors. This lack of stable personal identity not only is disorienting for the individual but presents very real problems for clinicians trying to develop realistic treatment plans.

Chronic patients are also bereft of the usual coping strategies available to normal adults. Not only are they unable to develop problem-solving and goal-attainment approaches on their own, but they are also without the range of psychological defenses, such as intellectualization, which many of us use comfortably to cope with anxiety. Instead, these individuals are routinely engaged in killing flies with machine guns, using a few extreme (i.e., psychotic) defenses to process relatively minor ambiguities and anxieties.

This particular set of vulnerabilities and deficits is probably no different for today's young adult chronic mental patient than it was for patients facing the world 30 years ago. However, the young adult chronic patient must wear these vulnerabilities in a changing mental health climate and a high-pressure social world, and must find a way to traverse the difficult stages of early adult life with this often inadequate equipment.

YOUNG ADULT DEVELOPMENT

While each of life's stages has its own tasks and potential pitfalls, the concerns of early adulthood, ages 20 to 40, are especially far-reaching. In his groundbreaking study of adult development, Levinson (1978) characterizes early adulthood as a time of great energy and capability, but also a time of great external pressure. The tasks of early adulthood include not only making choices about marriage, occupation, residence, and style of living, but also beginning to form a preliminary adult identity.

During this period of young adulthood, all of us struggle and experiment with the task of self-definition. These are the years during which adults separate from their families of origin, form new relationships, and achieve vocational success. Unfortunately, persons with chronic mental illnesses find these tasks more than they can manage. They routinely and repeatedly fail at familial separation, vocational choice, and interpersonal intimacy (Kanter, 1985a). Pepper et al. (1981) have described them as unable to make the transition from childhood dependence to adult independence.

Despite the mental illnesses that make it difficult for these patients to succeed at the tasks of young adulthood, they continue in many cases to see themselves as being no different from other young adults, and consequently to want the same things other young adults want (Pepper et al., 1981). Lamb (1982) has poignantly described the despair many of these patients feel when they face the transition from their 20s to their 30s and realize that they have failed to achieve even the most minimal life successes.

While it has always been difficult for chronically mentally ill adults to face the failures of unsuccessful young adult development, policies of institutionalization allowed them to retreat from adult pressures into a world of asylum care (Lamb, 1982). Current practices of deinstitutionalization offer no such escape. In fact, these policies may inadvertently force patients to return time and again to developmental tasks at which they have little hope of success.

GOALS AND VALUES OF DEINSTITUTIONALIZATION

The impact of the deinstitutionalization movement on today's chronically mentally ill adults cannot be overestimated. Not only does deinstitutionalization define certain policy initiatives that determine the nature and extent of service delivery, but it also both directly and indirectly espouses certain values that help define the milieu in which care will be rendered. Both at the practical level of policy initiatives and at the more abstract level of philosophy, deinstitutionalization has created a treatment environment that has inadvertently contributed to the phenomenon of the young adult chronic patient.

Deinstitutionalization not only resulted in many older, chronic patients being discharged into the community but it also limited the ease with which younger patients could gain access to inpatient care through practices of admission diversion (Bachrach, 1983). Additionally, deinstitutionalization has meant that hospital stays, when they do occur, are far shorter than in the past. These initiatives have resulted in the creation of what Pepper et al. (1982) have termed the uninstitutionalized generation: patients who for the most part have reached maturity and fallen ill since deinstitutionalization went into effect.

While few would argue for a return to institutional care, most would advocate for the comprehensiveness and coordination of services that resulted when all services were centralized under one roof (or at least one authority). With deinstitutionalization has also come decentralization of care, use of multiple providers, and fragmentation of services. While these deficits are bad enough in and of themselves, they are especially problematic for chronically mentally ill persons who deal poorly with stress and integrate experience with difficulty, if at all.

In addition to the practical policies of reducing inpatient beds, diverting

admissions, and shortening hospital stays, the deinstitutionalization movement has also advocated certain fundamental values. Bachrach (1984) defines
the humanizing of psychiatric care as the central goal of deinstitutionalization. Humanizing care has many practical implications for today's patients.
Rather than being warehoused in the anonymous institutions of the past,
patients are treated in environments that are more personal, closer to their
home communities (Stein & Test, 1982), and more respectful of their individual differences. While this is certainly a laudable goal, Minkoff (1982) has
pointed to at least one questionable outcome of this more individualized
approach. Under systems of institutionalization, patients were often treated
in a stereotyped and rote manner. While such behavior was in fact de-
humanizing, it was also clear and specific, and it defined the rules of normative behavior for patients. Under systems of more highly individualized
care, patients must define for themselves what they want and need. They are
encouraged, indeed expected, to be more active participants in planning
their own treatment. Such involvement is long overdue and generally to be
welcomed; however, it can be frustrating and confusing for patients who
really do not have the ego capacities to plan their own treatment in any
meaningful way. Such patients may feel angry at treaters who expect more of
them than they are capable of giving, resulting in some of the acting-out
behavior that has led to these young patients' being labeled as "difficult"
(Bachrach, Talbott, & Meyerson, 1987).

Deinstitutionalization, with the help of a series of court decisions
(Rachlin, 1983), has also ushered in the era of patients' rights. As opposed to
past generations of psychiatric patients, today's patients have the right to
treatment in the least restrictive environment and the right to refuse treatment. Perhaps more important than any specific right *per se*, these patients
have the subjective sense of having rights. Moreover, these new psychiatric
patients have grown up in the shadow of the civil rights movement and the
women's movement and know the language of personal rights and freedoms.
It is not uncommon for young adult chronic patients to present at clinics or
emergency rooms insisting on their "rights." Ironically, it may be this very
same behavior that results in their being labeled, somewhat pejoratively, as
demanding and entitled. Part of our difficulty in working with today's patients may well be that we are unused to dealing with patients who insist on
their own rights.

Finally, deinstitutionalization has advocated for the normalization of the
psychiatric population and the lessening of some of the stigma that accompanies mental illness. In many community-based programs enrollees are
referred to as clients, students, residents or members, rather than as patients. Certainly, in psychosocial programs it is not uncommon for staff and
patients to be on a first-name basis. Additionally, efforts are made wherever

possible to mainstream patients into resources designed for the general public rather than creating a series of separate but equal resources for mentally ill persons. Again, while these may be laudable efforts, they do have implications for patients' behaviors and may contribute to some of the attitudes attributed to young adult chronic patients. Frequently, these patients are described as denying their illnesses and rejecting patienthood (Pepper et al., 1981). While Pepper et al. (1981) agree that this avoidance of the stereotyped patient role is one of the sought-after outcomes of community treatment, it has other deleterious effects when patients refuse to take medications or to acknowledge their vulnerability to street drugs.

Deinstitutionalization has not only changed the locus and mode of delivering psychiatric care but it has also propounded a particular philosophy of care that advocates for care more focused on the individual, his or her rights, desires, and input. Such a milieu poses problems when patients have a fragmented or chaotic view of themselves and others. Under those circumstances, their participation may be chaotic, volatile, and confusing, charges often leveled against young adult chronic patients.

PRESSURES OF COMMUNITY LIVING

Deinstitutionalization accomplished two related but different outcomes when it made inpatient hospitalization less accessible to mentally ill persons. First, it denied them the structure and support available in a total care institution (Goffman, 1961) in which all services and resources were supplied by a consistent set of staff members. But second, it placed them in communities that were often the antithesis of the bucolic state mental hospitals. In the community—often a high-density, marginal urban environment—the chronically mentally ill person must contend with a variety of situational stresses (Pepper et al., 1981).

Living outside a total care institution requires that an individual be able to negotiate a range of routine tasks, such as shopping for groceries, doing laundry, riding the bus, talking to strangers, and managing money. Accomplishing these tasks and juggling the often conflicting demands of community living is typically more stressful than most patients can manage. It is important for clinicians to realize that patients often are not overwhelmed by the concrete task of grocery shopping *per se;* they are overwhelmed by the interpersonal hassles encountered in carrying out routine tasks—the woman at the checkout counter who wants to make conversation or the shopper who bumps into them on the way out of the store. Patients will often describe leaving their rooms as being akin to entering a war zone. Simple tasks become overwhelming and sometimes impossible as a result of the difficulty chronic patients have making decisions, setting priorities, and managing interpersonal distance.

Beyond their difficulties in managing community living in general, chronically mentally ill young adults experience additional stresses because they frequently participate in the culture of poverty (Friswold, 1987). Pepper and Ryglewicz (1984) have documented the history of vocational failure that often haunts young adult chronic patients. The vast majority who cannot work receive entitlement benefits. Unfortunately, these benefits do not allow individuals more than a subsistence level of functioning, and poverty carries with it additional stresses. Because they are economically deprived, chronic patients must live in run-down neighborhoods with higher crime rates and fewer city services. While poverty is difficult for non-mentally ill persons to cope with, it is doubly hard for mentally ill adults, who manage even minimal stress poorly. As one young woman rather desperately lamented, "It's bad enough being crazy; I can't handle being poor."

Chronic patients also experience stress when living in the community because many of the members of their support network are also mentally ill persons experiencing many of the same stresses and vulnerabilities (Harris & Bergman, 1985). It is not uncommon for a patient to have a friend who has been thrown out of the family home sleeping on the floor of his or her bedroom, or to have a friend in the hospital for suicidal or psychotic feelings. There are two consequences to having a support network dominated by other chronically mentally ill persons. First, one has the extra stress associated with having friends who are themselves crisis-prone and vulnerable to stress, and second, one's friends are less likely to be available to offer support if they are themselves in crisis.

Thus, while community living offers young adults with mental illnesses some obvious freedoms over institutional care, it also presents them with a variety of often intolerable stresses. These stresses result not only from the inherent hassles of city life but also from the reality that chronic mental patients have to contend with poverty and unreliable and volatile support systems. It is paradoxical that those members of our society least equipped to deal with stress often are confronted with overwhelming situations.

THE CULTURE OF THE 1980s

While it is certainly beyond the scope of this chapter to attempt an analysis of the multitude of factors converging to produce the cultural milieu of the 1980s, there are a few dimensions that have special relevance for this discussion of young chronic patients. The 1980s have been characterized as the "me generation," the "culture of narcissism" (Lasch, 1978). The popular press has highlighted the apparent turn from the social activism of the 1960s to the self-absorption of the 1980s.

Clinicians have described young adult chronic patients as "wanting what they want when they want it" (Bachrach, 1982). While it is certainly plausible to understand this demanding behavior as being the result of particular character pathology, it is also reasonable to assume that young adult chronic patients are, like other children of the 1980s, reflecting the values of their generation. Several years ago psychiatric emergency rooms and admissions wards saw patients who were the last burned-out remnants of the hippie generation (Harris & Bergman, 1983). These patients, who were used to living in communes and literally sharing the shirts off their backs, espoused a different set of values. Their pathology and their attempt to cope with the stresses of adult and community life were filtered through a different cultural milieu.

Additionally, one cannot talk about the decade of the 1980s without talking about substance abuse. Issues of use and abuse are frequently on the evening news as we hear about the latest epidemic to hit the streets. And not surprisingly, substance abuse is one of the main problem areas for young adult chronic patients (Bergman & Harris, 1985; McCarrick, Manderscheid, & Bertolucci, 1985; Safer, 1987). In their attempts to be like other young adults and to fit into difficult social situations (Bergman & Harris, 1985; McCarrick et al., 1985), young adult chronic patients frequently abuse highly toxic substances. Substance abuse among young patients is related not only to an increase in acting-out behavior (McCarrick et al., 1985) but also to increased incidence of rehospitalization (Safer, 1987). Unfortunately, because of their desire to avoid the stigma of mental illness, many young adult chronic patients prefer the label of substance abuser to that of schizophrenic (Pepper et al., 1981).

In order to adequately understand young adult chronic patients we must also understand the cultural milieu in which they have come of age and the peer pressures to which they are subject.

It is our contention that in viewing young adult chronic patients today we are not viewing a new clinical entity. Rather we are observing persons with severe and in many cases lifelong psychiatric impairment who are passing through the difficult developmental phase of young adulthood, while at the same time trying to cope with the pressures of community life in an era of social disinterest and heightened individualism, and with mental health services that are decentralized and often fragmented. It is in this context, and only this context, that we can understand the phenomenon of the young adult chronic patient. And it is in this context that we must develop treatment programs for patients. The question becomes not merely how do we treat young adult chronic patients, but how do we treat patients in the era of deinstitutionalization?

ASSESSMENT

As in the past, the development of viable treatment plans needs to begin with an adequate and relevant assessment of the individual. However, with the locus of the treatment now being in the patient's community rather than in the protected milieu of the state hospital, different variables must be assessed. The emphasis needs to be on functional dimensions of behavior (Pepper & Ryglewicz, 1984) rather than on traditional diagnostic categories, with a special focus on styles of interacting with others and on coping with routine and unpredictable occurrences. We have found the following dimensions to be especially relevant: extent and nature of overt symptomatology, ability to tolerate stress, overt resistance to the environment, level of motivation, extent to which interpersonal closeness is tolerated or sought, level of functioning, and extent and nature of social supports.

Overt Symptomatology. For patients to adapt to life outside an institution the issue is often not so much what their symptoms are but how annoying are those symptoms to the patient and those with whom he or she is going to be living. Take, for example, the case of two young male patients, both of whom feel compelled to spend their days walking. One walks at home, pacing back and forth in front of his mother all day. The other leaves the house in the morning, walks around the city all day, and returns home in time for dinner. In the first case the interference quotient of the symptom is quite high, while in the second case the symptom is tolerated by both the patient and his family.

Clinicians need to assess the extent to which overt symptoms will interfere with any of the principal tasks of community living, such as taking public transportation or working and living with others. Additionally, they need to evaluate how much stress the individual experiences because of the symptoms. Again, take the case of two young women, both of whom routinely experience auditory hallucinations. One is tormented by the voices, attempts to drown them out by taking drugs and drinking, and occasionally screams at them while walking down the street. The other woman considers the voices to be her friends and can occasionally be observed smiling or nodding to herself. The level of personal distress is very different in the two cases, and consequently the overt symptom needs to be assessed differently by clinicians.

Stress Tolerance. When patients were institutionalized in relatively low-stress environments, the question of their ability to tolerate stressful situations was frequently academic. When patients are placed in often stressful community environments, however, it may well be the most important question the clinician asks.

In fact, the question of stress tolerance is really three different but related questions. First is the question of what specific situations are stressful for the individual. While there certainly are some patients who experience the same high degree of anxiety in almost all situations, most patients experience anxiety or stress differentially across situations. It is important to differentiate stressful from relatively conflict-free areas of functioning lest patients be inadvertently subjected to experiences that might be experienced as intolerably stressful.

Second, it is important to ask both how debilitating and how pervasive the response to stress is. For example, the patient whose face twitches for a few moments when he or she feels anxious or stressed is quite different from the patient who responds to stress by stopping in his or her tracks and posing like a statue for hours. The extent of the response has obvious implications for treatment planning and potential success in a variety of life situations.

Finally, clinicians need to ask what mechanisms these individuals currently have in their repertoire for coping with stress. Unfortunately, many young patients cope with stress by self-medicating with drugs and alcohol, in which case the cure may be worse than the disease. While less debilitating, it is equally dysfunctional when a young male patient's only way of dealing with stress on the job is to run away. Clearly, some of the treatment for young patients must focus on the management of stress through medications to decrease their level of reactivity, by teaching them better coping strategies, and by designing environments for them that are less stressful.

Resistance to the Environment. Much of the difficulty young patients face in adapting to community living is a function of how resistant they are to influence or feedback from the environment. Researchers (Harris & Bergman, 1987a; Sheets et al., 1982) have identified subgroups among populations of young adult chronic patients who respond to treatment with passivity and compliance in much the same way that many older patients do. Not surprisingly, these are not the patients whom clinicians have labeled as the "bane and despair of our working lives" (Pepper et al., 1982). Rather, it is those young patients who must define themselves by saying no to the world who pose very real problems for clinicians.

For many young adult patients, the sense of personal identity is so fragile that the only way they can define themselves and avoid feeling impinged on by others is to take an oppositional stance. One young man who had a delusion that he was being controlled by machines from outer space automatically resisted any suggestion offered by his clinician or his family lest he relinquish what little control he had left over his own life.

Clinicians must assess the extent to which patients are resisting an idea because they really do not like it versus because they need to feel autonomous and independent of others. Clinicians need to be mindful not to steal patients' thunder by responding too enthusiastically to their tentative suggestions. What may result is that the patient will see the suggestion as the clinician's idea and will have to reject it in order to feel separate and independent. A series of such interactions can leave both patients and clinicians feeling frustrated and confused.

Level of Motivation. While the extent of overt resistance to the environment may correlate best with inability to function in a community environment, level of motivation is probably the best predicter of success. When assessing motivation, clinicians must also assess how realistic the goal is. One patient was highly motivated to return to college. He wrote letters to local universities, scheduled interviews, and filled out applications. Unfortunately, the goal was not a realistic one because he was unable to handle the interpersonal stress involved in being a college student.

Clinicians must also assess the extent to which a patient is genuinely motivated for a particular goal rather than merely imitating the goals of the clinician. Some patients will talk about wanting certain socially acceptable goals in order to please their clinicians. Generally, while these patients will sound as if they are motivated, they will rarely follow through on concrete behavioral assignments.

When patients are motivated, however, they can often overcome rather obvious obstacles in the pursuit of a particular goal. One young woman with a paranoid delusional system, intermittent auditory hallucinations, a series of physical handicaps, and a long history of revolving-door use of the state mental hospital wanted desperately to live in her own apartment. Her motivation enabled her to overcome her resistance to medications and her initial distrust of her clinician. An accurate assessment of a patient's motivation may allow a clinician to move forward with a plan that he or she might otherwise be hesitant to attempt. Moreover, by assessing what goals the patients have for themselves, the clinician may discover the basis of a working alliance with an otherwise recalcitrant or withdrawn patient.

Interpersonal Closeness/Distance. The extent to which patients seek out or avoid contact with other people is an important variable to assess when planning community treatment. While it may be relatively easy to minimize or even avoid having contact with others in a large institution, it is much more difficult to do so in the community where one must interact minimally in order to have basic needs for food and shelter met. Consequently, patients who are extremely fearful of others may go to great lengths to put distance between themselves and others. One patient reversed his sleep cycle in order to be up and active at night while the majority of the world slept. When he spent too much time with other people, he became alternately paranoid and homicidal.

While a need to maintain great interpersonal distance poses problems for community living, so too does the demand for too much contact and a failure to honor standard social norms regarding interpersonal space. Patients who manifest an excessive amount of contact-seeking behavior are often experienced by others as intrusive or pesty (Harris & Bergman, 1987a). Occasionally, patients experience so much anxiety when not receiving almost constant mirroring and validation from another person that they will invent reasons for contact. One patient made several trips to the grocery store, each time buying only one or two items, so that she would have a reason for interacting with other people.

Unfortunately, for some patients the need for contact is so great that they will precipitate a negative interaction in preference to no contact at all. Ironically, these negative encounters may make people more reluctant to interact with them in the future, and thus make it even harder to get the contact they so desperately seek.

Level of Functioning. Since community tenure requires some mastery of routine tasks of daily living, it is important to know whether or not patients have basic skills such as cooking, cleaning, buying groceries, managing money, and caring for their physical appearance. If skills are not present, then they may need to be taught. If, however, a patient possesses certain skills, but fails to use them, clinicians must look to issues of motivation, anxiety, or oppositionalism in order to understand the reason for the failure.

While level of functioning has obvious implications for how patients can cope with life outside an institution, it also has implications for their interpersonal relationships. When patients function poorly they often require more support and assistance from their friends and family. The need to provide concrete services over and above companionship, and comfort may prove taxing for network members and contribute to their own version of burnout. Additionally, when patients are unable to care for basic personal hygiene, they may offend and alienate potential resources, who become inclined to reject them before really giving them a chance.

Social Supports. When patients live in community settings they need a range of social supports in order to guarantee a basic quality of life. One needs other people, not only to meet instrumental needs for food, clothing and shelter, but also to address emotional needs for comfort, support, and advice. Clinicians must carefully evaluate not only the extent of network resources (i.e., who is available for what kind of support) but also the unspoken rules that govern network participation.

Studies of the support networks of young adult chronic patients (Harris & Bergman, 1985) reveal that, first of all, these networks contain fewer available members than the networks of non-mentally ill young adults. Many one-time network members either have grown frustrated and disillusioned over the years or have moved on to more successful and higher-functioning peer networks. Furthermore, many young patients are poor judges of what realistic resources do exist. Patients sometimes assume that old friends or distant relatives are available when in fact they are not. Others may overlook a potential source of support because they have not evaluated it accurately.

In addition to the somewhat objective assessment of network members, clinicians must also assess the less obvious rules that govern network behavior. Chronic patients often encounter great difficulty in interpersonal relationships because they misread the expectations and desires of other network members. Networks have expectations not only for what behaviors are desired but also for what behaviors will not be tolerated. In some networks there are many "do"s with respect to performance, governing a wide range of behaviors both inside and outside the network, while other support systems have few, if any, absolute requirements for membership. Other networks, in contrast, have a long list of "don't"s, behaviors for which members can be punished or even extruded. These expectations and proscriptions cover a span of behaviors ranging from overt psychiatric symptoms to financial contribution and work performance.

In addition to network rules, clinicians must also assess the level of stress apparent in a particular network and the patient's ability or inability to tolerate it. One young man routinely became highly symptomatic, often to the point of requiring hospitalization, after visiting with his extended family. Many of this patient's relatives were very successful professionals, and after a visit this young man's father would launch into an unfavorable and highly critical comparison of his accomplishments with those of his many cousins. Generally, networks that are either highly critical or overly involved tend to be stressful for patient members (Vaughn & Leff, 1976).

An assessment of relevant community variables, such as network support, level of functioning, tolerance of interpersonal closeness, level of motivation, environmental resistance, stress tolerance, and overt symptomatology, is necessary in order to plan noninstitutional treatment for young adult chronic patients. Assessment is, however, only the beginning of treatment planning. Beyond assessment, clinicians must have a set of guiding principles to assist in delivering community-based care.

CLINICAL PRINCIPLES OF TREATMENT

Bachrach (1982) has enumerated several principles of service delivery that need to be heeded in developing treatment programs for young adult chronic patients. These principles include comprehensiveness of services, linkages to appropriate resources, individualized treatment planning, flexibility of programs, access to hospital beds as part of the continuum of care, retention of appropriately trained staff, and attention to issues of cultural relevance. For the most part, these principles address planning at the systems level, and while they have implications for the clinical work of direct service providers, these implications need to be deduced. What is often needed by clinicians are principles that address, on a more individual level, their practical efforts with patients.

Accommodation versus Growth. Much has been said of the poignancy and frustration that accompany the juxtaposition of the words *young* and *chronic* (Pepper et al., 1981). We despair at the thought that people in their early 20s will be sick with a debilitating illness for the rest of their lives; but, for many young people chronic mental illness will be a lifelong struggle. Consequently, clinicians need to assess where patients and their support networks need to accommodate existing deficits, and where there exists the possibility for growth and change.

Accommodation routinely takes two forms. First, patients need to understand their illnesses and build in mechanisms of self-assessment and monitoring (Test, Knoedler, Allness, & Burke, 1985). By so doing they can develop strategies to compensate for ongoing deficits. For example, one young man experienced psychotic symptoms and a sense of fragmentation whenever he and his wife quarreled. He was unable to process her angry affect without decompensating. After several months of couples counseling, he learned to recognize a potential quarrel before it escalated and to get some needed distance from the situation by walking around the block a few times. These periodic walks were an accommodation to his underlying illness, which prevented him from processing affect in a more routine manner. It was a successful accommodation, moreover, since it allowed him to avoid the devastating consequences of a psychotic episode.

The process of accommodation may also take the form of finding or developing support networks that will tolerate existing symptomatology. One young man encountered much criticism from a succession of halfway houses because he was unable to begin his day before noon. He would be criticized for being lazy and oppositional and as a result would feel demoralized and inadequate and even less able to get up at 8:00 a.m. with the other residents. Eventually his placement would be terminated. Finally, his clinician found him a residential placement that allowed him to sleep late. This placement was willing to accommodate a rather long-standing symptom of the patient's illness, and while this accommodation has not resulted in any change in his waking behavior, it has resulted in his feeling less inadequate and demoralized.

Accommodation can thus focus on either the patient or his or her environment. In both cases the focus is on accepting and accommodating dysfunctional behavior rather than on changing it. During the treatment process clinicians need to balance accommodation and change. One does a disservice to patients by trying to change behaviors that are beyond their control to change (McCarrick et al., 1985). Similarly, however, one deprives patients of opportunities for growth by tolerating behaviors that can be changed. The real challenge in treating young patients is in knowing the difference between the two.

Developing Reasonable Expectations. Clinicians working with chronically mentally ill adults in the community face a set of contradictory premises. Operating under predeinstitutionalization assumptions, clinicians presume that when patients reside in the community, their psychiatric illness is stable and under control and they are both capable of living independently and motivated to do so. Regrettably, these assumptions, which might have been valid prior to deinstitutionalization, are no longer viable. Clinicians cannot safely assume that patients are stable or capable of independent functioning just because they reside in the community. In fact, deinstitutionalization policies have diverted from inpatient facilities patients who continue to be highly symptomatic.

Because of this somewhat paradoxical situation—namely, patients who reside in the community but are neither cured nor stable—clinicians are inclined to mistakenly develop unrealistic expectations for patients. Just because a patient is residing outside of an institution does not mean that he or she can ride public transportation, manage money, comply with medication schedules, or perform any of the host of other skills one needs in order to successfully live in the community.

With some subgroups (Sheets et al., 1982) of chronically mentally ill young adults it is relatively easy for clinicians to scale back expectations. Some patients, despite their youth, are passive and compliant and are highly identified with the patient role (Kanter, 1985b). These patients do best in low-pressure settings that are designed to meet their needs indefinitely (Meyerson & Herman, 1987). Since many of the patients in this subgroup have been ill since childhood (Harris & Bergman, 1987a), clinicians may find it relatively easy to establish modest expectations and realistic short-term goals.

For patients with good premorbid histories who currently deny that they are suffering from a mental illness and whose families still harbor hopes of a return to higher levels of functioning, it becomes much more problematic, but even more critical, for clinicians to set realistic goals. Unfortunately, despite their outward appearance of healthy functioning, such patients often have a recent history of social and vocational failures (Harris & Bergman, 1987a). Clnicians therefore need to be mindful of such patients' vulnerabilities without being so constrained by those vulnerabilities that they refrain from planning any challenging treatment activities.

Treating the Functional Adolescent. Despite the fact that many young adult chronic patients are in their late 20s or early 30s, many of them function emotionally as if they were much younger. Some are still caught in the rebelliousness that characterizes teenage years (Lamb, 1982). Others appear to need the external structure and support that teenagers receive when they live at home with their families (Harris, Bergman, & Bachrach, 1986). The obvious paradox of individuals with the maturity of functional adolescents but the chronological age and aspirations of adults makes treatment for these individuals challenging at best. Clinicians need to respect patients' age-appropriate desires for autonomy while also honoring their very real need for support and structure.

For most adults who do not develop a major mental illness there is a societally sanctioned period of transition between adolescence and adulthood during which time the individual lives with groups of his or her peers under the supervision of a responsible adult. These experiences usually occur at colleges or in military or volunteer corps and last from 2 to 4 years. During these times, young adults are free to experiment with a variety of personae and to engage in different kinds of relationships. All of this testing is done under the watchful eye of some adult leader who ensures that certain standards of behavior are not violated. Unfortunately, because of the often early onset of schizophrenia, patients often miss out on these transitional experiences.

We have suggested elsewhere that the development of a fraternal network for young adult chronic patients allows them such a transitional experience (Harris et al., 1986). In such a network there is both needed structure and opportunities for autonomous behavior. While age-appropriate acting-out is tolerated, there is peer pressure to control bizarre and dangerous behavior. Group cohesiveness is encouraged, and there is a frequent exchange of feedback and advice among network members.

In a similar vein, Pepper and Ryglewicz (1985) have suggested the formation of a "growth house" or developmental residence for young adult chronic patients. Such a facility would "provide family functions which the young adult has outgrown chronologically but not psychologically." It is important for clinicians to create such opportunities in which patients can gradually assume independent behaviors. Respect for the often rather lengthy transition from adolescence to adulthood can enable clinicians to provide patients with the opportunities they need for growth.

Balance Caring and Responsibility. It is important that clinicians develop caring and supportive relationships with the young adult patients with whom they work. Many of these patients have been buffeted between their own confused expectations and the equally unclear demands of the changing treatment system, and consequently need the continuity that comes from working with a stable and engaged clinician. While it may seem heretical to say so, this caring and concern needs to be tempered. It is indeed possible for clinicians to "care" too much.

It is not uncommon for clinicians working with demanding patients to extend caring to overinvolvement. Frequently, clinicians will appear to care more about the outcome of a particular intervention than about the patients themselves. This attitude of overconcern is dangerous from two perspectives. First, it lays the groundwork for a power struggle between clinician and patient. If a patient perceives that the clinician is overly invested in a particular outcome, then one way to separate from that clinician and achieve some autonomy is to oppose the outcome desired by the clinician. Additionally, this attitude of overconcern can lead to clinician frustration and eventual burnout.

Stein and Test (1982) have raised another difficulty when clinicians become overly concerned and inadvertently deny patients the opportunity to accept the consequences of their behaviors like responsible citizens. When clinicians try to protect patients from the impact of dangerous or foolish behavior they may, in the process, give them a distorted view of what the community will tolerate from its members. One young man, for example, refused to take medication for several months. His clinician worked with him in a consistent way to encourage him to comply with his prescribed medications but refused to issue any consequences for his noncompliance. On one occasion this man was engaged in a hostile tirade with his neighbors that attracted the attention of the local police. He attempted to excuse his behavior to the police by saying that he was a mental patient. Fortunately, one officer told him that was no excuse and he better learn to control himself if he wanted to stay out of jail. The next day this man came to the clinic agreeing to take medication. Concern that shields people from the consequences of their behavior may ultimately deny them the opportunity to learn from their mistakes.

Borrowing Ego Functions. Much has been written of the need for a working alliance with young adult chronic patients (Egri & Caton, 1982) in order for clinicians to provide, at least on a temporary basis, some of the ego functions impaired as a result of the individual's mental illness (Harris & Bergman, 1987b; Pepper et al., 1982). Clinicians may find themselves needing to take over activities of memory, future planning, and judgment. For some patients the need to borrow ego support will be temporary. For others, however, it will be more enduring and possibly lifelong.

This mentoring or ego-building function is perhaps best served by a clinician who functions as a case manager (Harris & Bergman, 1987b). Lamb (1982) has suggested that such a person not only coordinate and monitor services but also be available to help the individual process the difficult task of dealing with adult life with limited capacities. Using the case management relationship as a vehicle, the clinician can assist the patient in fortifying weakened ego capacities.

The present authors have gone a step further in suggesting that patients can internalize some of the integrative and problem-solving functions of the case management process itself (Harris & Bergman, 1987b). By so doing, patients develop capacities, heretofore absent, for coping with and assessing situations. This process of identification begins slowly, with patients initially imitating some of the reasoning of their clinicians but eventually coming to generate more integrated behavior patterns on their own.

Case management has typically been seen as a remedy for dysfunction within the treatment system. The case manager brings together fragmented services and negotiates the maze of multiple providers. Perhaps equally important, case management may be the treatment of choice for the intrapsychic fragmentation that besets the young adult chronic patient as well. A consistent and stable relationship with a clear-thinking clinical provider may enable patients to experience the structure and containment necessary for engagement in treatment and eventual growth—a type of structure previously only available as part of an inpatient hospitalization.

Finally, it is important for clinical case managers to assess the length of time for which particular patients will need to borrow ego functions. While for some group of patients this will be a lifelong requirement, it is certainly hoped that for many chronic patients a process of gradual weaning can take place. While it is problematic for clinicians to wean patients prematurely, it is equally troublesome for patients to be maintained in positions of dependency for longer than necessary.

Prepare for Life-Cycle Changes. Since the special demands of young adulthood are among the factors contributing to the phenomenon of the young adult chronic patient, it is reasonable to assume that when those demands are no longer operative a different set of clinical issues will surface. It seems a truism to state that young adult chronic patients will eventually become older adult chronic patients and that clinicians need to be prepared to help them confront different life-cycle issues (Gralnick, 1984).

Levinson (1978) maintains that, during middle adulthood, men take a step back and evaluate the state of their lives. They assess how successfully they have created a career, a love relationship, and a dream for themselves, and they come to terms with their real physical limitations and shrinking options for the future. If early adulthood has been marked by repeated social and vocational failures, as is the case for many young adult chronic patients, then clinicians can expect that middle adulthood may be a time of depression and despair as patients look back with pain and anger at their unrealized dreams.

Just as rebelliousness and expanded expectations are the markers of early adulthood, despair and hopelessness may well be the reactions of later adulthood. Clinicians must be prepared to help patients confront their realistic losses, but also to assist them in developing the needed rationalizations to go on (Harris & Bergman, 1984). Patients must be helped to see their successes as well as their failures, and to foster some hope for their futures. Without a positive view of the future, the risk of suicide is great (Harris & Bergman, 1984). One man in his mid-40s who had failed to develop a stable family life or career described himself as "obsolete" shortly before he took his own life.

Clinicians must be prepared with appropriate treatment interventions that will help patients to successfully confront the next set of life-cycle issues. Certainly, supportive counseling and psychotherapy might be useful interventions for confronting powerful affective responses. Similarly, supportive peer groups can be utilized to help people feel less isolated. On a more active note, clinicians will need to be aggressive about engaging patients in meaningful endeavors. Engagement and connection to others are clearly among those things that give meaning to life and make it worth living. For example, a small group of women in their late 40s, none of whom had married or had children, were brought together to form a support network for one another. By pooling resources they were able to rent a house together, thus giving them a sense of successful family life that would otherwise have been missing for them.

SUMMARY AND CONCLUSIONS

Treatment for chronic patients is more complicated than it was 30 years ago. When patients were chronically institutionalized, treatment options were few. Now, clinicians must develop treatments that not only accommodate to life-cycle issues but also take into account community stresses and the changing realities of the treatment milieu. In facing the challenges of the young adult chronic patient, we must realize that we are not encountering a new clinical entity, but rather are confronting the result of a complex interaction of cultural, social, and personal factors.

When we appreciate the complexity of the forces operating, we can begin to develop assessment strategies that take into account the demands of community living. Such community assessments can be useful in developing principles of treatment appropriate to the special needs of young adult chronic patients.

ACKNOWLEDGMENT

The author wishes to thank Helen C. Bergman, A.C.S.W., with whose assistance this chapter was written.

REFERENCES

Bachrach, L. L. (1982). Young adult chronic patients: An analytical review of the literature. *Hospital and Community Psychiatry, 33,* 189–197.

Bachrach, L. L. (1983). An overview of deinstitutionalization. *New Directions for Mental Health Services, 17,* 5–14.

Bachrach, L. L. (1984). The young adult chronic psychiatric patient in an era of deinstitutionalization. *American Journal of Public Health, 74,* 382–384.

Bachrach, L. L., Talbott, J. A., & Meyerson, A. (1987). The chronic psychiatric patient as a "difficult" patient: A conceptual analysis. *New Directions for Mental Health Services, 33,* 35–50.

Bergman, H., & Harris, M. (1985). Substance abuse among young adult chronic patients. *Psychosocial Rehabilitation Journal, 9,* 49–54.

Egri, G., & Caton, C. (1982). Serving the young adult chronic patient in the 1980s: Challenge to the general hospital. *New Directions for Mental Health Services, 14,* 25–31.

Friswold, B. (1987). Community living for the mentally ill: A case of illness or a case of poverty? *Coalition News, (Washington, DC), 2,* 3–4.

Goffman, E. (1961). *Asylums.* Garden City, NY: Anchor Books.

Gralnick, A. (1984). The young adult chronic patient: Review and critique of the literature. *Psychiatric Hospital, 15,* 199–204.

Harris, M., & Bergman, H. (1983). Youth of the '60s. *Hospital and Community Psychiatry, 34,* 1164.

Harris, M., & Bergman, H. (1984). The young adult chronic patient: Affective responses to treatment. *New Directions for Mental Health Services, 21,* 29–35.

Harris, M., & Bergman, H. (1985). Networking with young adult chronic patients. *Psychosocial Rehabilitation Journal, 8,* 28–35.

Harris, M., & Bergman, H. (1987a). Differential treatment planning for young adult chronic patients. *Hospital and Community Psychiatry, 38,* 638–643.

Harris, M., & Bergman, H. (1987b). Case management with the chronically mentally ill: A clinical perspective. *American Journal of Orthopsychiatry, 57,* 296–302.

Harris, M., Bergman, H., & Bachrach, L. L. (1986). Individualized network planning for chronic psychiatric patients. *Psychiatric Quarterly, 58*, 51–56.

Kanter, J. (1985a). Case management of the young adult chronic patient. *New Directions for Mental Health Services, 27*, 77–92.

Kanter, J. (1985b). Psychosocial assessment in community treatment. *New Directions for Mental Health Services, 27*, 63–75.

Lamb, H. R. (1982). Young adult chronic patients: The new drifters. *Hospital and Community Psychiatry, 33*, 465–468.

Lasch, C. (1978). *The culture of narcissism.* New York: W. W. Norton.

Levinson, D. (1978). *The seasons of a man's life.* New York: Knopf.

McCarrick, A., Manderscheid, R., & Bertolucci, D. (1985). Correlates of acting-out behaviors among young adult chronic patients. *Hospital and Community Psychiatry, 36*, 848–853.

Meyerson, A., & Herman, G. (1987). Systems resistance to the chronic patient. *New Directions for Mental Health Services, 33*, 21–33.

Minkoff, K. (1982). *Deinstitutionalization: Problems and prospects: Clinical implications for "new" chronic patients.* Paper, presented at the Institute on Hospital and Community Psychiatry, Louisville, KY.

Pepper, B., Kirschner, M., & Ryglewicz, H. (1981). The young adult chronic patient: Overview of a population. *Hospital and Community Psychiatry, 32*, 463–469.

Pepper, B., & Ryglewicz, H. (1984). Treating the young adult chronic patient: An update. *New Directions for Mental Health Services, 21*, 5–15.

Pepper, B., & Ryglewicz, H. (1985). The developmental residence: A "missing link" for young adult chronic patients. *TIE Lines, 2*, 1–3.

Pepper, B., Ryglewicz, H., & Kirschner, M. (1982). The uninstitutionalized generation: A new breed of psychiatric patient. *New Directions for Mental Health Services, 14*, 3–14.

Rachlin, S. (1983). The influence of law on deinstitutionalization. *New Directions for Mental Health Services, 17*, 41–53.

Safer, D. (1987). Substance abuse by young adult chronic patients. *Hospital and Community Psychiatry, 38*, 511–514.

Schacter, M., & Goldberg, W. (1982). GAP: A treatment approach for the young adult chronic patient. *New Directions for Mental Health Services, 14*, 85–89.

Schwartz, S., & Goldfinger, S. (1981). The new chronic patient: Clinical characteristics of an emerging subgroup. *Hospital and Community Psychiatry, 32*, 470–474.

Sheets, J., Prevost, J., & Reihman, J. (1982). Young adult chronic patients: Three hypothesized subgroups. *Hospital and Community Psychiatry, 33*, 197–203.

Stein, L., & Test, M. A. (1982). Community treatment of the young adult patient. *New Directions for Mental Health Services, 14*, 57–67.

Test, M., Knoedler, W., Allness, D., & Burke, S. (1985). Characteristics of young adults with schizophrenic disorders treated in the community. *Hospital and Community Psychiatry, 36*, 853–858.

Vaughn, C., & Leff, J. (1976). The influence of family and social factors on the course of psychiatric illness. *British Journal of Psychiatry, 129*, 125–137.

Index